Cultural Ontology of the Self in Pain

Siby K. George · P.G. Jung
Editors

Cultural Ontology of the Self in Pain

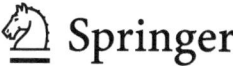 Springer

Editors
Siby K. George
Department of Humanities and Social
  Sciences
Indian Institute of Technology Bombay
Powai, Mumbai
Maharashtra
India

P.G. Jung
Department of Humanities and Social
  Sciences
Indian Institute of Technology Bombay
Powai, Mumbai
Maharashtra
India

ISBN 978-81-322-2600-0   ISBN 978-81-322-2601-7   (eBook)
DOI 10.1007/978-81-322-2601-7

Library of Congress Control Number: 2015945613

Springer New Delhi Heidelberg New York Dordrecht London
© Springer India 2016

Printed on acid-free paper

Springer (India) Pvt. Ltd. is part of Springer Science+Business Media (www.springer.com)

To Professor Goutam Biswas (1953–2012)

A thoughtful scholar of existential
phenomenology and contemporary
Indian philosophy, a fine exponent
of Rabindrasangeet; *above all, a friend*
and mentor to the two of us
and to many more, without borders.

Let me not beg for the stilling of my pain but for the heart to conquer it.

—Rabindranath Tagore

Acknowledgments

Our first thoughts to put together a collection of essays on pain was triggered by the invitation of Prof. Prafulla Kar to hold the third of the Enigma series Conference of the Balvant Parekh Centre for General Semantics and Other Human Sciences, Vadodara, India, of the year 2013 at the Indian Institute of Technology Bombay, with P.G. Jung as the conference coordinator. Some of the contributors to this volume presented papers at the conference on the theme "The Enigma of Pain." We are grateful to Prof. Kar and the Balvant Parekh Centre for the initial promptings.

We want to thank our contributors. Only six of the contributors presented papers at the original conference, and of them only four have given an updated version of the papers presented as chapters of this book. The other chapters were all written specifically for this volume in response to our 'note for contributors'. The chapters came in without much delay and the contributors, some of whom are well-known names in the field, showed exemplary collegiality and cooperation in responding to our editorial queries and revisions. As expected, some of those who promised to contribute later withdrew, and the fresh contributions were constrained by demanding deadlines. We owe them a special word of appreciation for meeting the deadlines without complaint and with the required rigour.

Our colleagues in the Department of Humanities and Social Sciences at the Indian Institute of Technology (IIT) Bombay and our Institute showed wonderful cooperation in the production and readying of this manuscript for press. Professional assistances and resources have never been wanting, whether it is about the Department or about the Central Library of IIT Bombay. We are grateful.

Shinjini Chatterjee, Senior Editor, Human Sciences, Springer, and Shruti Raj, Editorial Assistant, were extremely patient with regard to the unavoidable production woes of a collected volume. We could not keep several deadlines but Shinjini and her team at Springer, New Delhi, were extremely supportive, prompt and professional in their approach. We thank them.

This volume is dedicated to Prof. Goutam Biswas, a friend and mentor to both of us and to many more. He passed away while undergoing treatment in Chennai for cancer on 4 November 2012. Most affectionate friend and thoughtful philosopher,

'Goutamda' or 'Bulti' as he was affectionately called by his friends, was well loved by academics all over India. He mentored and encouraged young philosophers from all over the country. Age, rank and honorifics did not matter to him. An alumnus of HSS, IIT Kanpur, he wrote mostly on Martin Buber and Tagore. The "Other" was a constant concern of his philosophical musings. This was no accident. The most striking feature of Goutamda's character was a pronounced, rooted, generous cosmopolitanism.

Mumbai   Siby K. George
July 2015   P.G. Jung

Contents

Editors and Contributors

About the Editors

Siby K. George is Associate Professor of Philosophy at the Department of Humanities and Social Sciences, Indian Institute of Technology Bombay, Mumbai, India. He has previously been Lecturer of Philosophy at the Department of Humanities and Social Sciences, National Institute of Technology, Silchar, Assam. His area of research is twentieth-century Continental philosophy, and he writes on development, suffering, community, environment, selfhood, agency and the like from a critical-phenomenological perspective, paying special attention to non-western contexts. He is author of *Heidegger and Development in the Global South* (2015, Springer; series: Contributions to Phenomenology, 82). On the theme of pain and illness, he has published "Wellness in Illness" (*Samyukta: A Journal of Women's Studies* XI:2, 2011). His paper "The Affected Subject and the Case of Individuating Pain" is slated to be part of a forthcoming collection of essays on consciousness, subjectivity and otherness.

P.G. Jung is Associate Professor of Philosophy at the Department of Humanities and Social Sciences, Indian Institute of Technology Bombay (IITB), Mumbai, India. He is currently Fellow at the Indian Institute of Advanced Study, Shimla. His publications are largely in the field of philosophy of language, history of ideas, and the philosophy of everydayness. His two manuscripts, "Reading Wittgenstein all over again" and "Conceptualizing corruption through the corruptibility of the self", are currently being readied for publication.

Contributors

Douglas Allen is Professor of Philosophy and former Chairperson at University of Maine, USA, served as President of the Society for Asian and Comparative Philosophy and is Series Editor of Lexington's Studies in Comparative Philosophy and Religion. Author and editor of 15 books and over 150 book chapters and scholarly articles, he received Fulbright (1963–1964, 2009–2010) and Smithsonian (1992) grants to India, Maine Presidential Research and Creative Achievement Award, and Distinguished Maine Professor Award.

Daniel M. Becker is Director of the Center for Biomedical Ethics and Humanities, the Tussi and John Kluge Professor of Palliative Medicine, a Professor of Medicine in the Division of General Medicine, Geriatrics, and Palliative Care, and founding and current editor-in-chief of *Hospital Drive*, an online medical literary journal, at the University of Virginia, School of Medicine. He has distinguished publications of poetry and short fiction.

Shannon Hoff is Assistant Professor of Philosophy at the Memorial University of Newfoundland, St. John's, NL, Canada, and President of the Canadian Society for Continental Philosophy. She is author of *The Laws of the Spirit: A Hegelian Theory of Justice* (2014), with SUNY Press.

Phil Hutchinson is Senior Lecturer in Philosophy at the Department of Interdisciplinary Studies, Manchester Metropolitan University, UK. He is author of *Shame and Philosophy: An Investigation in the Philosophy of Emotions and Ethics* (2008, Macmillan). He is now working with clinicians and public health professionals to apply his work on shame in the context of clinical and public health. He also writes on Wittgenstein, the Philosophy of Social Science and the Philosophy of Health and Healthcare. Hutchinson is a regular contributor to *The Philosopher's Magazine* and maintains two blogs.

Kirsten Jacobson is Associate Professor of Philosophy at the University of Maine. She specializes in nineteenth and twentieth century Continental philosophy. Her published research has often focused on using phenomenology to conduct novel analyses of psychological and physiological illnesses ranging from spatial neglect to agoraphobia, and more generally to consider issues of "existential health."

Roman Meinhold (Ph.D., University Mainz, Germany) is Director of the Guna Chakra Research Centre, Graduate School of Philosophy and Religion, Assumption University, Bangkok. His areas of specialization include cultural critique, philosophy of art and culture, and philosophical anthropology. His publications deal with issues such as consumerism, environmental issues, eudaemonism, (pseudo-)therapy, and violence. He is author of *Fashion Myths: A Cultural Critique* (Transcript, Bielefeld, 2013).

Shefali Moitra retired as Professor of Philosophy from Jadavpur University, Kolkata. Her areas of special interest include philosophy of language, ethics, and feminist thought. She has published extensively and her books include *Feminist Thought: Androcentrism, Communication* and Objectivity and *Ujani Meye: The Life and Works of Simone de Be*auvoir (in Bengali).

David B. Morris is a writer and Emeritus Professor of English Literature at the University of Virginia. He has authored *The Culture of Pain* (1991), winner of a PEN prize and translated into German, Spanish, and Japanese; *Illness and Culture in the Postmodern Age* (1998), translated into German, Spanish, Portuguese, and Serbian; and numerous other research articles on the subject of pain.

Malem Ningthouja is currently Fellow at the Indian Institute of Advanced Study, Shimla. He holds graduate, postgraduate, and doctoral degrees in history from the University of Delhi. He is Founder and Chairperson of Campaign for Peace and Democracy, Manipur, and Member of the International Coordination Committee of the International League of People's Struggle. He is author of *Diametrical Nationalisms: Rulers, Rebels and Masses in Manipur* (2015), *India's War on Democracy: The Debate on AFSPA 1958* (2014), and *Freedom from India: A History of Manipur Nationalism* (2011).

John Russon is Professor of Philosophy at the University of Guelph in Canada. He is a specialist in Phenomenology, German Idealism, and Ancient Philosophy. His original works of philosophy include *Human Experience* (SUNY, 2003), *Bearing Witness to Epiphany* (SUNY, 2009), and *Sites of Exposure* (Indiana, 2015). He is also author of three books on the philosophy of G.W.F. Hegel.

Parinitha Shetty is Professor in the Department of English, Mangalore University, Karnataka, India. She presently works on missionary narratives, especially the history of the Basel Mission in the Canarese region. Her two representative publications are "Christianity, Reform and the Reconstitution of Gender: The Case of Pandita Mary Ramabai" in Journal of Feminist Studies in Christianity (2012), and "Missionary Pedagogy and Christianisation of the Heathens: The Educational Institutions Introduced by the Basel Mission in Mangalore" in Indian Economic Social History Review (2008).

R. Umamaheshwari is Fellow at the Indian Institute of Advanced Study, Shimla, India (for work on the project, "Reading History with the Tamil Jainas: Locating Identity, Memory and Marginalisations in Historiography"). She is author of *When Godavari Comes: People's History of a River* (*Journeys in the Zone of the Dispossessed*), 2014—which is based on the ongoing National dam-induced displacement project on Godavari River. She holds Ph.D. in History from Jawaharlal Nehru University, New Delhi. Umamaheshwari has been, for most part, an independent journalist-academic.

Chapter 1
Introduction: Cultural Ontology of the Self in Pain

Siby K. George and P.G. Jung

Abstract The term 'cultural ontology' evokes the sense that the social, political, religious and historical narratives and other cultural forces that are at play within the world one inherits exercise a sculpting power that shapes one's self, and this power is greater than the power that one has over them. The self thus formed is not an unchangeable substance but a non-substantial way of being or relating meaningfully to the world. The experience of pain is not an accidental element in the way of being of the self but is constitutive of the formation and being of the self. The process of meaning-making is intrinsically fraught with pain. Pain is at once aversive and necessary. This introductory chapter outlines the 13 other chapters of the book from the perspective of the cultural ontology of the self in pain, dividing them into three groups. The first set of essays deals with the various dimensions of the ontology of the self in pain; the second with the ethical, political and cultural angles, consequences and approaches to pain-experience; and the third with certain concrete contexts of the self in pain with reference to Indian social and political life.

Keywords Cultural ontology · Body-being · Representationalist · Antiessentialist · Meaning · Self

1.1 Cultural Ontology, Self and Pain

Beginning with Zborowski's pioneering anthropological work *People in Pain* (1969), literature on the cultural dimensions of pain has been common. Although empirically oriented works like Zborowski's have not been many (Encandela 1993),

S.K. George (✉) · P.G. Jung (✉)
Department of Humanities and Social Sciences, Indian Institute of Technology Bombay, Mumbai, India
e-mail: kgsiby@iitb.ac.in

P.G. Jung
e-mail: pgjung@iitb.ac.in

© Springer India 2016
S.K. George and P.G. Jung (eds.), *Cultural Ontology of the Self in Pain*, DOI 10.1007/978-81-322-2601-7_1

his contention that pain experience and expression have deep social and cultural underpinnings, and that people respond to pain not as bare, abstract individuals but as historical and cultural individuals (1969, p. 20) has informed subsequent understanding of pain.[1] This culturally informed approach complements the medical approach to pain and challenges the cognitive-scientific, physicalist, mechanistic, causal understanding of pain, leading to the ontological-literary-cultural and medical humanities writings on pain, placed at the interface of biology and culture (see Coakley and Shelemay 2007). Medical humanities today is replete with studies that exhort nurses, paramedics and physicians to recognize a holistic understanding and the cultural sensitivities of the sick body-being's experience and expression of pain for a more humane way of dealing with trauma, suffering and illness (see Carr et al. 2005). What is there in this book's essays that are not there in the profusion of material already available on cultural diversity in the experience of pain?

Elaine Scarry's *The Body in Pain* (1985) and David Morris's *The Culture of Pain* (1991) are two very differently oriented but landmark works in the culturally informed approach to pain. Scarry's frame of analysis is a political ontology of the world-shattering power of pain effected by its demonic inexpressibility—especially attached to such politically charged cruelties as torture and hegemonic silencing through oppressive domination—and the world-making power of human expression and creativity as a sort of inherently human, and therefore, ontological response to ineluctable pain that permeates existence entirely.

As a theoretically compact work, *The Body in Pain* does not look at the literature on pain that is not necessary for its tightly woven argument. Morris, on the other hand, seeks to puncture the thick walls of the physicalist's reductive paradigm by engaging with it and taking into account medical research on pain to emphasize the urgency to combine cultural understanding with "insights of numerous fields now separated by specialized vocabularies and divergent theories" (1991, pp. 6–7). Morris claims that "the experience of pain is not timeless but changing, the product of specific periods and particular cultures" (p. 4). In his *Illness and Culture in the Postmodern Age* (1998), Morris's term 'postmodern illness' stands for "our changed and still changing experience of human affliction" as distinctive as the cars and computers that define the postwar postmodern era are. He argues that these distinctive experiences of suffering in our era are products of the complex relations between biology and culture, wedded to the postmodern human's quest to live forever, something that *defines who we are today* (Morris 1998, p. 3).

Morris's argument is that the contemporary *self* is rather distinctive in comparison to *selves* of all previous historical eras and cultures. It is not that we can have an experience discretely separable from an unchanging core self, hidden beneath the folds of our transient thoughts. The self is *not* an unchanging substance but our *way of being towards* the manifold experiences that are always intentionally

---

[1]*People in Pain* is criticized for racial stereotyping, but Zborowski's conclusion that pain responses are culturally coded has found wide endorsement and the work is considered as the founding attempt to "the study of culture and pain" (Mander 2011, pp. 19–20; see also Morris 1991, p. 55).

already connected to a world. It is in this *being towards* that the self discloses itself as affected, oriented, composed and decomposed constantly by the forces of the world (that can be largely called 'cultural'), and it in turn affects, composes and orients its world. This disclosure highlights the fact that we are intentionally directed towards an already given world before we can objectively represent that world or its elements in consciousness. Our relation to the world, which *is* our being —given that there is no inner core to our being other than these relations—is not the mental representation of a discrete, subject-thing or *ego*. This antirepresentationalist strain current in recent continental and analytic philosophical traditions is reiterated elaborately in this volume too, as in Hutchinson's formulation of 'world-taking cognitivism' (see Chap. 8). Essential to this volume is the conviction that culturally given meanings inexorably impinge on self-formation, and among these meanings, culturally loaded interpretations of pain-experiences are constitutively central. This conviction is reflected in the essays of this volume and in a way also justifies its addition to the rich emerging literature on pain. Hence, the volume follows a non-substance ontology of the self, for which pain-meanings are central.

We contend that pain as an experience that inherently permeates our existence from top to bottom, is not peripherally but rather intrinsically constitutive and determinative of being a self. Explicitly articulating this conviction, Russon, in the ninth chapter of this volume asserts:

> Because our "selves" are not given in advance as ontologically independent components of our reality but are, instead, the cultivated ways we have of navigating the forces constitutive of our experience, the meaningfulness of our lives will always be embodied, will always rest upon the developed forms of our bodily engagement with the world. Our bodily organism and the physical world with which we interact bodily are inherently vulnerable to damage, however. For that reason, the meaningfulness of our lives will itself always be vulnerable *and therefore painful* (our addition in italics).

At the same time, we do not mean that ontology can be reduced to culture. Such a simple, unproblematic reduction of ontology to culture is problematic even for anthropologists.[2] By the invocation of the phrase 'cultural ontology', what we seek

---

[2]In a debate on the motion "ontology is just another word for culture" by the Group for Debates in Anthropological Theory in Manchester University in 2008, the motion was voted out. One of the supporters of the motion argued that the term 'ontology' captured what western anthropologists earlier understood as 'culture' of people different from the west, and in using the more philosophical term 'ontology', they "were trying to avoid the problems of representation" or of caricaturing the notions of reality of non-western peoples as merely 'cultural representations' of reality and not reality itself. Hence, the argument is, 'ontology' as a term comes to stand in place of the term 'culture'. Against this, one of the critics of the motion argued that 'culture' in fact *was* about representation and *cannot* circumvent the problems of representation. To interpret the understandings of peoples as 'culture' was "to relegate them to representations of a prior reality to which Western science claims privileged access." The term 'ontology' is "a way of accepting others' ability to inhabit wholly separate realities" (Rollason 2008). Another report of this debate is of Venkatesan (2010). The argument for the motion of this debate is discussed in detail in Carrithers (2012) and against the motion in Holbraad (2010). For an antirelativistic account of the antirepresentationalist ontological turn in anthropology, see Palecek and Risjord (2013).

to emphasize is the ontological point that the social, political, religious, and historical narratives and other cultural forces that are at play within the world one inherits, exercise a sculpting power that shapes one's self, and this power is greater than the power that one has over them. Our freedom to negotiate or reject some of these forces is a way of responding to them rather than inventing and inhabiting absolutely new cultural worlds. Thus, 'world' in this sense, again, is not an objectively present static entity but is rather a collective understanding of reality as a whole, accessed first and foremost through a non-representationalist processes of receiving and accepting phenomena in their meaningfulness. Without this primordial non-representationalist acceptation of our being in relation to the world, neither the representationalist objectifications nor the sciences as such are possible. What is meant by 'cultural ontology' here is the very ontological process of the non-representationalist reception of, or acculturation into, an already given world.

Within the modern representationalist paradigm, culture is construed as a facile representation of an unchanging, substantial, a priori reality. In contrast, what we seek to emphasize through the phrase 'cultural ontology' is the positioning of each 'world' as an authentic understanding of the meaningful being of reality that does not exhaust all its possibilities and shades. However, this does not mean that we wish to align ourselves with the Idealist's thesis that reality is mind-dependent. Rather, what we seek to underline is that the meaningful being of the manifold possibilities of reality are available to us only in the ways in which they are revealed to cultural worlds. Thus, they are not subjectivistic and willful appropriations or facile interpretations of human machination and intelligence[3] but are those available revelations of reality for humanity in context, which it always is. It is also these that inform the objectivistic and scientific interpretations of the world. Outside these ways and the expressive traditions that house them, the real *is* but not its meaningful being, as Heidegger contends in the assertion "[l]anguage is the house of being. In its home human beings dwell" (1998, p. 239).

Thus, by the phrase 'cultural ontology of pain' we refer to the mode of being of the self in pain, whether intense bodily pain, trauma or humiliation, that is in a significant sense affected ontologically by social and cultural forces that form the self. Speaking minimally, while it is debatable whether the structure of the self is

---

[3]While attempting a Heideggerian 'ontology of culture', McHoul (1999) observes that the advantage of such an understanding of culture is "it works with a radical requisitioning of whether everything that *is* is an object for a subject. That is, it works against the dominant, orthodox (but, for this reason, barely even mentioned) general picture of culture as being representationalist through and through. As Heidegger makes clear: Da-sein is not a simple objective presence (such as a human body or a person) with a representational capacity (consciousness, for example, or the capacity for thought) tacked on afterwards. It is not as if one simply placed an active circuit into an inert grey box. If this is so, Da-sein's equipmental being-with cannot be founded on such representationalist premises" (p. 103). Right from the beginning, humans are ways of being intentionally directed towards an already given world before they can objectively represent that world or its elements in consciousness. Our relation to the world, which *is* our being (there is no inner core to our being other than these relations), is not the mental representation of a discrete, subject-thing or ego.

totally reducible to these forces beyond one's conscious, willed control, the tremendous power exerted by these fluid forces upon our understanding of ourselves is undeniable. Thus the ontology of the self, minimally speaking, is not culturally neutral. If this contention of ours is granted, then it becomes important to understand, from a consciously articulated perspective of cultural ontology, that something as enigmatic, baffling and humbling as pain is in all its complexity, inscrutability and pathos, both self-destructive and self-formative, is absolutely central to and yet enigmatically disruptive of existence.

The essays of this volume, more than attempting to establish the impossibility of the culturally neutral ontological structure of pain, sheds light on the culturally imbued ontology of pain experience; how this structure gives us culturally variant experiences of and responses to pain; how meaningful it is to understand what cultural and social forces outside our control do to our pain experiences; how such understanding is necessary to deal with pain humanely and compassionately; and how our approaches towards painful experiences of others or ourselves become limited and even inhuman if we are blinded by the claims of a universal-univocal ontology of pain. However, no essay in this volume is straightforwardly a record of cultural diversity in the experience of pain like Zborowski's pioneering study.

These essays, in a way, deconstruct the reductive approaches to pain and contest reductive claims that seek to identify pain with "a neurobiological sensory function of the brain and spinal cord" (Woolf 2007, p. 27) or the idea that "all pains are physical and localizable and that all are created equal" (Hardcastle 1999, p. 7). The essays in this volume do not seek to understand pain, in Morris's caricatural phrase, as "an electrical impulse speeding along the nerves" (1991, p. 4). Morris attempts to break the myth of two pains, physical and mental—a result of Cartesian dualism—which is not the way many cultures, other than the modern, understand pain (1991, pp. 9–10). The essays of this volume too largely overlook the unthought division between mental and physical pain and consider all pains as pains of the whole embodied person so that one can consider intense bodily pain (for want of a better expression), shame, the sense of loss and traumatic personal and historical events under the same lens of pain. The essays bring to the fore the ambiguous and equivocal nature of pain: at once inescapable, fundamental and necessary for being human and at the same time harrowing, traumatic and aversive in its extremes. They recognize that eradicating pain and avoiding it at all costs does "not simply entail a radical rewriting of what it means to be human (and such rewritings have been part of human existence since its very beginning), but, rather, complete annihilation of perhaps not only humankind but of all sentient being" (Käll 2013, p. 1). Several essays of the volume (see Hoff, Jacobson, Meinhold and Russon) are on the ineluctability and positive necessity of pain. Although there is a distinctively personal element and pathos to pain, it is "also deeply entrenched with cultural, historical, political, social and symbolic meaning that both situates it in a specific time and place and at the same time removes it from being confined within the boundaries of individual experience" (Käll 2013, p. 1). The essays of this volume amplify these meanings of pain, and argue the case that these are not peripheral elements of pain but are rather integral and constitutive to it (see Allen, George,

Jung and Morris), and so understanding them as such is important to deal with extremely aversive pains (see Hutchinson, Moitra, Ningthouja, Russon and Umamaheshwari).

The essays in this volume are divided into three parts. The first group of essays argues the general case of cultural ontology of pain highlighting its various dimensions (Part I). The next group touches upon the ethical, political and cultural aspects of pain-experience (Part II), while the last group of three essays deals with pain-experiences in relation to concrete Indian social contexts: state-imposed torture, majority-imposed silencing of the historical memories and identities of communities, and transformation of the 'heathen' subject into modern and Christian one in the Canarese (Karnataka) region of India through the colonial Christian missionary narrative of suffering (Part III).

1.2   Ontology of Pain

In the first part of this volume, the ontology of pain is treated in its broad features, mainly by philosophers. The section begins with an essay on the history of ideas. While the force of the argument that modernity has made us detached subjects who 'calculate' the essence of all beings in discrete (often mathematical) forms/ideas is well-accepted today, it is not true that the enigmatic problem of pain was not central to modern ethical imagination. The political and ethical doctrine of utilitarianism can be looked at as the calculative orientation of modern imagination merging itself with the supposedly incalculable experience of pain, thus making it a truly 'modernist' understanding.

P.G. Jung's essay traces the link between the Humean-Benthamite utilitarian conception of pain and its historical predecessors (stoics, epicureans, Aristotle and Plato's Socrates). He argues that the experiential/phenomenal dimension of pain, rather than its singular and substantial essence or quiddity, can be traced even up to the beginnings of western moral philosophical reflections. Historically speaking, pain was always taken to be a more complex phenomenon than mere physical sensation, and thus the modern mainstream interpretation of it in terms of sensation within a causal-mechanical explanatory framework is an aberration. The difficulties the early writers faced in defining pain on account of its ambiguous nature—for example, the fact that the nature of some pleasures make their essence as pleasure equivocal—Jung takes as a sign of the pain-pleasure-complex's experiential thickness. However, notwithstanding the broader treatment of pain in its experiential thickness in these moral frameworks, the primary concern of the chapter is to highlight how these moral theories fell short in bringing to the fore the complex experiential texture of pain-experiences which we are now beginning to have a sense of, and which is the matter of concern in the essays of this book. In other words, the question that informs the essay is the failure of these moral theories, despite their central engagement with a thicker understanding of pain, to move towards a socio-cultural ontology of a being in pain. Jung contends that this failure can be seen to be hinged on the uncritical and constrictive assumption that pain is the 'contrary' of pleasure (the contrariety thesis), and the later acceptance of the impossibility of 'cognitive-error' in the experience of pain as pain (the naturality thesis). The moral frameworks that take pain to be cardinal to moral imagination, he argues, thus fail to develop a deeper understanding of pain-experiences on account of their pre-orientation towards the nature of pain as immediately given in its experience, and as conditioned on the contrary conception of pleasure.

Further, Jung contends that while these moral theories were perceptive of pain's experiential texture, they associated pain intrinsically with the individual's essence which is taken to have no social or cultural dimension. While the experiential richness of pain is acknowledged to be not merely a punctual sensation, this complexity is paradoxically taken to be arising out of a substantial, asocial and essentialist individuality. Since pain is the essence of an atomistic individuality, it is conceived as ceaselessly creating our world, considered as the sum total of substantial individualities. Thus, sociality has nothing to do with the phenomenality of pain; self as the underlying substance is the producer and experiencer of pain. This angle of the theories leading up to the modern understanding of pain, as highlighted in the second essay of this volume, thus opens up the space to appreciate the cultural thickness of pain lacking in the early moral theories of pain, which has important bearing also on the strategies for correcting the modern understanding of pain that this book's essays advocate. Indeed, it is only by relating the rich experiential dimension of pain with the cultural impingements on the formation of the self that experiences pain that we can conceive such powerfully painful experiences as stigma, humiliation, shame, political torture, or even the social response to illness.

If indeed it were true that pain is an experientially 'thick' way of being of the self towards the world that in turn affects self-formation, and if this way of being is constitutive for the self as most of the chapters of this volume argue, an extreme possibility of extreme pain then is, argues George in the third chapter, that it can lead to the shattering and destruction of the familiar, intimate self that one identifies with as 'mine'. Although there is no piece of experience that is as 'mine' as intense bodily pain, its extreme negativity, inexpressibility and aversiveness lead to the obliteration of our familiarity with ourselves and our world. It makes our being negatively strange to ourselves, and disrupts our meaningful projection of possibilities. When we cannot deal with our world and its possibilities meaningfully, in fact the 'I as being-in-the-world' turns into an extreme formulation of the Cartesian-type 'subject' without a world, engrossed in the extremity of its pain, unfree for possibilities and wrapped up in its worldless subjectness. Without our significant possibilities and our competence to deal with them, we lose ourselves. However, the antiessentialist notion of self that is thus at play in this understanding of the loss of self in intense pain immediately makes it evident that the self that can be lost can also be gained, recovered and reconstituted. Scarry has admirably argued that human creativity is at the centre of self-making and thus of self-recovery. However, George argues that in centering only on the notion of the 'artifice' as the pain-relieving, self-recovering, world-making phenomenon, Scarry falls for the modernist technological fascination and forgets the more fundamental aspect of human sharing and expression of pain to the other, which is the more ontologically authentic path to self-recovery.

An inescapable, terrorizing but invaluably instructive pain is the possibility of my absolute impossibility, the impending entry of my existence into nothingness with my death. Unlike most other pains that come and go in a sudden upsurge, death is with us throughout as the definite termination of existence, although indefinite as to when. Fateful illness can bring us face to face with the terror of death as it was for Tolstoy's Ivan Ilyich: "Morning or evening, Friday or Sunday— it didn't matter, it was all the same—grinding, agonizing pain, never for a moment relenting; an awareness of life hopelessly slipping away but not yet gone; the same terrible, relentless approach of hateful death..." (2008, p. 584). Martin Heidegger —whose unparalleled reflections on death invite us to receive, face and make meaningful the existential certainty, indeterminacy and pain of death—considered technological modernity as the very denial of death. "The self-assertion of tech- nological objectification is the constant negation of death. By this negation death itself becomes something negative..." (1971, p. 122). With the German poet Rainer Maria Rilke, Heidegger wants to "read the word 'death' *without* negation" (1971, p. 122) because existence itself is nothing but being possible. Possibilities of existence, however, are not created out of a magician's hat but are interpreted afresh each moment out of the store of the past or history. The most certain yet indeter- minate of these possibilities is death, painful and terrorizing, yet certain and ines- capable, and which stands at the core of our meaning-making project as its orienting limit and orbit. The fact of death is in fact irrelevant; what is relevant is our orientation towards death as the finite end of all possibilities of existence. Grasping death in this way makes us human, the fragile reed of Blaise Pascal, with our eyes open towards our glorious finiteness.

Kirsten Jacobson's chapter deals with how the pain of mortality can be trans- formed into 'a preeminent site for intimacy' by sharing, communicating and lis- tening to the many 'voices of the dying' and the vulnerabilities and terror associated with it. Jacobson's chapter is problematizing our contemporary culture of deathly silence surrounding death and the medicalized modern resistance to dying. As mortal beings we tend to turn away from our mortality. Ivan Ilyich thought that the syllogistic premise 'Caesar is mortal' "had always seemed to him to be true only when it applied to Caesar, certainly not to him" (Tolstoy 2008, p. 563). The ontological terror of death is, however, amplified technologically and institutionally by shielding us from facing this truth both when we are hale and healthy, and when we are ontically face to face with our demise. Jacobson's problem is this precluding of 'care' for our being through technologized aids and the modern hospital system. She refers to Heidegger, Rilke, the terminally ill philosopher Havi Carel, the Dutch phenomenological psychiatrist Jan Hendrik van den Berg and to the account of an anonymous dying nursing student. The nurse, for example, narrates the terror of nurses attending to her while dealing with the impending reality of her death. She observes that this is not only because they wanted to shelter her from the truth of death but guard themselves as well from the difficult truth of existentially grasping their own death. Both Carel and the nurse wanted their interlocutors to acknowledge and listen to their 'dying', which is but the ontically amplified version of every existence. Healthy facing up to our mortality, whether in terminal illness or generally as we live, makes it possible to be truthful and happy. In our constantly dying existence, filled with pain and pleasure, what is most crucial is the voices we speak to and listen to, and in death what comes to a halt is also the once heard and spoken to voice. This is why Jacobson argues that voicing and sharing the terror and pain surrounding the ontic possibility of death, which is ontologically certain already for everyone, is in fact responding to the utmost humanity of our sociality and intimacy—listening to in empathy rather than hiding from the terror of death.

The most essential aspect of pain is its "sheer aversiveness," says Scarry (1985, p. 52), and yet our cultures (*cultura*, *Bildung*, cultivation) teach us to welcome pain in rituals, therapies and art. Disciplining to be a 'cultivated' social being unmistakably involves suffering pain for the human being. Foucault teaches that a huge cultural change like historical modernity means nothing outside such painful disciplining to be a new type of humanity, which need not anymore mean the infliction of pain physically on the body; it, rather, means "a system of constraints and privations, obligations and prohibitions… an economy of suspended rights" (Foucault 1977, p. 11), which would itself be painful. However, modernity also means denial of pain, a 'culture of denial' of "the pain that power distorts and disavows" (Ramazani 2007, p. 7). David Morris writes that the secular-scientific modernity as epitomized in modern medicine "has eclipsed other systems of thought as almost to erase the memory that pain… once possessed redemptive and visionary powers" (1991, p. 125).

The cathartic, healing, redemptive power of pain, attempting to be erased by modern market, consumption ideology, technoscience, bureaucracy, globalizing currents, homogenization of nations/cultures and modern medicine, is not, however, fully erased and need not be, argues the chapter of Roman Meinhold. He throws light on our forgetting memories about the cathartic aspects of pain by calling to mind myriad cultural practices from different parts of the world, in the world's literature and works of art in general, and in psycho-therapeutic practices, which too are not specialized modern formal approaches but everyday practices like that of a father reinforcing and encouraging a child's pain-inducing angry behaviour by mimicking that very behaviour for the sake of producing the effect of revulsion to such a behaviour in the child for her to overcome it. 'Pain is treated with pain, but in a preventive way' as a therapeutic strategy of imitating the same phenomena (*imitation prominentis*), which is a case of cathartic *Aufhebung* (elimination), a 'homeopathic therapy'. Meinhold recommends the need to look beyond modern medicine for pain relief without denying the curative and palliative powers of it and without erasing cathartic pain from our cultural registers. The techno-modern world from which pain is camouflaged and absented, he seems to argue, is hyper-real and therefore unreal. The hyper-reality of such a world, however, dissimulates a painful world and disallows pain's legitimate reality. Pain hurts; denial of pain hurts all the more. Denial of pain accentuates what Scarry calls a second essential element of pain—its "inexpressibility" (1985, p. 19)—with costly emotional-personal and socio-political consequences.

In dealing with the cultural ontology of the self in pain, are we left only with the strongly antiessentialist claims, made famous in the twentieth century by the existentialist formulations of Heidegger, but especially by Sartre's pithy formula that "*existence* comes before *essence*" (Sartre 2001, p. 27)? Are all unqualified antiessentialisms relevant approaches to the problem of pain? Can there be cultural ontologies of the self in pain which are not strongly antiessentialistic? With Gandhi as his anchor, Douglas Allen's chapter answers these questions affirmatively. Summing up his decades of reflections on Gandhi, religion and politics, he caricatures dominant western and Indian philosophical trends as inordinately rationalistic and disinterested in concrete, lived experience such as pain.

For Allen, exceptions to this dominant trend include Marx, the phenomenologists and Gandhi. But Gandhi's approach here is notably distinct from that of the phenomenological existentialists because although he 'embraces a more open-ended, dynamic, relational, social ontology' of the self in place of tradition's essentialism, he considers the self that emerges out of relations—the relative self— as standing in opposition to the real, incorruptible and absolute self. In this he is with tradition. But unlike tradition, whether Hindu, Buddhist or western, the relative self is very important to Gandhi. Allen sees in the Gandhian formulation a middle path between the facile, fashionable relativism of the postmodern dissolution of the subject, which is effectively the new caveat for limitless free being, and tradition's rigid other-worldliness leading to absolute trivialization of concrete existence. Gandhi 'grants much more truth and reality' to relative being and considers human finiteness perpetually limiting a full grasp of the absolute. But the absolute nevertheless leaves its traces on the finite, relative self, which enters into our awareness and which we progressively come to understand as the absolute's mirror image, although we never make it to the full knowledge of its truth.

Truth and self are manifested in diverse, relative ways. This is the founding philosophy of Gandhi's strong pluralism and social engagement. But the criterion to know the many traces of the self and truth in our finite condition is the measure of nonviolence. Gandhi never denies pain's cathartic, transformative role especially when it involves voluntary suffering. A political fast for a morally sound cause is infinitely different from the sorrows of the hungry child. But otherwise, pain usually does violence to the self, to self-other relations, and especially to the dehumanized other in pain. The other's hunger and suffering has no justification as Levinas insists: "The Other's hunger—be it of the flesh, or of bread—is sacred; only the hunger of the third party limits its rights; there is no bad materialism other than our own" (1990, p. xiv). The other's pain and unfreedom is Gandhi's moral silver bullet, talisman, to measure one's steps in action, whether personal or political. Allen insists that such is the best possible way to the problem of pain, a way between antiessentialist absolutizing of the self's freedom and the essentialist absolutizing of the absolute self's otherness with no relative impingements left upon the world of experience. Even Buddhistic antiessentialism, the first of its kind anywhere in the world, in Allen's reading, did not face the problem of pain but passed it by. Gandhi's interesting middle path to the problem of pain as the realm of our committed engagements, regulated by nonviolence and an order of realities not fully knowable in our finite condition, which could in fact be a broader realm than Gandhi was willing to admit, still remains a charming metaphysics of action.

1.3 Culture, Politics and Ethics of Pain

Most of the chapters of this volume touch upon the culture and ethics of pain; however, the five chapters of Part II touch upon culture, politics and ethics of pain more pronouncedly. The chapters of this part start with a poem by Daniel Becker, a doctor-poet. The poem "Hurt" is a spirited meditation on both the person in pain who "curls up in a ball… teaching himself to disappear" and on the care provided to her/him in many contemporary medical settings. The poem vividly describes how pain hurts as seen through the eyes of those who provide care. And it is gently suggestive of how care providers themselves *could* hurt in giving themselves over to the solely professional approach, ruled by what David Morris in the first chapter of this section calls 'medical logos' as opposed to 'medical eros'. Becker is describing, no doubt, *about* pain as it unfolds before the eyes of those who treat the person in pain but is speaking more *to* the care provider herself not to be duped by "the patient satisfaction surveys that manage to equate good care with how easy it is to park." Treatment of pain cannot altogether escape causing pain but without an eye for suffering, a heartless, mindless, unfeeling professional approach helps feed rather than heal suffering. The objective approach to pain is necessary to deal with pain but it ought to be undergirded by the caring approach.

Following on from Becker's evocations, the first essay of the section is an able attack on the overtly rationalistic approach to health/pain care. As someone at the forefront of the humanities research on pain, David Morris in his chapter revisits the several shades of enquiry on pain that he has been championing for over three decades. Morris's interest and achievement has been to integrate the humanities narrative of pain with the medical rather than to emphasize their difference; however, his writings are buttressed with a gentle critique of the modernist, medicalized, physicalist, dualistic approach to pain.

In his chapter, Morris begins with differentiating medical logos from medical eros. Medical eros is desire expressed in a medical context. Desire, feeling and affection accompany and interpenetrate the experience of pain and illness. These are forces that directly affect our experience of pain and yet lie outside medical logos. He argues that medical eros takes us outside medical logos but towards ethics. Morris's central argument in the chapter is to suggest an integrative approach that takes medical logos and medical eros in their complementarity. Medical eros, suggests Morris, asks how narratives and stories 'go to work on us' in complementarity with medical logos. "Narrative bioethics in effect gives *medical eros* a significant role in protecting the sick and in redressing injustices that work special hardships on the ill." Race, caste, ethnicity, religion and gender have effects on pain treatment. Medical eros, through an attention to narrative, can reveal dimensions of pain and suffering that clinical logic and sound reason sometimes skillfully hide. Busting Scarry's 'unknowability-thesis' (1985, p. 51), Morris argues that "[i]n contrast to rationalist claims that another person's pain is always private and unknowable, which of course subverts the claim (to know) that it unravels consciousness, *medical eros* represents pain as more than strictly private, more than locked away in an unknowable single consciousness." Illustrating adeptly, Morris shows that medical practitioners, bound by the ethics of relieving pain and illness, are better served by medical eros in moments of conflicts rather than by medical logos and laws. Medical eros binds them to the claims of emotion and the power of the Levinasian 'face' in ethical decision making rather than to cold reason. Morris blends narrative, eros and ethics in the call to action to relieve pain in situations where reason is an obstruction. In the site of a fatal accident, for example, if we hesitate thinking of the quagmire of the law and rationalize, Morris's argument helps us see that we may prevent our ability and spontaneous ethical response or eros towards the Face.

Philosophers have responded to the cultural variance in responding to and expressing pain not by the concrete study of pain responses and the bearings of cultural notions on them but by explaining the ontological underpinnings of such a finding. They have done this sometimes by looking at particular emotional conditions that are painful and by showing how such pains can best be understood when we relate them to their context or world, from which they draw their import, rather than by explaining them as biological responses shared by animals in general or as cognitive propositional representations of aversive conditions. In this volume, Phil Hutchinson offers arguments from the standpoint of post-Wittgensteinian analytic philosophy for the case that we can understand a strong and universal emotion like shame best from a non-propositional and yet cognitive point of view. Philosophers inspired by the continental European tradition urge us to give up the term 'cognitivism' completely in relation to primordial phenomena like moods rather than consciously represented phenomena like statements (see Dreyfus 2004). Hutchinson, on the other hand, does not take cognitivism to mean mental or propositional representations, the aspect of cognitivism Heidegger and others attacked. Rather, cognitivism for him 'invokes no appeal to cognitive processes'. What he proposes is the idea of 'world-taking cognition' which preserves 'meaningful takings of the world operative sub-propositionally'.[4] Emotions like shame have an intentional relation to the world of its location. This relation is what he means by cognition.

Hutchinson had already argued in *Shame and Philosophy: An Investigation in the Philosophy of Emotions and Ethics* (Palgrave Macmillan 2008) that a concept like shame is different from one like fire on account of "the level of cultural specificity demanded, the number of concepts with which it can be internally related and the level of occasion sensitivity demanded for the internal relations to hold or

---

[4]When Hutchinson speaks about 'world-taking cognition', his moorings are analytical (Wilfred Sellars, John McDowell), but he records 'more than a passing similarity' to what he calls a 'fuller' concept of world in Husserl's notion of 'life-world' and Heidegger's 'being-in-the-world' (2008, p. 103, n. 44).

be active" (2008, p. 137). In the paper included in this volume, he has a twofold interest: (i) to add to the earlier argument that his concept of world-taking cognition has better explanative force in understanding the emotion of shame by referring to the perplexing phenomenon of placebo effect which too can be explained better as a meaning response, intentionally tied to the world, rather than as a result of conditioning or expectancy, and (ii) to argue that shame is a 'variety of pain experience', which is a meaning response tied to the world like the perplexing placebo effect. Hutchinson's argument is not at all that pain would be so culturally coded that the ache from a migraine possibly could be totally dissimulated as to appear a non-aversive experience for sections of humanity. Rather, his argument is fully with this volume's concern with cultural ontology of the self in pain. The argument is, we can understand the rich texture of culture-codedness in a powerfully revolting experience like shame, which is an experience of pain for an embodied and enculturated being, not by concentrating on the universality of biological responses or propositional cognition, but by paying attention to and, whenever necessary, deconstructing the 'culture codes' within which is couched the powerful forces of pain, more than its universal elements. Intrinsic to the universality of pain is its enculturated, world-taking cognitive fate. Without getting at pain in this way, the tremendous pathos and the cathartic power that pain brings cannot be properly grasped.

Suffering is not only inherent to a meaningful life; it is inherent to meaning as such. John Russon's chapter skillfully makes this argument and draws practical conclusions for contemporary medical care basing himself on Buddhist and phenomenological resources. It is well known that the Buddhist concept of suffering is a deeply ontological notion. The Buddha's teaching is not that human life is painful but that all is pain (*sarvam dukkham*). *Dukkha* is the nature of finite, relative reality. The Dhammapada, verses 277–279, make three sweeping ontological claims: "All created things are transitory… All created beings are involved in sorrow… All states are without self." After each of these affirmations, the refrain is: "those who realize this are freed from suffering. This is the path that leads to pure wisdom" (Easwaran 1996, pp. 162–63). Taking Merleau-Ponty's phenomenology of the embodied subject of agency as his starting point, Russon argues that meaningfulness for embodied subjects depends on embodied agency. The inherent limits of embodiment make meaningfulness itself vulnerable and so suffering is intrinsic to meaning. The self is not an independent substance, to teach both Buddhism and existential phenomenology, but is "the cultivated way of navigating the forces constitutive of our experience"; and so, meaning would always be intrinsically tied to our embodied, vulnerable, suffering ways of navigating our environment. *Dukkha* is ubiquitous. "Suffering takes as many forms as meaning takes." Suffering *is* meaning. All meanings *are* possibilities of pain.

Russon argues that understanding the ubiquity of suffering is important for appropriate, compassionate action in the face of suffering. The modern medical approach to suffering makes it a special testable and provable case of evil, which is to be gotten rid of, thus making the intimately meaning-making facets of suffering illegitimate and unknowable. The medical model also forgets the relationally structured individuality of persons, thus ignoring the social embeddedness of pain, leaving unattended the pain of separation, and coercing culturally embedded persons to suffer the alienation of becoming atomistic individuals. This approach, thus, detaches the embodied subject from the world, thrusting on her the 'disorders of dwelling', self-contained, impersonal and institutionalized existence as an individual atom of pain. Russon calls for alternatives that attest the alternative ontology of the person and reality found in Buddhism and phenomenology, as opposed to the ontology of mind-body dualism and individualism cultivated by the modern culture.

The emphasis on 'cultural ontology' in this book is not an endorsement of all culturally loaded understandings of pain. Some aspects of our being like our embodied agency are intrinsic to being in pain. To be in pain is to be embodied, although the meanings that we attach to embodiment do vary culturally. Nothing is pure matter for us, untouched by meaning. The body is even less so. A widespread, culturally loaded understanding of the body in pain that has haunted human communities across the globe is the perception that to be in pain is to be feminine, vulnerable, merely natural and uncultivated. The body "is not a pure symbol of contentless pain but an unconscious metaphor for the *mother's* sundered form, for the female materiality that 'delivered' us to pain, that propped our entire selfhood upon and against it" (Ramazani 2007, p. 43). Pain is gendered; the gendering of pain has consequences for sufferers, especially for women. According to Bendelow's sociological study, many people believed that "female hormonal and reproductive functioning and the role of motherhood were strongly felt to equip girls and women with a 'natural' capacity to endure pain, whereas there was no such biological preparation for boys and men" (Bendelow 1993, p. 289). She concludes that such gendered beliefs in fact lead "to inflicting or ignoring pain" (1993, p. 290).

Feminism has long known the many faces of woman's pain—structurally well entrenched, smoothly adapted, perceived as an unproblematic 'part' of nature. Shefali Moitra's chapter unwinds feminism's sustained encounter with the entrenched structures of woman's suffering, emphasizing all the way the structural depth of the production of the suffering feminine subject. But because of the structural depth of the gendering of pain and the play of power, intangible and systemic, Moitra's conclusion is poignant and weary. Feminism has not succeeded in transforming the suffering condition of woman although it is well-set to know and understand the many faces of woman's pain. The discourse of justice is Moitra's focus of attention, many sided and long winding. She rejects the justice of sameness/equality and of care. The justice of difference, which she accepts as significant, has introduced novel concepts, which receive no hearing in the face of deeply rooted patriarchy. The dispensers of justice are simply unequal to the task of understanding what it asks for and of acting appropriately, leading to absurd conclusions like blaming the victims of rape, so common in India. Feminism's fight against woman's pain does not yet have a language that entrenched patriarchy understands. Let us begin from the position of crippling pain is what Moitra wants to say as far as the question of dispensing justice to the woman in pain is concerned.

Describing this situation is as much part of the solution as whatever else needs to follow. It is where we must begin.

Pain is not univocally, uniformly aversive. We "need pain to stay alive" (Käll 2013, p. 1) and develop as responding and responsible social beings. However, modern cultures deny the need for pain learned in the crucible of centuries of accumulated, filtered human experience across cultures. Modern life powerfully proclaims to us that "pain is unnecessary and easily banished from our experience; and it is widely assumed that pain and suffering can lead to no positive outcomes" (Schleifer 2014, p. 3). This aspect of modernism is repeatedly critiqued and rejected in the essays of this book, especially those by Hoff, Jacobson, Meinhold, Russon and George. Robinson Jeffers, the American poet of inhumanism (the idea of decentering humans from getting smugly wrapped up in themselves) writes in his poem "The Artist": "I think/Peace marrying pain alone can breed that excellence/in the luckless race", and in his "The World's Wonders" we read: "...I have learned that/happiness is important, but pain *gives* importance" (Monjian 1958, pp. 25–26). Even as torture and cruelty, agony and affliction, are to be averted at all costs, the torments of angst that accompany disquieting existence and the aches that go with the exertions of the body in the face of the possibilities of existence are inescapable aspects of living with significant positive meaning. Pain is indispensible to cherishing the pleasures that life offers.

John Stuart Mill proclaims that in the case of modern humanity that can be directed to achieve its well-being through conviction or persuasion, "compulsion, either in the direct form or in that of pains and penalties for non-compliance, is no longer admissible as a means to their own good, and justifiable only for the security of others" (Mill 1991, p. 31). Mill's celebrated formulation of negative liberty based on the harm principle is absolutely central to the modern liberal idea of social life and of the person. Shannon Hoff argues in her chapter that concerns like that of Mill in fact have to be overridden in the actual practice of life in society because to teach the art of acting in consent, we need to form people without their consent. Transgression and conflict that cause pain in this process are never fully avoidable despite our liberal faiths. Further, "both to discover that one's present capacities need to be transformed, and to undergo activities that would lead to transformation, can be painful experiences." Since these are conditions of possibility for meaningful existence, it is unreasonable to structure personal, social and political life imagining that there cannot be pain; rather, pain is the 'happy fault' necessary to the formation of agency. Overprotecting children can turn out to be obstructive of their agency. In other words, Hoff is saying that the eagerness of liberal polity to secure pain-absent environments can itself prove to be reinforcing painful existence.

The liberal individual thus cultivated can suffer from the pain of exclusion. We develop our agency through interacting with our immediate world and suffering the pain involved in this interaction. Preventing this legitimate pain politically with the hallowed goal of forming the abstract individual, argues Hoff, pains us, for "when the explicit intersubjective affiliations constitutive of personal identity—whether social, cultural, or religious—are denied to us, we can experience pain." She relates such pain to the experience of colonization. Unmistakably, the political project of liberal individualism is Hoff's target of attack. If we become human through the unique interactions we are able to have with reality, removal of those interactions makes existence worthless and painful. Much has been written on the subject of the pain of what is denied by liberalism. Charles Taylor, who is at the forefront of this angle of critique, points out that mainstreaming atomistic individualism is "very often the source of difficult and painful intergenerational battles in immigrant families, just because these individualisms define the mainstream into which the children are being unavoidably acculturated" (Taylor 1991, p. 75).

While Hoff's and later Umamaheshwari's critique of what modernity excludes and overrides is significant and necessary, it is facile to think that modernity is a univocal frame of the pain of exclusion. Referring to the new genre of Dalit (erstwhile 'untouchable' in India's caste hierarchy) autobiographical literature that record personal pain as social critique, Sarah Beth Hunt notes that "Dalit autobiographies reconstruct the notion of pain as unnatural and the caste discrimination associated with such pain as something wholly un-modern by mobilizing 'modern' discourses of justice and human rights and depicting the nation as the guardian of the rights of its citizens" (2014, p. 184). Ramachandra Guha makes a similar point when he argues that it was modernity, not tradition that let B.R. Ambedkar rise from among the oppressed Dalit castes to become an icon of twentieth-century India and framer of the Indian Constitution (2006, p. 243). Our socio-political frames, whether liberal modern, traditional or postmodern, tend to conceal as much as they reveal, and among what they conceal are undoubtedly prominent the suppressed cries of pain and suffering of the weakest classes, castes and sections of society. Hoff's chapter takes our eyes to structural tendencies that are susceptible to produce and reproduce what Ashis Nandy calls 'institutional sufferings' (1978) within the liberal modern frame, which has in many ways become our unmistakable global fate.

1.4 Social Contexts of Pain

The Indian origin of this volume in the conference on the enigma of pain held in IIT Bombay (see the Acknowledgements and the last paragraph of this Introduction) also means that it has an obvious lack. There is no chapter in it that directly deals with the question of caste, quite a labyrinth of pain and suffering for millions of people in the Indian subcontinent even to this day, despite substantial legal, political and institutional ground gained in the postcolonial era. Cultural memories fraught with pain and shame, privilege and favour, still burn like undying embers. The more liberal democratic tradition yearns for the abstract casteless citizen in India, the more is the affirmation of caste identities. The pain of yesteryears, suffered silently and alone by communities and persons, is washed justifiably in the public eye of the modern Indian nation, eagerly premised on the equality of all its citizens. The commitment to correction of past suffering and equality of citizens is affirmed unequivocally in the Constitution, framed by an assembly of eminent citizens led by the Dalit icon of equality, B.R. Ambedkar. The symbolic meaning of the event of the Constitution regulates Indian nationhood, although the goal of reasonable equality stubbornly refuses to arrive. Dalit literature itself is said to be cast in the same mold as pain, bequeathed with the mission "to inform Dalit society of its slavery, and narrate its pain and suffering to upper caste Hindus" (Limbale 2004, p. 19) and other Indians.

This deficiency of the present Collection is nevertheless addressed partially by the chapter by Umamaheshwari on the suffering of people who are dispossessed of their land, home and livelihood by the acclaimed march of the juggernaut of modern development. The fact that people who are thus displaced in this and many other instances are India's Dalits and Adivasis (indigenous people or tribal communities) smacks of ethnic otherness. Umamaheshwari's chapter is also on the nearly 'absent' community of Tamil Jainas, whose painful past and history seem to have no place amidst the triumphalist histories of the glorious present, weaved around majority sentiment. Her aim is to give a poignantly authentic picture of the unnamable sufferings of dispossession, ironically sealed with the stamp of the modern nation's legal machinery, the pain of banishment of historical selves into oblivion and the mindless assimilation of these 'lost selves' into the 'self' swollen with the strength of numbers. She also wants to highlight that such pains are not registered, not chronicled; there is no therapy to cure victims of such pain, no measure to weigh their suffering. It is in the carefully choreographed absencing of these sufferings that the justice of the politics of democracy is realized. She hopes for a radical politics of reconstructing a polity that does not "constantly exclude". The chapter paints a pain that has no place in the pain literature. There are pains of the excluded, the nearly disappearing, the genuinely unseen, unheard pain.

An important argument of Elaine Scarry's *The Body in Pain* is that both the silencing of pain and the expression of pain can be used by tormentors to intensify pain. She notes that "the human attempt to reverse the de-objectifying work of pain by forcing *pain itself* into avenues of objectification is a project laden with practical and ethical consequence" (1985, p. 6). The consequence she has in mind in the book is of a significantly political nature. But the infliction of pain, the cause, in the political context is equally important. It is 'torture'. Scarry stresses that "torture consists of acts that magnify the way in which pain destroys a person's world, self, and voice" (p. 50), an act that creates the regime's power over the subject. But the destruction of voice in torture does not simply mean that the finding of the voice in torture is unproblematically heartening. "In compelling confession, the torturers compel the prisoner to record and objectify the fact that intense pain is world-destroying" (p. 29). Insignificant information is thus forcefully let out of the mouth of the tortured body as a part of torture and, paradoxically, in order to silence the victim.

Malem Ningthouja's analysis attests Scarry's seminal observations on torture in the context of India's northeastern state of Manipur, bordering Burma, where the armed forces special powers act (AFSPA), a draconian piece of legislation that bestows extensive and unaccountable powers on the armed forces, is complexly poised to purportedly secure citizens against rebel terror, to torture citizens under the pretext of terror, to feed rebel rage in that process and thus, ironically, to secure rebellion and terror for good. Ningthouja's aim is not to find solutions to this complex political tangle but to understand the dialectics of military torture flourishing on terror and rebel terror flourishing on state-sponsored torture. In fact, the aim of this author, for whom the tag 'activist scholar' fits the most among the contributors of this volume, is not even to understand the vicious cycle of the political dialectics of torture and terror, but to study how pain becomes the publicly memorialized event, a totally transformed event from the intensely private, unsharable and most lonely experience that pain is before it can become the commemoration of a people's sedimented memories of suffering. He has much to say on the various trails and tracks of the memorialization of tortured bodies, but perhaps the most significant part of what he says is that neither torture and terror nor the commemoration of torture is innocently emptied of all pain. Inasmuch as the dialectics of torture and terror negate each other and affirm their own necessity and reality, the embodied 'civil' subjects of torture and terror, the permanent sufferers in the politics of terror and torture, are poignantly poised as the redeemed by both rebel terrorists and statist torturers. Neither the condition of being with the State nor of being stateless takes them out of the banal reality of politically constructed suffering. Ningthouja, however, puts the onus expectably on the State, asking it the uncomfortable question whether fighting terror with torture, which then feeds terror all the more, has any democratic-political legitimacy.

Elaine Scarry asks whether "the mental, verbal, or material process of making the world is not held to be centrally entailed in the elimination of pain as the unmaking of the world is held to be entailed in pain's infliction?" (1985, p. 22). She argues, thus, that the body in pain is at the centre of creating the world for pain's relief, and destroying the world for its infliction. The creation and destruction of the world depends on whether or not imaginative objectifications of thought in verbal expression and matter in the making of artifacts are forthcoming. From the point of view of the cultural ontology of the self in pain, our most original making is self-making or self-formation. Self-making does not occur in unbridled freedom, understood as the existential will to spontaneously reject and accept. Rather, original self-formation unfolds in receiving, accepting and responding to the world more passively than actively, so that the active adult can enter into the finite freedom of choice and agency on the basis of an aboriginal reception. And yet freedom is not only based on passive reception but, paradoxically, also on subjugation and domination. At the centre of the child's life stands what is most unpleasant and thus painful—punishment and disciplining through punishment. The problem of pain is central to the aboriginal receptions and subjugations of the child.

But Michel Foucault has taught us to see in the history of punishment the ways pain circulates and dissimulates itself in the dexterous webs of power and politics in relation to that which is the source of pain: our body-being. He observes that "the body is also directly involved in a political field; power relations have an immediate hold upon it; they invest it, mark it, train it, torture it, force it to carry out tasks, to perform ceremonies, to emit signs" (1977, p. 25). What Foucault speaks about is not the production of individual subjectivity or subjectivity at all but the non-subject-like receptive-passive production of historical humanity at noticeable junctures and cultural locations in history. Pain—not necessarily physical sensation but the domination and disciplining of our body-being—is thus central to not only self-making, but also to the 'collective self' understood as that socio-cultural-historical space of meanings into which we enter passively at our aboriginal beginnings and make sense of ourselves and our world. Sometimes at crucial junctures of history, forces outside our control and those that repel, and sometimes forces that curiously fascinate and enchant, impinge on our historical selves and transform them for good. Colonization is certainly one such juncture of history. Gender, caste, race, faith—these are also such historical contingencies but more nebulously spread across the pages of history than something like colonization, which is more easily locatable historically. The problem of pain in such instances is probably invisible.

However, not always. Parinitha Shetty's chapter on the missionary narrative of pain, unmistakably grounded in *Discipline and Punish* and focused on the archives of the Basel Mission in the Canarese region of south India (Karnataka), looks at the Mission's hospitals in the region and what they did to the 'heathens' who took succour in modern medicine. What they received was relief from pain and illness, a new narrative of pain and a new profiling of the disciplined body, always disambiguating the 'power' of the new body-being they were invited to enter into and the perils of what they were invited to leave behind. Far from imagining pain to be the fully escapable existential contingent, the missionary narrative harped on its existential ineluctability and power to reform and save fallen (heathen) body-being. The cathartic power of pain described by Meinhold is repeated in the missionary narrative in its material and religious power to politically save heathens. The dual salvations of colonial Christianity and modern Enlightenment were deftly intertwined in the politics of liberating the body-being in the missionary narrative, especially marked in such spaces as opened up by the singular problem of sufferings wrought by caste rules to both the privileged and the disadvantaged castes. Caste rules forbade the Dalit to be treated by traditional medicine but the same rules forbade the upper castes to be treated by modern medicine for fear of pollution. The problem of pain was one of the powerful factors for breaking with tradition's inhumanity to the Dalit and the imprisonment into a thousand rules of purity and pollution it forced upon the privileged. Shetty's chapter attests the centrality of the problem of pain in the making and remaking of selfhood and identity, not only in the large canvas of giant historical frames like modernity but also in fringe frames like colonial Christianity, although not unconnected to the project of historical modernity, at least as far as the history of colonization goes. Shetty stresses the undeniable porosity of our selfhood weaved out of narratives of pain and power when she says, for example, that "converted native Christian was never completely free of the remnants of heathenism."

In the history of self-formation, thus, pain becomes cathartic, ambiguous and ineluctable, but as Umamaheshwari insists, the pain of forgotten and lost selves, denied historical memories, and power-induced historical transitions of communities is not an easily erasable page of history as we are learning each day in today's India. The questionings of Ningthouja, Umamaheshwari and Shetty force us into the unfamiliar territory of exercising, what Ashis Nandy calls, "a new skepticism in the case of the defeated cultures… [that involves] challenging a series of ideas—among them progress, rationality, development and modern science" (2002, p. 209) are central. The register of pain is a profitable lens to relook at these 'modern truths', although no simplistic hope of regaining lost selves and lost histories is a tenable approach to the register of pain if that register is not to repeat history and inflict further pain through the very lens of pain. The register of pain probably asks us to correct our present from repeating the pains of history and thus to imagine futures that will not escape pain completely but will negotiate suffering meaningfully and compassionately.

It must be mentioned that the theme of the present volume, 'Cultural Ontology of the Self in Pain', emerged after the presentations and deliberations of an earlier Conference on the theme, "The Enigma of Pain", organized in March 2013, by the Department of Humanities and Social Sciences, IIT Bombay, in collaboration with the Balvant Parekh Centre for General Semantics and Other Human Sciences, Vadodara, India, with P.G. Jung as the coordinator. Since only four of the 13 papers of this volume are revised versions of the papers of the conference, this book cannot be called a product of the conference; however, the conference provided the original motivation, both for the theme as well as for putting together the essays of this volume.

References

Bendelow, G. (1993). Pain perceptions, emotions and gender. *Sociology of Health & Illness, 15*(3), 273–294.

Carr, D. B., Loeser, J. D., & Morris, D. B. (Eds.). (2005). *Narrative, pain and suffering. Series: Progress in pain research and management* (Vol. 34). Seattle, WA: The International Association for the Study of Pain.

Carrithers, M. (2012). Ontology is just another word for culture: For the motion (I). *Critique of Anthropology, 30*(2), 156–68.

Coakley, S., & Shelemay, K. K. (Eds.). (2007). *Pain and its transformations: The interface of biology and culture.* Cambridge, MA: Harvard University Press.

Dreyfus, H. L. (2004). Taylor's (anti-)epistemology. In R. Abbey (Ed.), *Charles Taylor* (pp. 52–83). Cambridge: Cambridge University Press.

Easwaran, E. (Trans.). (1996). *The Dhammapada.* New Delhi: Penguin.

Encandela, J. A. (1993). Social science and the study of pain since Zborowski: A need for a new agenda. *Social Science and Medicine, 36*(6), 783–91.

Foucault, M. (1977). *Discipline and punish: The birth of the prison* (A. Sheridan, Trans.). New York: Vintage.

Guha, R. (2006). *How much should a person consume?: Thinking through the environment.* Ranikhet, India: Permanent Black.

Hardcastle, V. G. (1999). *The myth of pain.* Cambridge, MA: The MIT Press.

Heidegger, M. (1971) "What are poets for?" (1946), (A. Hofstadter, Trans.). In M. Heidegger, *Poetry, language, thought* (pp. 87–139). New York: Harper & Row.

Heidegger, M. (1998). Letter on "humanism" (1946), (F. A. Capuzzi, Trans.). In M. Heidegger, *Pathmarks* (W. McNeill, Ed.) (pp. 239–276). Cambridge: Cambridge University Press.

Holbraad, M. (2010). Ontology is just another word for culture: Against the motion (2). *Critique of Anthropology, 30*(2), 179–85.

Hunt, S. B. (2014). *Hindi Dalit literature and the politics of representation.* New Delhi: Routledge.

Hutchinson, P. (2008). *Shame and philosophy: An investigation in the philosophy of emotions and ethics.* Basingstoke: Palgrave-Macmillan.

Käll, L. F. (2013). Introduction: Dimensions of pain. In L. F. Käll (Ed.), *Dimensions of pain: Humanities and social science perspectives* (pp. 1–12). Abingdon, UK: Routledge.

Levinas, E. (1990). *Difficult freedom: Essays on Judaism* (S. Hand, Trans.). Baltimore, MA: The Johns Hopkins University Press.

Limbale, S. (2004). *Towards an aesthetic of Dalit literature: History, controversies and considerations.* (A. Mukherjee, Trans.). New Delhi: Orient Blackswan.

Mander, R. (2011). *Pain in childbearing and its control: Key issues for midwives and women* (2nd ed.). Oxford: Wiley-Blackwell.

McHoul, A. (1999). The ontology of culture—Way-markers. *Humanitas, (XII)*2, 88–103.

Mill, J. S. (1991). *On liberty in focus* (J. Gray & G. W. Smith, Eds.). London: Routledge.

Monjian, M. C. (1958). *Robinson Jeffers: A study in inhumanism.* Pittsburgh, PA: University of Pittsburgh Press.

Morris, D. B. (1991). *The culture of pain.* Berkeley, CA: University of California Press.

Morris, D. B. (1998). *Illness and culture in the postmodern age.* Berkeley, CA: University of California Press.

Nandy, A. (1978). Oppression and human liberation: Towards a third world utopia. *Alternatives, 4* (2), 165–180.

Nandy, A. (2002). *Time warps: Silent and evasive pasts in Indian politics and religion.* New Brunswick, NJ: Rutgers University Press.

Palecek, M., & Risjord, M. (2013). Relativism and the ontological turn within anthropology. *Philosophy of the Social Sciences, 43*(1), 3–23.

Ramazani, V. (2007). *Writing in pain: Literature, history, and the culture of denial.* New York: Palgrave-Macmillan.

Rollason, W. (2008). Ontology—just another word for culture?: The group for debates in anthropological theory, Manchester, 9 Feb 2008. *Anthropology Today, 24*(3), 28 & 31.

Sartre, J-P. (2001). Existentialism is humanism (1945). (P. Mairet, Trans.). In S. Priest (Ed.), *Jean-Paul Sartre: Basic writings* (pp. 25–57). Abingdon, UK: Routledge.

Scarry, E. (1985). *The body in pain: The making and unmaking of the world.* Oxford: Oxford University Press.

Schleifer, R. (2014). *Pain and suffering.* New York: Routledge.

Taylor, C. (1991). *The ethics of authenticity.* Cambridge, MA: Harvard University Press.

Tolstoy, L. (2008). "The death of Ivan Ilyich" (A. Briggs, Trans.). In L. Tolstoy, *The death of Ivan Ilyich and other stories.* London: Penguin.

Venkatesan, S. (Ed.). (2010). Ontology is just another word for culture: Motion tabled at the 2008 meeting of the group for debates in anthropological theory, University of Manchester. *Critique of Anthropology, 30*(2), 152–200.

Woolf, C. J. (2007). Deconstructing pain: A deterministic dissection of the molecular basis of pain. In S. Coakley & K. K. Shelemay (Eds.), *Pain and its transformations: The interface of biology and culture* (pp. 27–35). Cambridge, MA: Harvard University Press.

Zborowski, M. (1969). *People in pain.* San Francisco: Jossey-Bass Publishers.

Part I
Ontology of Pain

Chapter 2
Ontology of Pain in Moral Theories

Abstract Pain has been a central concept in moral theories, especially among those that take the conceptual pair of pain–pleasure as central to its very formulation. Thus in a way, they present to us a way of understanding the role of pain in its holistic avatar within the fabric of one's being as being-in-the-world. This essay first undertakes the tracing of this ontology of pain within such moral frameworks through a brief exegetical exercise that is intent on highlighting that the ontology of pain that emerges through these various moral theories is uniformly informed by the *principle of contrariety* and the *principle of naturalness*. The second part of the essay would, through broad strokes, bring to fore the implications of these principles upon the ontology of pain. Through this, it would highlight why the ontology of pain as conceived within these moral theories cannot naturally translate into a fully fleshed out discourse on the social ontology of pain and remain, at best, an asocial ontology of pain.

Keywords Epicureanism · Stoicism · Utilitarianism · Contrariety · Naturalness · Social · Asocial

I am grateful to Joseph Lobo and Shannon Hoff for their critical inputs.

P.G. Jung (✉)
Indian Institute of Advanced Study, Shimla, India
e-mail: pgjung@iitb.ac.in

P.G. Jung
Department of Humanities and Social Sciences, Indian Institute of Technology Bombay, Mumbai, India

2.1 Introduction: Towards an Ontology of Pain

The question 'what is pain?' is, by and large, a nineteenth century interrogative stance that emerges rather forcefully with the rise in the disciplines of Medicine and Psychology, and their claims to 'scientificity'. From the latter half of the nineteenth century this question is what translates into the fervent attempts to categorize the term and to sharpen its boundaries, so as to distill the metaphysical elements that it might share with its historical synonyms 'suffering' or even 'unpleasantness.'[1] For some, this delineation of the boundaries of the notion of 'pain', as Eric Cassel's work (2004) highlights, was based on the rise of the division between objective and subjective knowledge in the 'sciences', and the insistence that the predicate of 'certainty' was an exclusive characteristic of the former. For others, this delineation was necessary in order to provide a naturalistic ground for the developing domains of Medicine and Psychology.[2] For yet others, it was a prerequisite step that facilitated lucidity and precision to the positivistic discourse that came to be labelled as 'Philosophical psychology'. The importance of the notion for Philosophy of Mind can be gauzed from the fact that as late as 1967, Putnam asserts that "the typical concerns of the Philosopher of Mind might be represented by three questions: (1) How do we know that other people have pains? (2) Are pains brain states? (3) What is the analysis of the concept *pain*?" (1975, p. 429).

Such attempts to cleanse the notion of pain functioned to reduce it to its narrower connotation of 'sensations *of* and *in* the body'. The body was construed as the locus

---

[1]The term 'suffering' has a much broader connotation and cannot be unproblematically identified with the term 'pain'. For instance, a person with bodily deformity *may not* experience pain, but he/she *may* nevertheless be suffering. Simply put, following Eric Cassel, bodies are in pain while persons, notwithstanding its ambiguous connotations, suffer (2004, p. v). However, given the scope of this chapter in terms of its engagement with moral theories, the term 'pain' is used to stand for the term 'unpleasantness' to impart to it a broader connotation than its connotative identification with 'afflictions of the body'. In doing so, one can fruitfully speak of pain in terms of the 'pain of boredom', 'painful company', 'pain of guilt' and so on, and as there are unpleasant sensations, there are unpleasant memories as well. Here, 'pain' therefore means something that is 'unpleasant' as it captures the fundamental sense in which it is employed within the moral discourse that the essay engages with.

[2]The consequences of this dominant tendency, on the one hand has led to the steady *reduction* of the connotation of the term 'pain' to mean the mechanical, determinist, and law-governed representation of the complex system of nervous transmission from the site of injured tissues to the brain, within medical science. This representation of pain was far more materialistic and reductive than the one conceived by Descartes himself (see Morris 1994, pp. 12–13). Such a representation, however, was shaken, first by the phenomenon of pain without lesion, and then by the rise of knowledge of *chronic* pain. Though such reductive representation of the notion is now being seriously questioned, following the seminal work by Morris (1991), one cannot also ignore the rise of pain-scales, and algometry within the 'scientifically' oriented disciplines like psychology and psychophysics (see for instance, Noble et al. 2005; Melzack 1983). Needless to say, the term 'pain' has come to mean significantly different things for people engaged with it in different disciplines. In fact, the difference of the connotative aspect of the term 'pain' between the sciences and the humanities is so divergent in terms of the sense signified that many a times what is common is merely the term. This *oneness* of sense can perhaps be sought to be addressed, as suggested by Boddice, by "training of the ear and of the pen" (2014, p. 2).

of 'objective claims'[3] and consequently medicine, in its bid to 'objectivity', becomes fundamentally engaged with the category of 'disease'. This turn towards confining 'pain' to bodily sensations within the discourse becomes the dominant mode, and not surprisingly so, from the nineteenth century onwards, since this bias was then bolstered by fresh discoveries pertaining to the intricate mechanisms of the nervous system and with the refinement of the stimulus-response framework within Psychology. With this prevailing tendency, 'pain' was sought to be distinguished even from its broader correlate 'unpleasantness'. One cannot miss to note this tendency in the journal articles and reviews engaging with the notion during the late nineteenth century.[4] In some cases, as with the 1895 review article of Sidney E. Mezes, one can see the explicit demand, with a sense of urgency, that the term 'pain' be restricted to mean "an unpleasant sensation, either of touch or systemic, of abnormal intensity" (1895, p. 46), emphasizing that

> Pains arise in the case of burns, lacerations, bruises, the crushing of any part of the body, neuralgia (*not nervousness*), toothache, inflamed tissues, etc., etc. Pains, that is, in strictness are a *class of* highly unpleasant sensations located quite definitely in the body'. (1895, p. 22; emphasis mine)

Although the reductive physicalist's insistence on the objectivity of pain is still a dominant mode (see for instance, Hardcastle 1999), there has nevertheless been a steady rise of a voice within the discourse that decries the legitimacy of this reductivist insistence. The last few decades has seen a forceful emphasis on the ways in which the subjective and the socio-cultural aspects undergird the varying meanings that 'pain-experiences' come to acquire, highlighting how pain-experiences defy the reductivist's neat mechanical and 'objectivistic' explanatory structures of pain and its affects.

In the light of the above, how do we place moral theories that take the notion of pain as cardinal? These moral frameworks clearly take the notion to signify more than what the reductive physicalist would agree to, but at the same time, they do not manage to explicitly embed the notion inalienably within the realms of the subjective and the socio-cultural. Within these moral frameworks, the question 'what is pain?' becomes an exploration that seeks to address the existential question of pain in its phenomenality. Here querying the *whatness* of pain, takes a tacit turn to an engagement with its *whyness*, seeking to make sense of it in terms of its existential function. The distinctiveness of such an orientation emerges in terms of the interpretation that one provides to the term 'being' in the phrase 'being in pain'. The former orientation of 'whatness' takes the term 'being' to be a verb, while the latter

---

[3]This was one of the crucial reasons for the interest in 'phantom limbs', for it set to seriously challenge this identification by highlighting the experience of pain in the absence of its bodily correlate that could act as its locus. Phantom limbs thus challenged the very idea that there could be no pain without lesion.

[4]From the range of conceptually oriented scholarly articles available on the notions of pain and pleasure, one can see that it was a theme of great interest from the late nineteenth century. For instance, see Brinton (1876), Stanley (1889), Marshall (1889, 1891, 1895), Bain (1892), Nichols (1892a, b), Hutchinson (1897), Anonymous (1921).

orientation of 'whyness' treats it as a noun. Consequently, in the former orientation, to raise a question of *whatness* in relation to 'being in pain' is to primarily raise the question 'what is it to be in pain?' or 'what does it mean to say I, or someone, is in pain?' Thus, the explorative attempt of such an orientation is to address the phenomenality of the *state* of being-in-pain. In contrast, the latter orientation takes the interrogative stance of addressing, not the *state* primarily, but rather the phenomenality of pain in relation to the *being* of the person who is in pain. It is in this primary relation of pain to the *being* of a being-in-pain, rather than to a state in which the being happens to be, that the latter orientation can be said to be an *ontology of a being in pain.*[5] Interrogating pain in terms of its *whyness* in relation to *being* has had a significant import on the discourse on morality and has lent it a distinct trajectory. As we shall see, it is along this trajectory that the ontology of pain first finds its precursor in classical moral theories. Moving beyond the binary lens of pain as a 'sensation' and as a 'feeling'/'disposition', these moral theories can be seen as implicitly explicating the role of pain in its holistic avatar within the fabric of one's being, and as a being-in-the-world. Within this orientation, the question of 'whatness' of pain is not neglected, but simply put under the purview of what I call the *principle of familiarity*[6] where the unmediated subjective familiarity with pain in terms of its 'thatness' becomes the ground of knowing *what it is,* and hence, is taken to sufficiently answer the substantive question pertaining to its *whatness.*

Thus, the attempt to elicit an ontology of pain is, in a way, to *re*think the trajectory of the notion in its varying formulations in the dominant moral theories that take pain as an axial category, and to trace its conceptualization through them, charting out its legitimate existential sense. Of course, the tracing of such an ontology of pain within the dominant moral frameworks is an extrapolation, given that these theories were not explicitly engaged in formulating ontologies of pain. This essay precisely makes such an attempt to foreground the ontology of pain in these theories through a brief exegetical exercise, with the intent of highlighting that the ontology of pain that gets sketched through these various moral theories are

---

[5]The literature on 'pain', following the popularity of the two seminal works, that by Scarry (1985) and Morris (1991), in my reading can be precisely categorized along this division. While both Scarry and Morris seek to argue against the narrow envisaging of pain in strict medical terms, the former seeks to do so by exploring the question of 'what is the import of pain to my *being*' while the latter seeks to open up the medical discourse to the question, 'what is the import of my *being* to pain?'.

[6]The 'principle of familiarity' was also invoked by psychologists and 'medical professionals'. Instantiating the invocation of this principle, Thomas Lewis, who was closely associated with both, the field of medicine, as well as psychology, begins the Preface of his *Pain* by declaring that "[r] eflection tells me that I am so far from being able satisfactorily to define pain, of which I here write, that the attempt could serve no useful purpose. Pain, like similar subjective things, is known to us by experience and described by illustration. The usage of the term in this book will be clear enough to anyone who reads its pages; to build up a definition in words or to substitute some phrase would carry neither the reader nor myself farther..." (1942, p. v).

uniformly informed by the 'principle of contrariety', and the 'principle of naturalness'. Given the constraint of space, my brief concluding section will indicate the implications of these two principles for the ontology of pain.

2.2 Part-I

2.2.1 In the Socratic Thesis...

The first interrogation of pain in this modality comes to us in Plato's *Philebus* which offers the Socratic view that "when the harmony in animals is dissolved, during such time there is both a dissolution of their natural state and a generation of pain... and the restoration of harmony and return to nature is the source of pleasure" (31d; 32d–e). Further along the Dialogue, Socrates accentuates this view to Protarchus when he remarks:

> I have often repeated that pains and aches and suffering and uneasiness of all sorts arise out of a corruption of nature caused by concretions, and dissolutions, and repletions, and evacuations, and also by growth and decay... And we have also agreed that the restoration of the natural state is pleasure (42c–d).

The Socratic view presented here by Plato, which later serves as the grounds for the distinction between the Epicureans and the Stoics, foregrounds a particular modality to look at pain that is in resonance with the Hippocratic view that pain is a signifier pointing to an individual's condition in relation to what is *natural*.[7] The *Philebus* thus renders a diagnostic value to the notion of pain, more or less in the same vein as does the Hippocratic view.[8] Further, within Greek thought, what a sign signifies (*sēmainon*) could only be deciphered within the larger, tacitly held, *world-view* or the idea of a *cosmos*. Thus, the *Philebus* in its diagnostic approach portrays pains and pleasures as indicators of one's conformity or digression from one's ordained place within the *cosmos* predetermined by the nature of one's *being*. Clearly then, here, the denotative power of the term 'pain' transcends the narrow confines of pointing to something in and of the physical body.

Further, the fact that Socrates in *Philebus* upholds that one could have pleasures of recollection from memory (33c; 36b) or the storehouse where past sensations are preserved (34a); and the Socratic division of pain into "pain of the soul *alone*"

---

[7]Hippocratic medicine is structurally grounded within the triadic notions of *disease*, the *patient* and the *physician*, or what is often referred to as the 'Hippocratic Triangle'. Within Hippocratic medicine, as Rey emphasizes, the patient's description of his pain is of "greater significance than in other concepts of medicine" (1995, p. 20), and that within the Hippocratic system "pain signifies... which is certainly not to be taken as an isolated symptom but rather as part of an overall picture of how the patient looks, what his behavior is like compared to how he generally behaves, his stools, urine, sweat, etc." (p. 20).

[8]The construal of pain in this manner is what would be later picked up by Epicureans and extended to its logical entailments.

(like fear and anxiousness) which are produced by expectations, and the "pleasures of the soul *alone*" produced by hope (32c), is a clear indicator that the notion of 'pain' as outlined in the *Philebus* is not confined to the bodily or physical pain in either of its modern categorization—*chronic* or *acute*. In fact, given the five-sense-organs framework within which they largely conceived sensations, and given the diverse functions that they allocated to the sense of touch, pain was more closely seen, within the thought schemas of the Greeks, in terms of its relation to the soul through the lens of passions, rather than an explicitly reductive correlate to what we would call 'sensation' today.

This broadening of the notion is more clearly discerned within Aristotle's nuanced formulation of sensation in psychophysical terms, under the rubric of the hylomorphism that pervades his works, especially in his articulation of the key notion of *phantasia*—anotion that was to find a cardinal position in the doctrines of the Stoics. As Modrak elaborates, the perceptual faculty for Aristotle was not merely confined to sense perception but was rather seen as grounding our broader capabilities such as our ability "to imagine, to dream, to remember" and more importantly, it was seen as intricately woven with our ability to "engage in goal-directed behavior" (1987, p. 2). This, therefore, essentially positioned 'sensation', and there by 'pain' as a notion within the legitimate concerns of a moral framework in the Greek thought schemas in general. The psychologist Karl Dallenbach in his 1939 conceptual review article suggests that it was precisely this influence of Greek thought "on philosophical and scientific thought" that "delayed the recognition of pain as a sensory quality" (p. 331).

It would not be far off the mark to suggest that what contributed to this non-identification of pain with a narrower connotation of 'sensation' in Greek thought was the way in which sensations were understood through the 'five-senses'. Their 'sensory framework' makes the rigid identification of pain strictly as a 'sensation' commonsensically problematic, since unlike other sensations, pain does not confine itself to any of the five-sense-organs as such, nor does it indicate a distinct sense organ for itself. Thus, the mode in which the ontology of pain is sketched in the *Philebus* is more holistic in its orientation to one's *being* as such, rather than the modern day shaping of the notion in strict mechanical and physiological terms. Pain as outlined in the *Philebus,* thereby provides us a broader mode of conceiving it in terms of a diagnostic mechanism that is indicative of one's deviation from, or conformity to, the path that is natural to one's *being*. Within the Socratic thesis, pain is thus construed as a *relational* notion that is indicative of the movement of one's being towards degeneration from what is 'natural' to it, irrespective of whether we take the Socratic hedonism as outlined in the *Protagoras*or his apparent non-hedonistic position in the *Gorgias*.

Further, the notions of 'degeneration' and 'restoration' are broader in their scope as far as the Socratic usage is concerned, for it includes not merely the bodily affections like hunger and eating (*Philebus*, 31e), or thirst and drinking, or heat and cooling (32a), but also the recovery of lost knowledge or sensations (34b). Notwithstanding the fact that it might be contentious to hold, as Rudebusch's does, that the Socratic thesis on pleasure is to be read as an engagement with an exclusive non-sensate notion of pleasure (see 1999, pp. 65–96) or a *modal* account of pleasure-pleasure as a mode of activity that orients the agent's being in a particular way (5); and notwithstanding the philosophical nuances involved in the various positions of pain that can be drawn out from these Dialogues, at the very least, it could be consistently held that the Socratic notion of pain pertains to the state of one's *being as such* and not merely to the physical body; and is essentially relational insofar as it is conceived primarily in terms of an activity or a process in relation to a being's natural state.

2.2.2 *In Nicomachean Ethics…*

Aristotle in his *Nicomachean Ethics* rejects the idea of conceiving pleasure strictly in terms of a 'coming-to-be' (1152b; 1173a–b) or as a state that comes about through the overcoming of a deficiency. In doing so, he does appear to distance himself from the Socratic position that relates the nature of pain and pleasure with each other and conceives them in terms of the notions of 'degeneration' and 'restoration', respectively. However, we must note that Aristotle's discomfort with the 'coming-to-be' modality of framing pleasure is precisely that even such a perspective bases itself primarily upon the pleasures concerning the body like those related to thirst and hunger, where the pleasure of replenishment is necessarily preceded by the pain experienced through a lack (1173b). For him, such a formulation articulates the nature of pleasure that holds in these cases as universal, and that it does so at the cost of ignoring those pleasures that are painless, and thus do not conform to such an articulation. Aristotle argues that such an approach dilutes the distinction between an "activity" or a process that gives us pleasure by virtue of replenishment and restoration and a "state" of pleasure (1152b–1153a) where no such prior demand of replenishment or pain-experience is required. Although for Aristotle, the necessity to maintain this division arises by virtue of the fact that the blurring of this division would lead to an over-emphasis on the bodily pleasures given that they neatly categorize themselves in the former kind, what it highlights for us is the fact that within Aristotle's formulation, pain, as is in the Socratic thesis, is still conceived *through* pleasure and not in isolation from it.[9]

   Although Aristotle's division of pleasure does confine pain to the realm of 'pleasure activity', he does agree that within this realm of pleasure, we do experience pleasure through a process of replenishment. Thus 'pain' as deprivation or deterioration is necessarily connected to pleasure; the latter emerging precisely

---

[9]Further, his argument that conceiving pleasure strictly in terms of a 'coming-to-be' would fail to accommodate pleasures, like those of "contemplation", "learning", and "the pleasures of smell, and many sounds, sights, memories and hopes as well", on the ground that these are "painless pleasures" for "no deficiency of anything has arisen, of which there might come to be a replenishment" (1173b), rather resonates the Socratic classification of "pleasures and pain of the soul alone" in the *Philebus* (32c) instead of positioning itself in stark contrast to it.

through an overcoming of the former.[10] Further, though in Aristotle's formulation, a 'pleasant state' does not presuppose pain-experiences, it does not completely exclude pain as such either. He abrasively states that "people who claim that the person being tortured, or a person who has fallen on very bad times [pain as deterioration], is happy if he is good [a pleasant state] are... talking nonsense" (1153b). This strongly suggests that though pleasure can be independent of pain in terms of a 'pleasant state', the ontology of pain in Aristotle is nevertheless, in some indirect way, still related to these states as a precursory requirement insofar as a 'pleasant state' presupposes that pains be overcome or that the 'incidentally pleasant' be restored first.

Further, Aristotle can still be read as upholding, though in a nuanced manner, the relational aspect of pain as seen in the Socratic thesis, where pain is construed in terms of the state of one's being and in relation to an activity or a process against the horizon of our ordained natural state. The centrality of the notion of 'impediment' in Aristotle's attempt to define pleasure in terms of completion of an activity as "an activity of one's natural state...that is unimpeded" (1153a), and his effort to make this definition generic and applicable to both the pleasures pertaining to the senses as well as those of "contemplation" and "thought" (1174b–1175a) highlights, an orientation that is similar to the one adopted within the Socratic thesis, notwithstanding its differences from it. Thus Aristotle too renders the notion of pleasure, and thereby derivatively the notion of pain, a much broader scope by positioning it essentially in relation to an activity of a doing-being and considers pain-experiences within the larger landscape of such experiences qua our being.

The ontology of pain thus far sketched addresses the question of pain, in terms of its role or place in affirming and conforming the nature that is peculiar to our *being* as humans *as such,* and grounds pain within the larger domain of *doing*, that is, within the realm of goal-oriented activities. This, as we have stated earlier, render the notions of pain and pleasure a position of cardinality within moral discourse. Within such a framework, the notion of pain becomes synonymous with the *unpleasant,* and the *feeling* or the experience of pain or *unpleasantness* is seen in an inalienable relation to the realm of *being* and *doing*. However, within this very ontology of pain, Aristotle's *Nicomachean Ethics*, in tune with that which is suggested in the Socratic thesis too, explicitly closes off the possibility of an ontology of pain that is independent of its relation to pleasure. Particularly, Aristotle's explicit formulation of the division between that which is 'incidentally pleasant' and that which is 'naturally pleasant', clearly confines the conceptualization of any ontology of pain as being possible only when conceived in relation to pleasure. Given that the realm of pain is confined to the sphere of the incidentally pleasant alone (since only the incidentally pleasant emerges as a 'coming-to-be' through an act of restoration or through a negation of pain), the possibility of any ontology of

---

[10]For Aristotle, these pleasures are, however, 'remedial' in nature and are 'incidentally pleasant' and are not to be confused with the 'naturally pleasant' which is the mark of a 'pleasant state'. The latter is "pleasant by nature" and produces "action in a healthy nature" in contrast to the former which merely restores it to a state of healthy nature (1154b).

pain that is unrelated to pleasure is thus foreclosed. This closing of the possibility of a discrete ontology of pain in the Socratic thesis, and more forcefully in Aristotle's *Nicomachean Ethics*, is of grave consequence to the very modes in which pain comes to be subsequently conceived.

2.2.3   Ontology of Pain as Negation

Both the Socratic and Aristotle's thesesplace the notion of pain centrally within a moral discourse, yet in them, the ontology of pain emerges *only* as the mirror negation of the ontology of its counterpart—pleasure. In them, the ontology of pleasure does not merely inform the ontology of pain but rather defines it. The ontology of pain here is but an inferential ontology that is sketched out via negativa. Thus, though it frees the notion of pain from the narrower modern connotation as *sensation*, which seeks to grasp it solely in terms of its pragmatic biological function of aversion from bodily harm, it nevertheless does not move towards a fuller articulation of the potentiality that is thus opened up by this freeing of the notion. This freeing of the notion of pain can itself be read as being incidental and brought about by virtue of the fact that the notion of pleasure refuses to contain itself within the bounds of 'sensation'.

Thus, the principle of contrariety, which was the central principle among the early Greek cosmologists, and which finds a modern voice in Hegelianism, is the principle that frames the notion of pain–pleasure here. Although the invoking of this principle is evident throughout the *Philebus* and explicitly so in the Socratic treatment of the possibility of an intermediate state between that of pleasure and pain (43eff.); one of the most articulate invocations of the above principle occurs in the *Phaedo* where Socrates, reflecting upon this relation of opposition between pleasure and pain, observes:

> How singular is the thing called pleasure, and how curiously related to pain, which might be thought to be the opposite of it; for they are never present to a man at the same instant… their bodies are two, but they are joined by a single head… as I know by my own experience now, when after the pain in my leg which was caused by the chain, pleasure appears to succeed…. (*Phaedo*, p. 60)

The principle of contrariety opens up a peculiar possibility, namely, that of relating in an intelligible and harmonious manner, two relata of opposite natures in a singular plane of relation. Socrates metaphorically puts this across as being akin to the joining of two bodies with a single head. The enabling of this peculiar possibility of bringing together relata of opposite natures renders it as the favourite principle among the early Greek cosmologists, and one that is most thoroughly and emphatically employed by Aristotle. The development of his logic is grounded through and through in this principle. The Cartesian dualism too, as Ryle emphasizes in his *The Concept of Mind*, is based on the tacit employment of the principle of contrariety. Aristotle's employment of the principle in his engagement with the notion of pain is undeniable throughout the *Nicomachean Ethics*, but its invocation is explicit in his brief explication of the notions of pain and pleasure as providing the needed conceptual grounds for the notion of "punishment" (1104b), and even more so when he holds that the objects of choice, namely, "the noble, the useful, and the pleasant" stand in a relation of contrariety with "their contraries, the shameful, the harmful, and the painful" (ibid., also see 1154b, 1175b).

Invoking the principle of contrariety in making sense of the notion of 'pain', in an important sense, impoverishes the possibility of its exploration since it comes to be conveniently framed as the 'absence' of pleasure.[11] Thus the exploration of pain comes to be reduced to an exploration of *that which is absent*, namely, pleasure; and pain, within such an enframement, comes to be essentially seen and understood *through* the lens of pleasure. Its nature, function and its relation to our *being* cannot be construed independently without the mediation of the nature of pleasure. The ontology of pain under the light of the principle of contrariety thus becomes an inferential ontology. Further under the ambit of the principle of contrariety, pain-experiences come to be essentially framed as negative experiences, though the possibility of their employment or their appropriation towards a positive end is acknowledged and fruitfully employed as well.

2.2.4   In the Epicurean Formulation...

This inferentialontology of pain, as deciphered above within the Socratic and Aristotle's theses, forms the archetype for the later sketch of the ontology of pain, and is clearly traceable in the Epicurean formulation. The Epicurean articulation, though distinct from the Socratic and Aristotle's formulations, can still be read as a fuller mapping out of the terrain of pain-experiences within the dominant purview of the principle of contrariety. The principle of contrariety here explicitly governs the conceptualization of the notions of pain and pleasure, and further secures these two notions in an inalienable relation of a twin pair: 'pain-pleasure'. It is within the Epicurean thesis that we find, for the first time, a sustained effort to place the twin notions in the highest cardinal place within the domain of ethics. Furthermore, it is in the Epicurean doctrines that the structure of the inferential ontology of pain that is implicitly present in their predecessors' theses finds an avenue for a fuller articulation in their identification of 'good' with that which is 'natural' to one's being and the 'good' being explicitly dictated by the twin notions. In other words, the Epicurean discourse is the first in the history of ideas that consciously attempts to formulate the notion of pleasure as the ultimate human *telos* and given that the Epicurean discourse conforms to the principle of contrariety, it too, thereby, posits pleasure as the negation of pain. Volitions, which are indicative of our conscious

---

[11]In a sense, this is akin to the impoverishment of aesthetics that comes about when one treats shadows as an 'absence' of light, as highlighted by Tanizaki (1977).

goal-oriented actions, for the Epicureans, are necessarily governed by the primordial and inviolable dictates of securing pleasure (*hedone*) for one's self. It is this inviolable nature of our volitions that necessitate any conception of good to be inevitably related to pleasure. The congeniality of a choice towards the securing of one's pleasure, which is but the negation of one's pain, thus becomes the yardstick for every judgment concerning the good within the Epicurean discourse. Epicurus is explicit in his words of advice to Menoeceus;

> For it is to obtain this end that we always act, namely, to avoid pain and fear... For we recognize pleasure as the first good innate in us, and from pleasure we begin every act of choice and avoidance, and to pleasure we return again, using the feeling as the standard by which we judge every good... (*Epicurus to Menoeceus*: [cited henceforth as ME], pp. 31–32).

Thus, the Epicurean formulation naturalizes the ontology of pain by positioning pain and pleasure as the originary or the primordial affections that are natural to us, and thus by the same stroke, they pave the way for the possibility of formulating a naturalized ethical discourse that would later come to be fully explored and exploited by the likes of Hume and Bentham. But the connotation of the terms 'pleasure', as evoked in the Epicurean discourse, is much more sophisticated and nuanced than a simplistic allusion to the satisfaction of one's appetites of the senses and the flesh, and does not entail the identification of the 'good life' as an unbridled partaking and promoting of the enjoyment of a subjective feeling brought about by the satisfaction of the choices that afford them. Thus, in tune with their predecessorial formulations, neither pleasure, nor pain (which is treated as its contrary), is confined to the experiences of the flesh alone.

Even though the Epicurean doctrine inverts the predecessorial formulation that *virtue* is what imparts pleasure to the fact of acting virtuously by conversely upholding that virtue is the negation of pain (or that it is the resultant pleasure that determines certain actions as virtuous), it still conceives of pleasure and pain in the light of 'right understanding' of desires[12] and as being rightfully in need of mediation through a conscious exercise of the prudence in our choice to either pursue or avoid them. Epicurus thus warns Menoeceus:

> ...And since pleasure is the first good and natural to us, for this very reason we do not choose every pleasure, but sometimes we pass over many pleasures, when greater discomfort accrues to us as the result of them: and similarly we think many pains better than pleasures, since a greater pleasure comes to us when we have endured pains for a long time. Every pleasure then because of its natural kinship to us is good, yet not every pleasure is to be chosen: even as every pain also an evil, yet not all are always of nature to be avoided.

---

[12]The Epicureans distinguish desires into two major classes: one that is *natural* and the other that is *vain* or empty. The class of natural desires is further divided into two classes, namely, *necessary natural desires*, and the class that lacks this necessity. Depending upon what these desires are necessary for, the class of necessary natural desires is further divided into three kinds: desires that are necessary for happiness, for the repose of the body, and the third for life itself. Although Epicurus is not explicit about the hierarchy of these desires, it is clear that the hierarchy moves from those necessary for life itself, to those that pertain to the body and happiness, with desires that are empty or vain placed at the lowest rung of the scale.

Yet by a scale of comparison and by the consideration of advantages and disadvantages we must form our judgment on all these matters... (ME, p. 32).

The *prima facie* paradoxical Epicurean thesis that even though pleasure is the highest good, not all pleasures are to be chosen, is better made sense of, if we bear in mind that Epicurus, under the influence of Aristotle's thesis, sought to distinguish *kinetic*pleasures from *static* or *katastemaic* ones. Furthermore, the Epicurean formulation is also under the influence of Aristotle's thesis that choice and action unfold in the direction of a *telos* or a final state that we *ought* to move towards. These bring forth the implicitly operative thesis that the good life is not a chaotic fulfilment of desires, or a whimsical pursuit of pleasures, but is rather that which is to be achieved through a deliberated strategy of attaining a state of pleasure that is an *end-in-itself,* thus rendering prudence as a virtue that is inalienable from a good life. Epicurus' advice to Menoeceus thus runs:

> When, therefore, we maintain that pleasure is the end, we do not mean the pleasures of profligates and those that consist in sensuality, as is supposed by some who are either ignorant or disagree with us or do not understand, but freedom from pain in the body and from trouble in the mind. For it is not continuous drinkings and revellings, nor the satisfaction of lusts, nor the enjoyment of fish and other luxuries of the wealthy table, which produce a pleasant life, but sober reasoning, searching out the motives for all choice and avoidance, and banishing mere opinions, to which are due the greatest disturbance of the spirit.
> Of all this is the beginning and the greatest good is prudence... for from prudence are sprung all the other virtues, and it teaches us that it is not possible to live pleasantly without living prudently and honourably and justly, nor, again, to live a life of prudence, honour, and justice without living pleasantly. For virtues are by nature bound up with the pleasant life, and the pleasant life is inseparable from them. (ME, p. 32)

The passage clearly suggests that for Epicurus, the most pleasant state is not a state of accumulated pleasures achieved through the satiation of our sensuous desires as such. It is rather a state which is pleasant by virtue of *aponia* (freedom from bodily dis-*ease*) and *ataraxia* (freedom from mental dis-*ease*), that is, as Cicero puts it in his *De Finibus Bonorum et Malorum* (*On Ends*) [cited henceforth as DeFi.], a state that is marked by a "complete absence of pain" (DeFi., Vol. I, p. 38).

The Epicurean adherence to the principle of contrariety as the overarching principle governing the very ontology of 'pain-pleasure' relation is clearly manifested in their non-recognition of a neutral state that is marked neither by pain nor pleasure. It is the upholding of the principle of contrariety as the governing principle that permits the Epicureans to assert that a complete absence of pain would also consequently entail a 'complete absence of pleasure'.[13] It is this firm adherence

---

[13]Although the absence of pain entails an absence of pleasure, given that the recognized *telos* of human life within the Epicurean formulation is a *desirable* state, *pleasantness* must be predicated of it. Such 'pleasantness' though distinct from the *kinetic* pleasure that is experienced in the negation of pain, must nevertheless be a pleasant state. It is the recognition of this tacit demand grounded in the nonnegotiable relation between *desirability* and any conceived *telos* of one's existence that forces the Epicureans to enigmatically uphold the 'state of complete absence of pain'

to the principle of contrariety, by virtue of which the Epicureans are perhaps, by far, the staunchest polarizers of the 'pain-pleasure' duality. For within the Epicurean framework, pain is explicitly seen as the precondition for the possibility of pleasure. Thus, in a sense, the Epicureans uphold the primacy of pain over pleasure given that within their conceptual frame, the latter is essentially the fallout of the removal of the former and hence presupposes it. Hence, if pleasure is but the 'negation of pain', an absence of the possibility of negating any pain given its 'complete absence' would also lead to a state, that is paradoxically, not pleasant. Epicurus enigmatically declares that "we feel pain owing to the absence of pleasure; but when we do not feel pain, we no longer need pleasure…And for this cause we call pleasure the beginning and end of the blessed life…" (ME, p. 31).

In other words, their notion of pleasure, both *kinetic*as well as *katastemaic*, highlights the belief that while the ontology of pain is firmly grounded in the *actual*, the ontology of pleasure finds its locus in the domain of the *potential*. This entails that for the Epicureans, all desires for pleasure are ontologically tied to pain and that the satiation of these desires come about solely through the removal of pains that ground them. Thus within the Epicurean formulation, the negation of pain *is* pleasure. This renders them rather close to the Buddhist ontology of pain.[14]

(Footnote 13 continued)

as being marked by *ataraxia* and *aponia,* while at the same time as being *pleasant*. It is also for this reason that the division of pleasure into the two classes of *kinetic* and *katastemaic* becomes central in the Epicurean doctrines. This division is made clearer in *De Finibus Bonorum et Malorum,* where Lucius Torquatus, an Epicurean, clarifies the division to Cicero, who is unwilling to accept the Epicurean identification of pleasure with a state of complete absence of pain. Torquatus explains that the highest good which could be negatively characterized as the complete absence of pain, and positively as a state of *aponia* and *ataraxia* is a case of 'static' (*katastemaic*) pleasure, comparable analogically to a state of pleasure when one experiences no thirst at all that demands to be quenched, while the pleasures that one experiences from the satiation of anticipated or intended desires are 'kinetic' and can be compared analogically to the pleasure experienced when one drinks when thirsty (DeFi.: II.9). Torquatus' explanation is rooted in the Epicurean thesis that the highest good cannot vary in intensity or degree and is "the limit and highest point of pleasure" (DeFi.: I.38–39); a state that does not seem to hold true for pleasures emanating from gratification, given that one can re-project the limit of one's desire to be gratified and thereby redefine the degree to which it is gratified either in terms of its intensity or its degree. The highest pleasure, on the other hand, that ensues from the complete removal of pain is a state of *ataraxia* and *aponia*, which the Epicureans, therefore, hold to be a state that cannot be conceptually improved upon through an act of reinventing the limit of one's feeling of a *lack* of anything, and therefore, the state too dissolves any possibility of reinventing the limit of one's feeling of being satiated.

[14]The Buddhist perspective, irrespective of the various sectarian affiliations, is firmly rooted in the fundamental belief that existence *is* suffering (*duḥkha*) and that the ultimate telos of human life, that is *nirvāṇa, lies in the cessation of this suffering (duḥkhanirodha).*

2.2.5 Pain and the Principle of Naturalness

Although the Epicurean thesis is responsible for casting the notion of pain to a cardinal position within moral discourse, the ontology of pain that can be elicited from within their ethical formulation is a rigidly constrictive one owing to their staunch adherence to the thesis of an inalienable relation between pleasure and pain, which is itself construed under the influential purview of the principle of contrariety. Thus the Epicurean formulation emphatically forecloses any possibility of an opening up of the structures for a discrete ontology of pain that is not routed through an ontology of pleasure. In other words, the Epicurean doctrine poses an even grimmer possibility for an ontology of pain that is not inferential via negativa than that which is pictured within Aristotle's formulation.

Furthermore, in the upholding of the primordiality of pain and pleasure as originary affections, the entailing corollary thesis, viz., of an inherent natural capacity in us to discern the nature of affections and the impossibility of any incorrect identification of pleasure *as* pleasure and pain *as* pain, also comes to be consequently upheld within the Epicurean framework. Thus, it not merely secures the principle of contrariety, but in addition, it fundamentally promotes the legitimacy of identifying pain and pleasure as originary affections that are *natural* to us. And therefore, by virtue of their immediate accessibility, any possibility of error in our discernment of pleasure *as* pleasure and pain *as* pain is foreclosed.

This invocation of legitimization of the *natural* by virtue of its *immediacy* is what, I call, the invocation of the *principle of naturalness*. The *principle of naturalness* is upheld in the Epicurean doctrine to primarily assert the primordial nature of pain and pleasure, and thereby to uphold the cardinality of the conceptual pair within moral discourse by virtue of it being *natural* to us. However, in doing so, it also tacitly positions these notions as those whose conceptual clarity cannot be further improved upon. The *giveness* of these affections that is ensured by the Epicurean *principle of naturalness* also implies that these cognitions are never marked by any ambiguity or vagueness insofar as their cognition is concerned. Thus, within the Epicurean framework- though one could legitimately raise questions that pertain to the function of these affections, their categorizations, and our responses to them- the question of *whatness* of that which is signified by the terms 'pain' and 'pleasure' would be a completely superfluous one. The *principle of naturalness,* by relating the *natural* with the *immediately given*, further legitimizes the inferential ontology of pain as the *natural mode* of engaging with the notion of pain. In other words, the principle of naturalness, when held together with the principle of contrariety, as in the Epicurean engagement, renders the very relation of contrariety posed between pain and pleasure as *natural,* and as the only legitimate mode of construing an ontology of pain.

Although it is evident that the principle of naturalnessas invoked in the Epicurean doctrines is grounded on the understanding of *nature* as it figured in the Presocratic cosmologists, it must be conceded that the Epicureans contributed in a significant way towards its revival by prominently foregrounding the cardinality of the value of 'nature' and the 'natural', and its necessary relation to the notion of the 'good' through their engagement with the conceptual pair of 'pain-pleasure' in their ethical discourse.[15] It is in the wake of this revived interest in the Presocratic cosmological doctrines, and especially in those propounded by the Presocratic metaphysical atomists, that the doctrines of both the Epicureans and the Stoics emerge. However, despite their common ground, the divergent positions adopted by the Epicureans and the Stoics on the 'pain-pleasure' pair are well-known. The crucial difference between the two lies in the fact that unlike the Epicureans, the Stoics do not hold the primordiality of pleasure and pain as central ethical categories within their ethical formulations. It must, however, be recognized that the basis of this difference lies precisely in the fact that both uphold the principle of naturalness. It is this insistence in the doctrines of the Stoics, as noted by Diogenes Laertius in his *Lives of the Eminent Philosophers* (cited henceforth as DL), upon the inalienability of the 'good' from that which is 'natural' that pivotally punctuates their discourse. It highlights their firm conviction about the commitment of natural beings to their own preordained nature and, thereby, to Nature itself.[16]

2.2.6   In the Stoic Formulation…

The Stoics, despite their differences with the Epicureans, are in complete agreement with the latter insofar as the legitimacy of this identification of the 'good' with 'that which is natural' is concerned. The stoic discourse in its finer nuances unfolds precisely from this thick assumption of the *principle of naturalness*. In other words,

---

[15]It is this ontological trait of the inalienability of a being from Nature, or what is natural to its being and attunement with the rhythm of Nature, that forms the ground for all variants of the 'cradle argument'.

[16]This of course assumes that the nature of particular things is in some way uniform so as to ensure a harmonious nature as a whole, which is to say that the varieties of natures of particular beings reconcile and manifest the neat Nature of the whole, or explicate the cosmic nature as such. This seamless blending of the anthropic into the cosmic is a central feature of the Stoics as well as the Epicureans. The Stoics, as Long stresses, firmly held that "from the long-term point of view nothing… is independent of Nature's ordering… From the perspective of the part, poverty and ill-health are unnatural to mankind. But such an analysis is only made possible by abstracting human nature from universal Nature. From the perspective of the whole even such conditions are not unnatural, because all Natural events contribute to the universal well-being" (p. 180), even if it runs counter to the human perspective. One must note that for the Stoics it is "the harmonizing of the dissonance, not the creation of dissonance" that is the primary task of Nature. Addressing this issue of the accommodation of distinct and sometimes contrary particular natures within the universal nature in the discourse of the Stoics, Long remarks that, "…[i]t is difficult to resist the conclusion that the Stoics' desire to attribute everything to a single principle has produced a fundamental incoherence… But to this they would reply that the harmony of the universe as a whole is something which transcends any attempt to view the world from the perspective of a particular part [and that if] … we view Nature's activities as contradictory this is due to the limitations of human vision" (p. 182).

the explorative efforts of the Epicureans, and the Stoics, to bring forth a naturalistic ground for ethics concurrently become the very ground for embedding the *principle of naturalness* within the structures of an ethical discourse, even if it be that such a foregrounding can be interpreted to be epiphenomenal to their project. It is hard to contest that the ethical is deeply grounded in the category of 'nature' in Stoicism.[17] The identification of the 'good' with 'nature' runs consistently throughout the discourse of the Stoics, starting in the fragmentary works of Zeno (who proclaims that the end of life is to strive for a living that is in agreement with nature) to the later matured thesis of Chrysippus of Soli (who claims that the end of life is to strive for a living that is in agreement with nature) (DL VII, pp. 86–88). It is the Stoics' amalgamation of the Socratic insistence with Aristotle's teleological approach that results in their primal thesis that *virtue is natural to us*. The doctrines of the Stoics can be read as the unfolding of the Socratic insistence on the immanence of virtue, and the pursuit of the good as being the *telos* that is fundamentally natural to us, under the purview of the principle of naturalness. In essence then, the principle of naturalness, in the hands of the Stoics, translates into the formulation of their cardinal thesis that the fundamental structuring of Nature is such that the good for one's own being is immediate. For them our being is driven by a 'primary impulse' to conform to its own particular nature in preserving the constitution of its being *qua* Nature (DL VII, pp. 83–86), though they uphold reason in lieu of the Epicurean 'prudence' as the primary discerner of 'what is, in fact, natural.'[18] One can discern the play of the principle of naturalness within the discourse of the Stoics in their adherence to the thesis that values are of value insofar as they promote a "state of mind which tends to make the whole of life harmonious" (DL VII, pp. 104–106)

---

[17]The emphasis on 'nature' as a philosophical category within the doctrines of the Stoics and the Epicureans is also, as Inwood suggests, a move to satisfy the philosophical urge of stability, a characteristic that is taken to be the hallmark of any sound philosophical paradigm by the Greek thinkers (1985, p. 224).

[18]Ethical perversion, for the Stoics is thus symptomatic of dissonance between human nature and Nature brought about by undisciplined impulses (*oikeiosis*) that either misleadingly seem geared towards our primary impulse, or move away from our primary impulse, which is to be in harmony with one's true nature that is pervaded by Nature itself. The Stoic, as Inwood reads, thus understands the unnatural, or the irrational, as a case of *oikeiosis* emerging from misunderstandings (1985, p. 184). Therefore ethical perversions for the Stoics result from 'falsehoods that extend to the mind' and are the root cause of passions or emotions, which are but perversions that emerge, as Zeno claims, by virtue of 'an irrational and unnatural movement in the soul' (DL VII, pp. 110–112). It is this discerning of what is really choiceworthy that is the hallmark of a wise man. It is this perceptiveness on his part that rescues him from the infirmity that arises out of an error of discerning that which is natural and thus choiceworthy, that is sought to be highlighted in the declaration of the Stoics that 'the wise man is passionless' (DL VII, pp. 114–117) and can never err (DL VII, pp. 121–123). The centrality of Reason for the Stoics emerges precisely due to the fact that the route to the discernment to what is natural is through it alone. Reason is thus seen as the supervening craftsman that enables the agreement of human beings with their true nature that is in resonance with the immanent order of Nature. The primordial inalienability of the virtuous from Nature is reinforced by the Stoics' insistence that "when a rational being is perverted, this is due to the deceptiveness of external pursuits or sometimes to the influence of associates. For the starting points of nature are never perverse" (DL VII, pp. 88–90).

and accordingly, the 'good' comes to stand for an "aptitude for one's proper function" (DL VII, pp. 100–102).

However, pleasure and pain for the Stoics, in contrast to the Epicureans, arise precisely due to the grave deficiency on the part of an individual to discern what is natural to its being,[19] thus giving the *principle of naturalness* and its relation to pleasure and pain a peculiar twist. They argue that the Epicureans miss the finer fact that pleasure "never comes until nature by itself has sought and found the means suitable to... [our] existence or constitution [and is therefore] an aftermath comparable to the condition of animals thriving and plants in full bloom" (DL VII, pp. 86–88). The Stoics thus object to the Epicurean identification of a mere byproduct (pleasure/pain) that comes about in the pursuit of the goal, with the goal itself, which is to be in harmony with one's nature. However, in taking pleasure and pain to be a supervening product in our pursuit and attainment of what is, or is not natural to our very being, they nevertheless confer an indirect naturalness to the

---

[19]Given the close relation that was sought to be established by the Stoics, following Zeno's *Exposition of Doctrine*, between what they considered as the three principal parts of philosophy, namely, the logical, the physical and, the ethical, first explicitly demarcated by Xenocrates [Zeno's discourses at the Stoa following that precise order as we are informed by Diogenes Laertius (DL VII, pp. 39–41)], the naturalistic grounding of the ethical in their hands pivotally depended upon the epistemological positions (DL VII, pp. 48–51) that followed from their adherence to the principles of metaphysical atomism. Hence, in the discourse of the Stoics, the ethical is deeply grounded in their understanding of the nature of the knowing subject and the modes of knowledge production. This epistemic emphasis thus catapults the theory of senses to a place of primacy within the discourse of the Stoics, much prior to the position of cardinality conferred to them during the modern period by thinkers now categorized as 'Empiricists' (Hume in particular, who was familiar with their works). This epistemic grounding of the ethical is highlighted by the central position occupied by the doctrine of presentation (*phantasia*) and sensation (*lekta*) in their discourse and its relation to their atomistic metaphysics (see DL VII, pp. 43–54). This can also be read alternatively from the point of view of the primacy of logic within Stoicism, which they hold to be the underlying structure, the "bones and sinews", the protective "shell" or "fence" (DL VII, pp. 39–41) that makes possible the access to, and the flourishing of, truth and the grasping of nature as such, be it within the province of Physics or Ethics (VII, pp. 81–83). If one bears in mind the fact that the logic, at the least for the Stoics, did not confine itself to its present day narrowly delineated province of propositions, and argument forms, but denoted a much broader domain of the science of the study of *logos* or the study of the rational order of the cosmos or nature, along with the art of articulating the same in speech. Thus, it is useful to remind ourselves, as suggested by Inwood, that for the Stoics, "speaking well also meant speaking truly and virtuously" (p. 226). Thus, the discerning and disciplining of the movement of reason is an essential precondition for the attaining of true presentations of nature without precipitancy of the mind's *assent* to sensations (DL 46–48), which is to say the acceptance of the mind to take the sensations as faithful representations of the object or nature. And given that our actions are governed by sensations or what we make of presentations, "unless we have our perceptions well trained, we are liable to fall into unseemly conduct and heedlessness" (DL VII, pp. 46–48). Hence, for the Stoics the wise man is synonymous with a true dialectician (DL VII, pp. 81–83). Following Ian Mueller, Ianwood remarks that for the Stoics, "logic had both an epistemological and a moral significance... [for]... it helps a person to see what is the case, reason effectively about practical affairs, stand his or her ground amid confusion, differentiate the certain from the probable, and so forth" (p. 229).

experience of pain and pleasure (DL VII, pp. 94–97).[20] It is this entailment of the naturalness of pain and pleasure, bereft of the ontologically primordial force of *ought* in governing our actions that gives rise to an air of insipid *givenness* of pain and pleasure within human existence. It is by virtue of this denial of *any* prescriptive force to pain and pleasure in the doctrines of the Stoics, unlike in the doctrines of the Epicureans or their predecessors, that ultimately grounds the attitude of the Stoics' *indifference* to pain and pleasure.

It is this indifference towards pain and pleasure that comes to be the dominant prescribed attitude towards pain during the early period of the Roman Empire, which can well be said to have adopted Stoicism as its 'official' philosophical position following the likes of Seneca, Epictetus, and Marcus Aurelius. Highlighting this attitude of indifference propounded by Stoicism, Aurelius in his *Meditations* recommends:

> Let the part of thy soul which leads and governs [the rational part] be undisturbed by the movements in the flesh, whether of pleasure or of pain and let it not unite with them, but let it circumscribe itself and limit those affects to their parts. But when these affects rise up to the mind by virtue of that other sympathy that naturally exists in the body which is all one, then thou must not try to strive to resist the sensation, for it is natural: but let not the ruling part of itself add to the sensation the opinion that it is either good or bad. (1940, Book V, p. 26)

It is in this rendering of the Stoics' attitude of *indifference* towards pleasure and pain, within their ethical doctrines, in contrast to their hitherto conferred cardinal position as the locus of the ontologically primordial force of *ought,* that brings about an important turn in the historical trajectory of the ontology of pain. Through their assertion that the experience of pleasure or pain is in itself not a mark of being in accordance, or in dissonance with what is natural to us in the larger schema of Nature, the discourse of the Stoics relegates the pursuit of an ontology of pain to a position of marginality, if not to a position of redundancy, within the domain of the ethical, while upholding both the principle of naturalness,as well as the principle of contrariety.[21] Furthermore, the Stoics' thesis of *givenness* of pain within human

---

[20]The Stoics' denial of pleasure and derivatively of pain is a nuanced rejection and cannot be treated as a wholesale one. That is, what is rejected in Stoicism is the Epicurean positioning of pleasure as the primordial goal of life's pursuit and not the experiencing of pleasure itself. For the Stoics, in its former positioning as a goal, pleasure is symptomatic of lack of mediation of impulses by reason, and thus is indicative of disease that the mind is capable of falling into, just as the body is susceptible to diseases like "gout" and "arthritis" (DLVII, pp. 114–117). It is the disease of the soul when its impulses transgress into the domain of irrationality and transform itself as an "irrational appetency" or desire or craving (DLVII, pp. 112–114). Thus, pleasure is but the pursuit of an "irrational elation at the accruing of what seems to be choiceworthy" when in fact it is not, and conversely, pain or grief is "an irrational mental contraction" (DL 117–119), which for the Stoics are both marks of perversion of one's being. However, as a supervening byproduct, they do hold, 'joy', as a 'counterpart of pleasure' which is a 'rational elation' of being in harmony (DL 114–117) with one's nature and thereby with Nature as such.

[21]The mode of 'contrariety' is one of the six modes of meaning or sense production within their epistemological apparatus, the others being, "direct contact, resemblance, analogy, transposition, [and] composition" (DL VII, pp. 51–52).

existence renders it natural, while at the same time, without much significance. It is this unique blend of upholding the naturalness of pain while at the same time denying it much signification that opens up the possibility of providing it significance.

Such a construal of pain when placed on an explicit plane of theological transcendence is what allows for the Christian interpretation of its signification, and the Christian attitude towards pain during the mediaeval times, treating it as a divine sign of exclusive happiness in the hereafter. It is this interpretative turn made on the plane of theological transcendence, *sans* the axial role of reason, that precisely enabled the Christian discourse to project a new mode of engaging with the thesis of the *givenness* of pain, which as Perkins (1995) argues, prevailed and led to the steady growth of Christianity. Further, given the close affiliation between the Stoics' thesis of the *givenness* of pain and the recognition of the givenness of evil in the world, the ontology of pain gets comfortably conflated with the ontology of evil within the Christian theodicy, and with it the notion of evil too comes to be construed under the dictates of the logic of the principle of contrariety. It is this recognition of the givenness of evil in the world when seen against the horizon of the principle of contrariety that provides the germane grounds for the rise of privation theories of evil in Christian theodicy, beginning with Augustine who saw in the privation theory the only possible mode of accounting for the problem of evil. Although it cannot be doubted that Aquinas' formulation of the privation theory of evil in his *Summa Theologica* is more nuanced; since it explicitly invokes the idea that privation is not identical to a mere absence or the negation of a presence, but rather is to be conceived as an absence of that which is naturally due to the nature of a being (1952, Part I. Ques. 48. Art. 5), it too is rooted on the givenness of evil in the world and is dealt with in the horizon of the principle of contrariety.

Notwithstanding the fresher interpretations provided to the notion of pain in terms of its significance to one's 'being-in-pain' within the Christian theodicy, the overarching ontology of the 'divine', however, completely subsumes the ontology of pain. Here, the 'being', as well as 'pain', of the 'being-in-pain' comes to bear an ontological import only within the logic of the ontology of the 'divine'. Thus the metaphysical concerns of theology further suffocate the possibility of a discrete ontology of pain by subsuming it completely within the bounds of signification that could be afforded to it within the broader contours of religion.

2.2.7 The Revival in Hume and Bentham

The ontology of pain findsa forceful attempted return into the domain of 'secular' discourse of the ethical through the writings of those like Hume and Bentham. Hume, in an important respect, revitalized the importance of the conceptual 'pain-pleasure' pair. While still engaging with the intricate relationship between pain and evil and their centrality to the foundations of religion and to theodicyas such (see Hume 2007a, Parts IX and X; also his manuscript titled, *Fragment on*

Evil; Hume 2007b), he nevertheless managed to place pain and pleasure once again in a cardinal position within ethical discourse by arguing for the primordiality of passions over reason within the sphere of human actions.[22] Hume writes: "there is implanted in the human mind a perception of pain and pleasure as the chief spring and moving principle of all its actions" (1911, Book I, Part III, Sect. X).

However, given the initial lack of interest in his works and thereby its constrained dissemination, it is only through the works of Bentham that the primordiality of the conceptual pair of pain–pleasure comes to be popularized.[23] The axial role of this conceptual pair in Bentham's *An Introduction to the Principles of Morals and Legislation* is evident from the fact that it begins with the proclamation of the primordiality of pain and pleasure as the "two sovereign masters" that solely govern "what we ought to do, as well as to determine what we shall do" (1932, p. 1). Bentham's writings are suggestive of a 'social' ontology of pain given the fact that his 'Principle of Utility'was not merely meant as a guide for the pursuit of an individual's virtue, but rather was extended as a legislative principle of social and political governance. In this sense, Bentham clearly opens up the ontology of pain to a broader domain of the socio-political, from the narrower confines of a Greek framework of virtues that is primarily centred upon the individual.[24] This move was hitherto not achieved by the virtue-ethics orientations that were available within the dominant ethical discourse operating with the pain–pleasure pair. Bentham, in this regard, goes further than Hume, for he does not merely revive the primordiality of the notions of pain and pleasure(subsumed in his works under the category of "interesting perceptions") (1907, Chaps. V, I). In his works, one can read the movement of the ontology of pain from the purview of a *being-in-the-natural-world* to a domain of the *being-within-the-social-world*. It is in Bentham that the

---

[22]Although it is evident that Hume was influenced more by the doctrines of the Stoics than by those of the Epicureans, insofar as his epistemology is concerned, his extensive elaboration of the psychological machinery of human beings that positions *passions* as the primordial ground of the will is starkly Epicurean in its outlook (see *A Treatise of Human Nature*, BK II, Part III, Sect. III). However, Hume's treatment of pain and pleasure as the primordial grounds of our actions is more intricate and nuanced than the Epicurean account. Hume's division of pain and pleasure in terms of an *experience* of pain and pleasure *vis-à-vis* an idea of pain experience, and the differing impact of these on us (see 1911, BK I, Part III, Sect. X), and his elaborate framing of his nuanced *double theory of passions* in terms of this division in Part I, Book II of *A Treatise of Human Nature*, clearly illustrate this.

[23]Bentham's *Principle of Utility* is resoundingly close to one of Hume's own notes on Bayle (Mossner No. 19), now available to us as *Hume's Memoranda*. Hume notes there, "[m]en might have been determined to avoid things harmful and seek the useful by the augmentation and diminution of pleasure as well as by pain...." (2007c, p. 107).

[24]Although Bentham's categorization of pain and pleasure and the discussions revolving around it centre on the individual, we must note that Bentham conceives the term community as a *fictitious* term (1907, Chap. I. IV) or a "noun-substantive which is not the name of a real entity, perceptible or inferential... a conception of which can be obtained by consideration of the relation borne by it to a real entity..." (1932, p. 12). For Bentham, the interest of community can only be grasped through the concrete interest of the individual, and hence the community can only be understood through the reality of the individual.

conceptual pair of pain–pleasure gets represented as notions that move beyond the individual, and as having direct social import. Bentham's work seeks to underline how the *social-space* as such is fundamentally governed by 'interesting perceptions' or by the 'pain/pleasure' pair, and how one could possibly legislate the individual within a social order through them. This turn that Bentham gives to 'interesting perceptions' liberates the ontology of pain from its ordained position within a strict discourse of the ethical, moving it to a cardinal position in the socio-political domain. However, having said that, despite his elaborate classifications of the varieties of pain and pleasure as 'efficient causes or means' of actions, Bentham still hazily conceives of the conceptual pair in a relation of contrariety insofar as he conceives pleasure as "immunity from pain" (1907, Chaps. III, I) which is also evident in his definition of *utility* which places the two notions in a stark relation of contrariety (1823, Chaps. I. III). Bentham clearly conceives of pain as not merely governing the *being* of the individual but the social as well. But given that Bentham primarily conceives the *being* of the social (taken in the sense of a community) as being wholly derivative from the *being* of the individual, he falls short of exploiting the entailments of his own thesis. It is well-known that Bentham conceived the individual and the social in terms of a conceptual unity, where to imagine one was to imagine the other. The ontology of pain that can be traced in Bentham's work fails to conceive of the social *as such* and therefore within the Benthamite formulation, it would be impossible to imagine the social *as such* as having any impact upon the *nature of pain*. It is this impenetrable nature of pain, fundamentally seen in its corporeality, which makes it impervious to any alternation in its nature, and that leads him to argue for the foundational role of the *physical sanction* as the ground over the *moral*, the *political* and the *religious* ones (1907, Chaps. III, XI). This unalterable nature of pain, as he conceives it to be, is of consequence to his ontology of pain, when we recall that the *principle of naturalness* is upheld by Bentham as the first principle in relation to pleasure and pain. This essentially means that the nature of pain is *a given* for Bentham with no possibility of alteration, and that nature, given his adherence to the principle of contrariety, is to generate an *aversion* towards it. Simply put, for Bentham, pain can change the modality in which a being engages with the world, but the modality in which the being engages with the world cannot change the nature of pain.

This is not to highlight the comparatively trivial point that Bentham conceives the engagement of the social being as completely regulated by the experiences and expectations of pains and pleasures, but rather to emphasize the fact that pain is fundamentally conceived of in its corporeality by Bentham. His ontology of pain conceives the nature of pain to unfold *only through* the concrete individual. It further foregrounds the fact that given the unalterable nature of pain within the Benthamite framework, to grasp the nature of pain in one of its manifestations is to understand the nature of pain in its entirety. The *religious*, the *moral* and the *political* structures within Bentham's formulation are merely regulative channels of exploiting the *singular* nature of pain, viz., its aversive nature, for the establishment of order in the society or to fashion the behaviour of the individual by acting as a deterrent force (1907, Chaps. III, I). These *sanctions* of legislation are not, in

Bentham's formulation, constitutive mechanisms of pain-production, but merely regulative ones. The Benthamite formulation even in its richness thus impoverishes the ontology of pain by conceiving the triadic relation between pain, the individual, and the social as merely flowing in a linear, singular direction. In it, the only response to pain is to avoid it and the only function of pain is to deter, even if this deterrence in some rare cases takes on the form of ensuring a positive action like forcing someone to speak the truth by inflicting pain (torture).[25] In Bentham, the ontology of pain thus becomes the ontology of the relation between the individual's will and the social order. Bentham does recognize the fact that pain can transgress the bounds of the personal into the broader space of the social, as is highlighted in his classical utilitarian move of broadening, the scope of his principle of utilityfrom the individual to the community. However, his ontology of pain fails to explore the modalities in which one could expand the domain of play of pain from the 'personal' to the 'social' by precisely working through the space that is opened up by the structure of the 'inter-personal' often evoked by pain-experiences, either in a mode of 'closing off of the other' or 'closing off from one's self', or in a mode of 'calling unto the other'.

2.3 Part-II

2.3.1 Conclusion: Moral Theories and the 'Asocial' Ontology of Pain

Pain, as conceived of within these moral theories, can thus be seen as consistently construed in an inalienable relation with pleasure under the overarching principle of contrariety. Thus, notwithstanding the broader and thicker signification that they impart to the notion of pain, they nevertheless approach it through a preconceived lens that shades it through, and against, the nature of pleasure. This, thereby, brings about a foreclosing of the possibility towards any form of discrete ontology of pain within these moral theories. For instance, given that they conceive of the pain–pleasure pair in light of the *principle of contrariety,* the complex and enigmatic act of voluntarily welcoming of pain and its function therein, be it in its religious or spiritual manifestation, or in masochism, would be, with a single stroke, reduced to a case of ulterior pleasurewithin the reductive modality of these moral discourses.

Further, within these theories, pain emerges against the principle of naturalnesswhich is co-opted as its other horizon of unfolding. It thus comes to be treated as a *fact,* either mental or physical, that in its originary stance, pertains and confines itself to a *subject* that is immediately conscious of pain and its nature. And given that the notion of pain that is invoked within these theories are embedded with a

---

[25]Bentham, while expressing his view on torture, justifies its use in rare cases (see Twining and Twining 1993, 519ff.).

framework dominated by ethical concerns, they thereby construe pain through a *singular function*, namely that of its import upon the ethicality of an individual. The issue here is not that the ontology of pain within these moral discourses assumes the primacy of the *subject* in pain in their discourse. In fact, from the first law of *pathei-mathos* (learning through suffering) of Aeschylus' Zeus to the present day discourse on pain, the centrality of the *subject* emerges rather forcefully and places the *subject in pain* at the very centre of any ontology of pain. In fact, the very experience of pain, and the primacy of the *subject* in pain (seemingly impervious to any conceptual manoeuvre of isolating pain as such from the structure of its experience, and thereby its interwovenness with the experiencer), is what grounds the preponderating modality through which the notion of pain is explored, and sought to be made sense of, since antiquity. Bluntly put, pleasure and pain is a predicate of the living and thus seems to invoke the representation of an inalienable relation of pain to the *subject in pain* in its phenomenality. However, the ontology of pain within these moral discourse centres upon a particular kind of subject, namely, the 'ethical'. The ontology of an 'ethical-being-in-pain', here, is taken to stand as the proxy for a 'being-in-pain' *as such*. Thus the depth and the intricacies of the ontology of pain in these theories come to be intrinsically woven with the scope of the ethical framework itself, consequently making it fall short of attaining its fullness. Of course, it would have been an unproblematic truism if this reductive construal of pain, in its terms of its singular import on the ethical, was to simply mean that an ethical theory construes the individual *as* ethical. But the problematic curtailing brought about here, by such a reductive construal of pain that is suffused solely in terms of its ethical import and necessarily anchored in a 'particular ethical subject', is in terms of the nature and the very *significance of pain,* which it drastically alters. These theories completely appropriate pain-experiences towards a singular import upon the individual. The reductive ontology of pain in these moral theories fails to address and accommodate the diverse modalities through which pain makes our world, and we in turn, the world of pain. In this regard, they immiserizes the ontology of pain. After all, pain-experiences are not merely significant to the individual in terms of its ethical import. It, in many ways, as highlighted by Scarry, constitutes the very nature of the individuality of the individual. In fact, in some cases of extreme pain, it may be the grounds for the very loss of individuality itself.

Further, the anchoring of pain in the concrete 'ethical subject' brings about a notion of pain that is essentially corporeal, where pain-experiences can only be construed in terms of a particular 'subject in pain'. 'Pain', within the ontology of pain in these moral theories, deny any 'abstract pain' that is unrelated to a particular individual; 'beyond' and 'without' a *particular subject*. It is this lacuna that forecloses the possibility of construing any genuine notion of 'pain of a community'. Thus, the ontology of pain within the moral discourse falls short of a social ontology of pain. Although they do acknowledge the relation that obtains between pain and the 'social', this construal is essentially meditated by an embodied particular subject in pain, who then in turn, is either rooted within the woven bounds of a society or a culture, and is thus *necessarily* the metaphysical basis for it (as epitomized in Bentham). For instance, within the virtue-centric theories, the ontology of pain remains tightly constrained within the bounds of the 'individual' and fails to transcend it, and to raise itself to the level of the 'social'. Even within the richer ontology of pain in Bentham, the 'social' dimension of pain is as good as absent given that the 'social' is seen as no more than an aggregate of 'individuals'.

More importantly, the 'other' in pain here can only be construed in terms of an unproblematic comparison with the 'I', and the *other in pain* merely is the image of the *self in pain* with no distinctness in either its structure or in its function. Within these frameworks, the pain of the other is real only in the precise modality in which it affects the self. No pain of the *other* can be a pain that the 'I' is alien to; and more problematically, no pain is unique to the *other* by virtue of *being* precisely that specific other. Given the presupposition of the universality of ethical prescriptions that ground these theories, the ontology of pain within them forecloses all possibilities of any pain that is not open to universalization. The modalities and the nature of affectivity of *seeing* the other in pain is literally immiserized by equating it with *other* as the *self in pain* that is just another.

The forestalling of any possibility of an 'abstract pain' that is 'beyond' and 'without' a *particular subject* also entails the abjuring of the possibility of any 'collective memory' of pain as such, and consequently precludes the possibility of a 'socio-cultural' ontology of pain. It thus fails to see the possibility of pain without *particular owners* precluding all incorporeal 'floating collective memories of pain'[26] which is the central pillar of a cultural ontology of pain.

Given the horizon of the *principle of naturalness* against which these theories unfold, the ontology of pain that can be deciphered within these moral theories, therefore, take the *subject* who experiences the pain as its intended object rather than 'pain' itself. They are consequently incapable of envisaging a discourse that could emerge in an engagement with pain *as such*, like the thick discourse on pain that follows from the realization of, what Scarry marks as (1985, 162ff.), the 'objectless' nature of pain. Thus, ontology of pain within these moral theories in its failure to push this centrality of the 'particular subject' to the background fails to foreground the socio-cultural aspects of pain-experiences, through an evasive act of foregrounding without negating the *subject* as such, and thus remains at best, an asocial ontology of pain. Notwithstanding the experiential richness of pain that is acknowledged in these theories to be not merely a punctual sensation, this complexity is nevertheless taken to be arising out of a substantial, asocial and essentialist individuality. Thus, sociality has nothing to do with the phenomenality of pain and the self as the underlying substance is the sole locus of pain. Here, pain

---

[26]It must be noted that 'collective memory' is not 'collective' because it is shared; rather it is precisely because it is 'collective' that it is shared. It is not that one must, as a 'particular subject', have a pain-experience that has been had by others as well that comes to constitute a 'collective memory of a pain-experience'. Rather, it is in the partaking of the particular subject in this collective memory of a pain-experience that enables one to experience it.

never transcends the self, is never vague and ambiguous, and is devoid of the mystery and the enigmatic structures in which it makes our world and we, in turn, make our world of pain.

References

Anonymous. (1921). The physiology of pain. *The British Medical Journal, 1*(3146), 571–572.
Aquinas, T. (1952). *Summa theologica* (Fathers of the English Dominican Province, Trans., and revised by D. J. Sullivan). Chicago, IL: Encyclopedia Britannica.
Aristotle. (1966). Ethica Nicomachea (W. D. Ross, Trans.). In W.D. Ross (Ed.), *The works of Aristotle* (Vol. IX of XII Vols. Set). London: Clarendon Press.
Aurelius, M. (1940). The meditations of Marcus Aurelius Antoninus (G. Long, Trans.). In W. J. Oates (Ed.), *The stoic and epicurean philosophers: The complete and extant writings of Epicurus, Epictetus, Lucretius and Marcus Aurelius* (pp. 491–587). New York: Random House.
Bain, A. (1892). Pleasure and pain. *Mind (New Series), 1*(2), 161–187.
Bentham, J. (1907). *An introduction to the principles of morals and legislation (1823)*. London: Oxford Clarendon Press.
Bentham, J. (1932). The theory of fictions. In C. K. Ogden (Ed.), *Bentham's theory of fiction* (pp. 7–156). London: Kegan Paul.
Boddice, R. (Ed.). (2014). *Pain and emotion in modern history*. Hampshire, UK: Palgrave-Macmillan.
Brinton. (1876). On pleasure and pain. *The Journal of Speculative Philosophy, 10*(4), 431–435.
Cassell, J. E. (2004). *The nature of suffering and the goals of medicine* (2nd ed.). Oxford: Oxford University Press.
Cicero. (1999). *De Finibus Bonorum et Malorum (On Ends)* (cited as *DeFi*). (H. Rackham, Trans.). London: Harvard University Press. Reprint of Second edition (1931) by Loeb Classical Library (Vol. 40).
Dallenbach, M. K. (1939). Pain: History and present status. *The American Journal of Psychology, 52*(3), 331–347.
Epicurus. (1940). Letter to menoeceus (cited as ME) (C. Bailey, Trans.). In W. J. Oates (Ed.), *The stoic and epicurean philosophers: The complete and extant writings of epicurus, epictetus, lucretius and marcus aurelius* (pp. 30–33). New York: Random House.
Hardcastle, V. G. (1999). *The myth of pain*. Cambridge, MA: The MIT Press.
Hume, D. (1911). *A treatise of human nature* (1738) (Vol. 2). London: Everyman's Library.
Hume, D. (2007a). Dialogues concerning natural religion (1776). In D. Coleman (Ed.), *Dialogues concerning natural religion and other writings* (pp. 3–102). Cambridge: Cambridge University Press.
Hume, D. (2007b). Fragment on evil. In D. Coleman (Ed.), *Dialogues concerning natural religion and other writings* (pp. 109–112). Cambridge: Cambridge University Press.
Hume, D. (2007c). From Hume's memoranda. In D. Coleman (Ed.), *Dialogues concerning natural religion and other writings* (pp. 105–108). Cambridge: Cambridge University Press.
Hutchinson, W. (1897). The value of pain. *The Monist, 7*(4), 494–504.
Inwood, B. (1985). *Ethics and human action in early stoicism*. Oxford: Clarendon Press.
Laertius, D. (1995) *Lives of the eminent philosophers (1925)* (Vols. I & II) (R. D. Hicks, Trans.). Cambridge, MA: Harvard University Press.
Lewis, T. (1942). *Pain*. New York: Macmillan.
Long, A. A. (1986). *Hellenistic philosophy: Stoics, epicureans, sceptics*. London: Duckworth.
Marshall, H. R. (1889). The classification of pleasure and pain. *Mind, 14*(56), 511–536.
Marshall, H. R. (1891). The physical basis of pleasure and pain. *Mind, 16*(63), 327–354.
Marshall, H. R. (1895). Emotions versus pleasure-pain. *Mind (New Series), 4*(14), 180–194.

Melzack, R. (Ed.). (1983). *Pain measurement and assessment*. New York: Raven Press.

Mezes, S. (1895). Pleasure and pain defined. *The Philosophical Review, 4*(1), 22–46.

Modrak, D. K. W. (1987). *Aristotle: The power of perception*. Chicago, IL: University of Chicago Press.

Morris, D. B. (1991). *The culture of pain*. Berkeley, CA: University of California Press.

Morris, D. B. (1994). What we make of pain. *The Wilson Quarterly, 18*(4), 8–16, 18–26.

Nichols, H. (1892a). The origin of pleasure and pain – I. *The Philosophical Review, 1*(4), 403–432.

Nichols, H. (1892b). The origin of pleasure and pain – II. *The Philosophical Review, 1*(5), 518–534.

Noble, B., Meldrum, M., Have, T. H., Seymour, J., Winslow, J., & Paz, S. (2005). The measurement of pain, 1945–2000. *Journal of Pain and Symptom Management, 29*(1), 14–21.

Perkins, J. (1995). *The suffering self: Pain and narrative representation in the early Christian era*. London: Routledge.

Plato. (1961). Phaedo. In *The four Socratic dialogues of Plato* (B. Jowett, Trans.). Oxford: Clarendon Press.

Plato. (1964). Philebus. In *The dialogues of Plato* (Vol. III) (B. Jowett, Trans.). Oxford: Clarendon Press.

Putnam, H. (1975). *Mind language and reality: Philosophical papers* (Vol. 2). Cambridge, UK: Cambridge University Press.

Rey, R. (1995). *The history of pain* (L. E. Wallace, J. A. Cadden & S. W. Cadden, Trans.). Cambridge, MA: Harvard University Press.

Rudebusch, G. (1999). *Socrates, pleasure and value*. New York: Oxford University Press.

Ryle, G. (2009). *The concept of mind (1949)*. London: Routledge.

Scarry, E. (1985). *The body in pain: The making and the unmaking of the world*. Oxford: Oxford University Press.

Stanley, M. H. (1889). Relation of feeling to pleasure and pain. *Mind, 14*(56), 537–544.

Tanizaki, J. (1977). *In praise of shadows*. (T. J. Harper & E. G. Seidensticker, Trans.). Bradford, UK: Leete's Island Books.

Twining, W.L., & Twining, P. E. (1993). Bentham on torture. In B. Parekh (Ed.), *Jeremy Bentham: Critical assessments* (Vol. II) (pp. 512–565). London: Routledge.

Chapter 3
The Familiar Stranger: On the Loss of Self in Intense Bodily Pain

Siby K. George

Come, you, you the last I recognize,
Incurable pain within the web of flesh…
Totally pure, totally unplanned, free of the future,
I climb on the tangled pyre of suffering,
certain of never getting anything back
for this heart whose reserves are gone.
Am I still the one who, unrecognized, burns?
I bring no memories here.
Life, life. To be outside it
While I burn. No one knows me.

—Rainer Maria Rilke.

Abstract The self is not an unchanging substance but a way of being that can be destroyed and regained. As the embodied and narratively sedimented way of being toward other persons and the world as such, the identity of the self is a thickly layered and dynamic formation of meaning. One of the enigmatic experiences that can trigger the loss and destruction of the self is intense bodily pain. Destruction of the self in pain comes to mean that one is weary with one's being, leading to the experience of selfhood in its worldless bareness. The worldless self, thrown up by intense bodily pain, is an extreme form of the 'I' that is a stranger even to oneself, having to persist without the intimate layers of meaning associated with the 'I myself.' Hence, the layers that vest the self with meaning and significance like the world and other persons become unmeaningful in intense bodily pain. The damage that totally aversive pain inflicts upon the self is often short-lived, but it can also be terminal, permanent and sometimes lastingly self-diminishing. Human culture as such and the caring gesture of others can be seen as two specific ways of assisting persons to regain their lost selfhood. The chapter develops these themes with reference to the philosophical works of Martin Heidegger, Emmanuel Levinas and Hannah Arendt, the last poem of Rainer Maria Rilke named "*Komm du…*" and Elaine Scarry's *The Body in Pain*.

Keywords Self · Loss · Recovery · World · Artifact · Caring

S.K. George (✉)
Department of Humanities and Social Sciences, Indian Institute
of Technology Bombay, Mumbai, India
e-mail: kgsiby@iitb.ac.in

© Springer India 2016
S.K. George and P.G. Jung (eds.), *Cultural Ontology of the Self in Pain*, DOI 10.1007/978-81-322-2601-7_3

51

The loss of self in intense bodily pain is one of the most enigmatic of experiences because pain individuates the self to the extent of totally shutting out her/his world of significance. Pain unveils the insufferable, intolerable, destroyed self. The self thus individuated is a stranger even to her/himself, a not-self, an unrecognizable phantom self without its rich layers of associations and meanings. Rilke, therefore, asks in the above lines: "Am I still the one who, unrecognized, burns?"[1] The self in intense bodily pain is the 'I', no doubt, but the "I" who is a stranger even to oneself, and hence the 'familiar stranger'; the "I", who is a stranger to the extent of being a "not-I", a lost "I".

The loss of self in acute and chronic suffering and pain (Scarry 1985; Charmaz 1983, 1991; Smith and Osborn 2007) and in trauma (Stolorow 2011, p. 55; 2007, p. 20) has been documented in the literatures of sociology, anthropology, psychology, psychoanalysis, and literary studies. Some of these accounts are well informed by philosophical perspectives in genuinely interdisciplinary ways (see Stolorow 2011, 2007). In this chapter, my aim is to look at the loss of self in intense bodily pain, whether acute, chronic or terminal, from a mainly philosophical vantage point.

In the first section below, referring to Elaine Scarry's thesis of world-destruction in intense bodily pain in her admirable *The Body in Pain* (1985), I argue that the disruptive dimensions of intense bodily pain can come to mean the destruction of selfhood per se in various degrees, although the experience of the loss of self itself and its intensity and impact may have largely cultural underpinnings. In the second section, I initiate a complementary reading of the ontologies of human existence of Martin Heidegger and Emmanuel Levinas, on the basis of which I can describe an understanding of the self that is destroyed in intense bodily pain. My claim here is that what Scarry describes as destroyed in pain is not merely the world of the self but the self itself. In the third section, I move to a phenomenological description of the destroyed self as such, and in the final section, I briefly dwell on the role of human and technological agency in self-recovery.

3.1 Pain and the Loss of Self

The strong distinction between physical and psychological pain has the Cartesian privileging of the mind over the body as its basis. Literature dwells deeply on psychological suffering (Scarry 1985, p. 11), but the English language that gave words to the tragedy of King Lear, complains Virginia Woolf, "runs dry" when a sufferer tries to describe a headache (2002, pp. 6–7). What separate somatic and

---

[1]Rilke's final poem "*Komm du…*" was composed in 1926 from his deathbed "two weeks before an agonizing and untreated ("I want my own death, not a doctor's") leukemia killed him" (Rilke 2010, p. 98). I may also add that my own disenabling experiences of pain and incapacity while undergoing an autologous bone marrow transplant for multiple myeloma in 2011 permeate this study.

psychic pains are the sensations and experiences they educe. One does not deploy one's powers of sobbing in sadness and smiling in happiness, notes the ecophenomenologist David Abram, like a commander piloting a ship. I am indistinguishable from these powers "as my sadness is indistinguishable from a certain heaviness of my bodily limbs" (1996, p. 46). Focus on intense bodily pain—for want of a better term—in recent philosophy of pain is necessitated by the privilege accorded to psychic pain by tradition and literature.

The pain of a dagger spearing through the skin or a nail piercing the foot is sensually different from the gripping trauma that takes over me in a tragic loss. Grief may weaken the body and may lead to passing out, but the sensual details of grief are qualitatively different from the pain of a finger jammed in a door. Grief is not burning, smarting, stinging, throbbing, hurting in localized points of the body like the nail under the foot. The experience of a bone marrow transplant patient, collapsing into a hopeless self-obsession triggered by bouts of vomiting, diarrhea, insomnia and delirium, is predominantly an experience of the totally wearied body-being. Watching someone torturing a dear one is traumatic and affects the body-being but it still is not torture; there is nothing that pierces or strikes one's body from without or within in that instance. An absolutely aversive violation of the body in an illness, attack or accident induces pain that is also psychic but it is predominantly taken by the sufferer as an affliction of or infliction upon the body. In separating the bodiliness of an affliction like an aching tooth or an infliction like torture or rape from the affectedness of the ordeal of having to witness a dear one being tortured, we still need to stress that it is always the whole body-being that is in pain, and not an artificially separable mind or body.

Something that separates intense bodily pain from intense psychic pain, though not absolutely but only in terms of degree and sensual detail, is the destruction of the world of meaning of the victim of pain. In intense trauma, too, the world of the self becomes meaningless and "incommensurable with those of others" (Stolorow 2011, p. 55) but not completely destroyed and disrupted. Destruction of the world of the self would mean existential disruption or utter inability to project possibilities to make one's existence meaningful (see Morris 2008). Neither past nor future is significant in intense bodily pain, which is totally occupied with the present moment and the body. Scarry writes about this aspect of intense bodily pain in these words:

> Pain begins by being "not oneself" and ends by having eliminated all that is "not itself." At first occurring only as an appalling but limited internal fact, it eventually occupies the entire body and spills out into the realm beyond the body, takes over all that is inside and outside, makes the two obscenely indistinguishable, and *systematically destroys anything like language or world extension that is alien to itself* and threatening to its claims. Terrifying for its narrowness, it nevertheless exhausts and displaces all else until it seems to become the single broad and omnipresent fact of existence. (1985, pp. 54–55; my emphasis)

Scarry describes as 'totality' the power of intense bodily pain to comprehensively seize hold of the body-being of its victim, and for her this characteristic of pain is central because her study is preoccupied with the way pain makes and unmakes the world of the victim. In the first part of her study, Scarry shows torture and war to be literally and metaphorically destroying the victim's world of meaning and her language. Pain destroys word and world.

According to Heidegger's existential ontology, meaningful existence unfolds temporally as "[t]his past, to which I can run ahead as mine" (1992, p. 12E). Human existence is "primarily being possible", and as such it is constantly projecting possibilities of being upon its past or history, thus making the present real. This structure of existence also means that, in the words of Charles Taylor, "we grasp our lives in a *narrative*... that from a sense of what we have become, among a range of present possibilities, we project our future being" (1989, p. 47). Accordingly, in intense bodily pain, the temporal structure of existence collapses into the 'now', shrinking the rich history- and possibility-driven structure of the existential space of meaning to the 'terrifying narrowness' (Scarry 1985, p. 55) of the present and the body. Intense bodily pain, thus, leads to total existential disruption and world-destruction.

However, Scarry's world-destruction-thesis regarding intense bodily pain appears to be more than that. She points out that confessions mediated through torture are betrayals of "oneself and all those aspects of the world—friend, family, country, cause—that *the self is made up of*" (1985, p. 29; my emphasis). If so, what is destroyed in intense bodily pain is not merely the world but the self as such. The subtitle of *The Body in Pain* can equally be "the making and unmaking of the *self.*" Destruction of the existential experience of the world of the victim of intense bodily pain amounts to *destruction of the self as such.* Scarry's arguments are undergirded by this thesis, which she, however, does not fully clarify because her preoccupations are different: to show how intense bodily pain destroys the world of meaning we narratively erect in our expressive traditions and how human culture as such is premised on the underlying possibility of remaking the world liable to be destroyed by pain.

In an attempt to strengthen this contention, I now want to dwell on the notion of the self along with Heidegger and Levinas in an attempt to understand the destruction of the "self" as such in intense bodily pain rather than destruction merely of the "world" of the self. I shall argue that the self, destroyed in intense bodily pain, is a many-layered way of being.

3.2 The Losable and Makeable Self

The human self is losable, destroyable and recoverable because, unlike the Cartesian the thinking-thing, it is not an imperishable substance, an objective presence, a self-thing attached to accidental properties like body and its sensations, but instead "a way of Being" (Heidegger 1962, pp. 153, 312). Similarly, being not-self/inauthentic, too, is a way of existing. The self of everyday existence is said to be not "I myself" but "the they" because the socially leveled everyday way of being a self does not own up existential possibilities as specifically "mine". Even an inauthentic self is mine but not owned up specifically as mine. As a way of being, existence is not understood on the basis of a steady, unbroken, unattached "I-awareness", but on the basis of a mattering/caring and thus unsteady/broken way of being in relation to a world and understanding that world, which involves at the same time also *"a self-interpretation"* (Heidegger 1992, p. 8E). Every understanding is at the same time a self-interpretation and a world-interpretation. Existence is a projective understanding which stretches itself toward the future in order to make its own the possibilities of its past. Self-constancy can be existentially thought only in terms of the anxious anticipation of authentic being oneself as opposed to the lack of self-constancy in inauthentic disowning of the possibilities of the self (Heidegger 1962, p. 369). Because selfhood is a way of being, it can be lost and gained, disowned and owned up again, destroyed and made whole.

A substance-ontology, on the other hand, does not understand selfhood as losable and makeable. What is lost and remade are accidental peripherals, dissociable from the self-substance. Accordingly, pain does not substantially affect the self-substance, which is outside the rules of change and history, sensibility and meaning-making. The self in such a view is the unchanging substratum of all accidentals that appear and disappear. But from the perspective of non-substance ontology, what is destroyed and remade is not a marginal aspect of an elusive core self, but what constitutes that self's very way of being.

The receptions that I passively undergo in my early years help form the self. These receptions are ontological rather than ontic and concrete because they lie beneath all my conscious and concrete existential projections. They form the basic, but fluid, layers of my conscious historical existence. Between the conscious and the unconscious lies a whole realm of pre-reflective, mattering understanding and meaning that constitutes and deconstitutes the self constantly. This is the realm where human life gets sedimented as "being-in-the-world," an irreversible, ontological entanglement with the world. Self and world are not two entities, subject and object, but "belong together" in the basic constitution of human existence (Heidegger 1988, p. 298). Without the invisible background of the world in this sense, no meaningful understanding is possible. While human existence unfolds ordinarily in this manner of getting lost in the social world of our concern, existential angst about not being true to our own/authentic self-interpretations can push us into modified but more individualized ways of situating ourselves understandingly in relation to the world. Even in the sheerest case of individualization, the world is ineluctably tied up with self-interpretation. It is when we begin human ontology from the mistaken assumption of a "worldless I" and try to provide it with a world of objects that we plunge into explanatory difficulties about justifying the world (Heidegger 1962, p. 363). The Cartesian separation between the inner and the outer is thereby collapsed and human existence is understood as transcendence toward the world. Transcendence means "to *understand oneself from a world*"; existence "always already means to step beyond or, better, having stepped beyond" (Heidegger 1988, p. 300). Existence is already moodily attuned, understanding and falling being-in-the-world; existence can become a self only inasmuch as it always already has a world of significance.

The "world" in *Being and Time*, thus, is this relational space or totality of significance, composed of things invested with cultural layers of meaning and people bound together by history, language and narratives of significance, within which are nurtured, whether for good or ill, the being or meaning of the things and ideals of the community as such. Of course, human existence or selfhood is null and groundless because the social space of meaning that gives it stability and a sense of permanence is shot through with contingency and finitude (Aho 2009, p. 15). This space of significance is transformable across history. Human existence is not an objective presence but a dynamic temporal unfolding of an understanding of reality in relation to a concrete historical world. It "*is* this happening of understanding, and existence refers to the unique way that a human being understands or interprets his or her life within a shared, sociohistorical context" (Aho 2009, p. 13). One is not born with this understanding but grows into it through a process of acculturation, on account of which one is able to interpret oneself and *be* that self. Human existence is *mineness* that stands out into its world of meaning. Without the sociocultural space of meaning that stamps mineness with significance and identity, ek-sisting or ecstatic projection would become impossible.

However, it is not merely the world of meaning constitutive of selfhood that is destroyed in intense bodily pain; the very embodied agency of the self is disrupted and severely impeded (see George 2011). The impediment to embodied agency in intense bodily pain is as severe as to make embodied existence meaningless. Levinas observes that in intense nausea "there is nothing more to be done, or anything to add to this fact that we have been entirely delivered up" (2003, pp. 66–67). Levinas remarks that embodied agency is so severely impeded in intense nausea that we are no more ashamed to be helpless.

Hence, the insights of Heidegger about existence, summed up in the hyphenated phrase "being-in-the-world", are insufficient to understand the destruction of the self in intense bodily pain. Heideggerian conception of existence cannot be understood primarily as embodied agency, which according to him is derived from being-in-the-world (see Heidegger 1987, p. 196; Aho 2009, p. 3). In a similar vein, he speaks of sexual difference too as derived and existence as such as "asexual" (1984, pp. 137–139), which Derrida denounces as the confirmation of "all the most traditional philosophemes, repeating them with the force of a new rigour" (1983, p. 79). If embodiment and sexuality are derived from abstract intelligibility without considering how intelligibility itself is informed by embodiment and sexuality, we are reconfirming the Cartesian separation of body from mind, a consequence Heidegger did not want to attest. As situated transcendence toward the sociohistorical space of meaning, it does not make sense to say that this transcendence comes before embodiment and sexuality. The self in pain is the embodied, sexed being-in-the-world, which experiences pain in terms of embodied, sexed, world-oriented meanings. Meaningfulness as such is entangled with embodiment, sexuality and several other determinations of the identity of the body-being. Merleau-Ponty's phenomenology discerned that existence "understood concretely, is inseparable from this particular body and from this particular world" (2012, p. 431). When Heidegger says that sensitivity and insensitivity to pain are based on the understanding of being (1987, pp. 221–222), we must hear in that statement the cultural ontology of the self in pain in its totality.

The loss in intense bodily pain is the loss of the world of meaning and impediment to embodied agency. However, the world that is destroyed in intense bodily pain is primarily a world that we share with others. The loss of our shared being with others is a significant blow to our body-being because there is something uniquely special and precious about our embodied, sensual exposure to otherness, which Levinas like no other has brought to light. Already within selfhood, there is a work in progress that goes counter to *ipseity* (I-ness) by way of transcendence toward the other person. Because ethics is primarily this going beyond the self in selflessness, Levinas sees selfhood itself as aboriginally entangled in ethics. And because selfhood itself is this intertwinement with otherness, Levinas's later texts like *Otherwise than Being, Or Beyond Essence* (1974) has a distinctively Heideggerian sense of transcendence (Fagenblat 2010, pp. 104–105), which in his case speaks about the predilection for human otherness in our self-understanding. The exposure to otherness is not neutral for Levinas. It is substitution for the Other or "Other in the same" (Levinas 1998a, p. 25). This phrase means that selfhood is always already impinged by human otherness without the ego's will or choice, without the possibility of recollecting the origin of impingements within the temporal flow. Substitution unsettles the self's ipseity in response to human otherness, which is why it is the condition for ethical phenomena like sacrifice and compassion. He speaks of the ethical self as menaced and persecuted by otherness; that is to say, the unhistorical impingements of otherness upon the self are like blows received without choice. The impingements mould the self always already as ethical. But Levinas conceives the ethical self as worldless, unhistorical and unsituated as opposed to Heidegger; history, world and culture are later than ethical selfhood in Levinas's scheme. Leaving aside this problem, we can look profitably at his account of selfhood as exposure to otherness complimentarily with Heidegger's in order to understand the loss involved in intense bodily pain.

For Levinas, the ethical exposure to otherness arising out of the selfhood substituted for the Other is language in its aboriginal form. Language or expression in this sense is "saying"; it is openness of the self toward, and for otherness, before the utterance of words. Words, which reduce, freeze and inevitably betray the saying in some way, are the "said". Saying is not voice or verbal sign but exposure, gesture, proximity, contact, touch; it is the expression of escape from own Being toward the Other. Answer to the saying is responsibility. I do not say to the Other that I *am not*, but that I *am only* as transcending the "I" and saying to the Other (Levinas 1998a, pp. 48–49). The loss of self in intense bodily pain is self-destructive primarily because it individuates the self to the extent that our shared exposure to otherness, ethical selfhood as saying, is rendered meaningless.

Furthermore, Levinas points out that without conceiving the self as exposed, exiled and ousted, we cannot make sense of pain and pleasure. The self understood as the detached interior region can neither connect with, nor experience, the outside as pleasurable or painful. The self understood as the detached navigator of body and the affect fails to account for the significance of pain and pleasure as constitutive elements of being human. It is because the self is ontologically already an opening, an exposure, a wound, that it can suffer pain and enjoy pleasure. The exposure and woundedness of selfhood is "the caress in which pain arises." Pain and suffering, and even "the risk of suffering without reason" is the very meaning of the affected, exposed structure of the self (Levinas 1998a, p. 50). Both pain and pleasure are conditioned on our embodied, affected selfhood, our being-in-the-world. Being the affected self means "to enjoy and to suffer by the other" (Levinas 1998a, p. 90).

Taking Heidegger's and Levinas's phenomenology of selfhood complimentarily, we get a clue to what is lost in intense bodily pain. What is lost is the significance of our temporal projection into the world of meaning and our sensual openness for otherness. If our embodied exposure to other beings like us is the primary site of our selfhood and the condition for our experience as sufferers and enjoyers, intense bodily pain deprives us of this very condition of being human and a self. As Russon remarks, embodiment means that we are "sensitive to our environments… As bodies, we are in touch with others in the richest and fullest sense of being 'in touch with'" (2003, p. 22). Intense bodily pain brings embodied agency to a halt; embodied projection of meaningful possibilities is met with severe impediments. We are not spirits entrapped in bodies but embodied, sentient beings transcending toward otherness as such, both human and nonhuman. In intense bodily pain what is destroyed is the self understood as sensually porous, other-directed being-in-the-world. That which is experienced as lost in the most extreme moment of sentience—intense bodily pain is the sensuous awareness of a meaningfully recognizable "I". Hence Rilke's question: Am I still the one who, unrecognized, burns?

Coming back to Scarry's thesis of the destruction of the world in intense bodily pain, we must reiterate that what is destroyed in pain cannot merely be the world of the self but *the self as such* as being-in-the-world. If we continue to speak of a world that is unmade by torture, we are continuing with the self and world dichotomy. That which is unmade by torture is the self as such, and not merely the world about which we care because the bearer of intense bodily pain is an unrecognizably individuated self without the world of meaning that constitutes the self. That which is thus lost/destroyed is the self in the sense of the 'I' as inextricably bound up with a world. To this extent, Scarry's talk about world-destruction in pain, and the body in pain as the ground for the making and the unmaking of the world does not escape dualism. That is why she has no interest in the cultural ontology of the body in pain, although what she describes in relation to Judeo-Christian scriptures and the texts of Marx as essential responses to the body in pain in the western tradition cannot be understood except through the theoretical lens of the cultural ontology of the self in pain. The major expressive traditions of the self-making and self-unmaking powers of pain of different cultures are so varied in their mood and meaning that they in fact give rise to very different forms of self-making, self-unmaking and pain. Even as Scarry agrees that the self is *made up* of all that is meaningful (1985, p. 29), her descriptions about world-destruction suggest a residual self-essence that is still left after the "world" is destroyed in an instance of intense bodily pain like torture.

3.3 The Self Destroyed in Pain

The shattering of word and world in the darkest moments of excruciating pain is destruction of the self as such because the self is a many-layered way of being. Destruction and loss of self in pain is a positive existential condition that phenomenologists have occasionally described. I now relook at some of these descriptions in an attempt to positively characterize the self, destroyed in intense bodily pain.

In her *The Human Condition* (1958), Hannah Arendt writes that intense bodily pain, the most intense feeling we know of, is the most private and least communicable of experiences. Arendt's context is a discussion on the public realm or the common, wherein even our most intimate experiences receive a public reality so that we are assured of the reality of what we intimately see and feel, indeed the reality of the self and world, which thus leads to the strengthening of the intimate, private realm itself. But intense bodily pain, argues Arendt, cannot be dressed up for public consumption; it cuts us off from reality to the extent that once intensity disappears it is quickly forgotten in an attempt to get back to reality. Getting back to reality after its denial in intense bodily pain seems to be a natural course of human behavior. It reassures us that we are real rather than the unreal self of intense bodily pain (Arendt 1998, p. 51). Arendt points out that nothing "ejects one more radically from the world than exclusive concentration upon the body's life, a concentration forced upon man in slavery or in extremity of unbearable pain" (1998, p. 112).

But, paradoxically, the self of intense bodily pain is more starkly real than the everyday self. In the moment of its intensity, bodily pain creates an unbridgeable chasm between self and the world. In this sense, pain is the most private of experiences, absolutely subjective and unable to take expressive form within the world of things and others. Pain individualizes the self to that extent where nothing else exists but the victim's bare self, ipseity. Arendt refers to Rilke's phrase in the final line of "*Komm du...*" to say that in the most radical moment of selfhood, wrought by intense bodily pain, "I am no longer 'recognizable'" even to myself (1998, p. 51). So Rilke asks whether the one who suffers and burns is still the 'I' and why is the 'I' so unrecognizable? Because all memories dry up in that moment, because all reserves of the heart and being are gone, intense bodily pain is not only aversiveness to a sensation, but to 'self' itself. Pain rends my being open because it is the incommunicable myself. Though I have a mother or a wife, or an intimate friend, near my bed of pain, all of them turn strangers in a moment of excruciating bodily pain. That moment individuates me and takes me to the land where I am alone, but the 'self' that I encounter in that land is a stranger even to myself. I am not recognizable even to myself; my being is aversive to myself. The self is still the 'I' and to that extent familiar, but is also stranger with the world and embodied agency destroyed. The self in intense bodily pain is the *familiar stranger*. "Even though it occurs within oneself," says Scarry, "it is at once identified as 'not oneself', 'not me'..." and the object that gives pain, an enemy who inflicts pain, a disease that afflicts me, a terrible tragedy that befalls me, is also "'not me,' 'against me'" (1985, p. 52). The self in intense bodily pain is familiar as the 'I' and strange as the 'I' who is not-self.

Intense bodily pain is nauseous because as Levinas writes, nausea "amounts to an impossibility of being what one is" and in it "we are at the same time riveted to ourselves, enclosed in a tight circle that smothers" (2003, p. 66). On the one hand it is the experience of 'pure being', the 'I' alone, cut off from the world of significance and of others, and on the other, the pure I that nausea presents to me is a meaningless I, unrecognizable and strange. Intense nausea throws social customs, shame and proprieties of behavior to the wind. The social customs we normally respect and abide by are unmeaningful in nausea. Virginia Woolf also points out that there is a childish outspokenness in illness; "things are said, truths blurted out, which the cautious respectability of health conceals" (Woolf 2002, p. 11). Levinas points out that 'shameful manifestations of our body' in conditions like nausea may be more carefree than in morally wrongful actions. The 'very fact of having a body, of being there' itself might come to be a flaw in nauseous states and 'shame appears purified of any admixture of collective representations.' He refers to nausea in solitude without the presence of any caregiver or companion and even there the nauseous person is "still 'scandalized' by himself" (Levinas 2003, p. 67). Indeed, Levinas shows that the presence of another might be desirable in such cases because then the nauseous self becomes the ill subject of treatment. On the other hand, nausea in solitude brings to the fore the pure, naked being of self, bereft of all meaning and recognition. Levinas muses that utter shame and nausea are similar in their revulsion with being oneself. Wanting to evade and escape one's being, unsuccessful as it turns out to be, is central to intense bodily pain.

Scarry emphasizes the death of speech in torture, the active annihilation of language. She carefully ties this active murder of voice to the elimination of word in intense bodily pain. "Physical pain is not only itself resistant to language," she reminds, "but also actively destroys language, deconstructing it into the pre-language of cries and groans. To hear those cries is to witness the shattering of language" (1985, p. 172). But what she has in mind here is a larger destruction, not merely word, but also world: "Intense pain is world-destroying" (Scarry 1985, p. 29). She refers to the common phrase about intense, though momentary, pain: I saw stars. In that moment one forgets one's world of meaning. By actively inflicting pain, a torturer destroys the world of the tortured twice, in the pain itself and in the confession obtained, a betrayal. Again, intense pain destroys time, the victim's stretch of unified self-awareness. It is this crucial disruption of the ecstatic unity of temporality that makes the self unrecognizable in intense pain. If the self is linguistically structured, as both Heidegger and Levinas discern, then what is destroyed by the destruction of speech is the self itself. The destruction of word, world and time is in fact the destruction of self as sensually open, linguistically and temporally structured, embodied being-in-the-world.

In intense bodily pain, selfhood is radicalized by its absence, by its strangeness to itself—unrecognizable and totally other—because selfhood is mineness tied to a world in advance. David Biro, a physician and patient who underwent a bone marrow transplant, writes that "pain severs our engagement with the world and thrusts us inward… In pain we are alone" (2010, p. 47). Being alone without the world and without embodied agency, selfhood is radicalized as bare and naked. It is the mere "I", which it is not in the everyday and the authentic modes of being. The layers of significance that produce selfhood suddenly vanish and one cannot relate with others although relation is desired more than at other times. Incapacities and the withdrawals of the circle of significance radicalizes the I as I, which becomes unbearable and unrecognizable. In intense bodily pain we are not even ourselves as meaningfully understood but strangers even to ourselves, the familiar stranger.

Much has been written on the gradual loss of self in chronic pain (Charmaz 1983, 1991; Gotlib 2013). In the anti-Cartesian ontological tradition, the self is not only transcendence or exposure toward the world and others in terms of embodied agency, but also in terms of the self as an unfolding story, a narrative identity (Ricoeur 1992), "a narratively constituted, changeable, and fluid notion of who one is" (Gotlib 2013, p. 47). Charles Taylor observes that Heidegger's understanding of "the inescapable temporal structure of being in the world" in *Being and Time* also suggests a narrative notion of selfhood (1989, p. 47). In chronic pain, notes Gotlib, the victim substitutes a "familiar and *previously reliable* self," a self thought to be one's proper identity, with a less desirable and improper self. She emphasizes that the narrative history of the self is not altogether obliterated in chronic pain but is reconstituted in reaction to pain as an identity that does not want to know itself or be known by others, "a self centered on the urgency of fear, on the loss of the familiar, and on an uneasy acknowledgement of its own emergence" (Gotlib 2013, p. 49). This, however, is not the case with intense bodily pain, whether brief or long. The narrative unity of the self is broken and totally obliterated in such pains and the ruptured "I" is not recognizable to the self.

Is self-obliteration in extreme bodily pain unique? How do we distinguish it, for example, from orgasmic self-obliteration? Orgasmic self-obliteration is a forgetfulness of self with extreme pleasure.[2] It is the excess of pleasurable sensations obliterating the pleasure-pain mélange that gives rise to the embodied, narratively united being-in-the-world. Self-obliteration in intense bodily pain is a positive 'destruction' and excess of being in its negation. We use the term 'destruction' to indicate an intolerable condition, a condition that devastates the person to the extent

---

[2]According to the Tibetan Buddhist tradition, "subtler levels of mind manifest during uncontrolled processes as in fainting, going to sleep, ending a dream, experiencing orgasm, sneezing, and dying" (Hopkins 1998, p. 251). This tradition does not speak of these states as the loss of self for well-known reasons, but as steps in the movement towards deeper levels of consciousness. Blissful orgasm, for example, is a technique in the tantric traditions of the East for achieving the mind of clear light. "The pleasure of orgasm is so intense that the mind becomes totally fascinated and entranced with pleasure such that both the usual conceptual mind and the appearances that accompany it melt away, leaving the innermost mind in its pristine state. In orgasm, the phenomena of ordinary life that are so concrete and solid that they seem to have their own independent existence melt into the expanse of the reality behind appearances" (Hopkins 1998, p. 253). Notice that the destruction or melting away of what we have been calling the self (being-in-the-world, exposure to and substitution for otherness, embodied agency and narrative identity) is considered here as revealing the reality behind appearances.

that she/he is no more that same person in a negative sense, either for a brief period or for a longer duration. The intense bodily pain that Rilke underwent during the last stage of his untreated leukemia was a self-destroying pain that prompted the poet to ask 'am I still the one, unrecognized, burns?' The heightened sensations that give rise to the two kinds of self-obliterations are totally different: one is extreme pleasure and self-gratification; the other is extreme pain and self-destruction.

However, we experience pains differently in accordance with the cultural–historical trails that form our self. This emphasis is widely accepted since the first ever anthropological study on pain (Zbrorowski 1969). The emphasis is repeated by Morris (1991) from a different disciplinary terrain—literary and medical knowledge about pain. Do the experiences of the destruction of the self in pain also vary culturally? During the brief period of invalidity and utter helplessness after bone marrow transplant, the biggest difficulty I had was in negotiating my cultivated identity as an academic and my traditional rural Malayali-Indian identity. According to the latter I was prompted to wail and be expressive about my condition and demand the right to be cared by my wide circle of relatives and friends, but according to the former I had to be restrained, dignified and trusting in the logic of medical isolation. What I managed to do in fact was probably a mixture of the two, although at the most hopeless moment when the veil fell, I think I was the latter to the surprise of the doctors and the nurses. Kathy Charmaz remarks that chronically ill Americans suffer the loss of self on account of the assumptions of independence, hard work and individual responsibility they have inherited from the Protestant Ethic. "With such values, the chronically ill question their own self-worth and view their developing limitations as losses" (Charmaz 1983, p. 169). Caregivers think of chronic illness as a temporary disruption that can be overcome by acute care. Hence, they don't pay attention to pain as such leading to further loss of self. Even in intense bodily pain which destroys the self, the expressions of the loss of self with the body and language as the site are very varied. As long as the body and language are sites of culture, expressive traditions will vary. The intensity of the loss of self itself varies culturally. Cultures that emphasize independence and freedom are more likely to feel that the self is destroyed with intense bodily pain. Similarly also in cultures which abide by the retributive notion of 'karma' (Burley 2013). Burley observes that these conceptions cannot be changed by arguments and rationalizations but "only by one or other party in the debate undergoing a change of perspective so transformative that it would amount to a change in form of life" (2013, p. 159). However, I presume that all cultures, irrespective of expressive traditions, come to feel the destruction of the self in intense bodily pain. And inasmuch as the loss is real only in our embodied, expressive being, the loss of self itself is cultural. There is no internality to this loss outside the exteriority of being embodied and human.

Intense bodily pain is an internally diversified category. The thesis of destruction of the self in intense bodily pain might look trivial and overblown when we consider cases like a nail accidently piercing the foot or the little finger jammed in the door. Such cases immediately prompt us to juxtapose self-amnesia in orgasm or sneezing with self-destruction in intense bodily pain. However, the meaning of the thesis of self-destruction in intense bodily pain changes considerably when we consider torture, which for example, Scarry has analyzed with exemplary skill, gaining wide acceptability. The intense pain and insult suffered in the Auschwitz concentration camps, described again most insightfully by Victor Frankl, is another example of the meaning of the thesis of self-destruction in intense bodily pain. Frankl narrates that those among the prisoners who lost faith in the future suddenly gave up and "let himself decline and became subject to mental and physical decay" (1985, p. 95) in the face of intense inhuman pain. Of course, Frankl's theory is that even in intense bodily pain the destruction of self could be prevented through the projection of meaning. According to him, this alone could explain the "paradox that some prisoners of a less hardy makeup often seemed to survive camp life better than did those of a robust nature" (1985, pp. 55–56). Intense chronic bodily pain that accompanies some illnesses and persistent pains of unknown causes are other examples. While some experiences of intense bodily pain destroy our sense of self completely, a chronic bodily pain, as Charmaz shows, changes self-understanding negatively, and to a certain extent, unrecognizably. Short durations of intense pain can also be self-destroying, at least for that duration.[3] Sometimes self-destructions in intense bodily pain are so completely damning, as in the case of Rilke in the last stage of his life or some people in the Auschwitz concentration camps, as described above. But pain can also lead to self-diminution. Lawrence Langer's *Holocaust Testimonies: The Ruins of Memory* (1991) discusses the painful memory/history that haunts Auschwitz survivors. In some cases, the question is not one of the totally destroyed self, but of the self, diminished and disfigured, by the inerasable memory of pain. The diminished self "lapses into a bifocal vision, as its past invades its present and casts a long, pervasive shadow over its future" (Langer 1991, p. 172).

---

[3] A prominent understanding of the Alzheimer's disease is in terms of the loss of self (Capps 2008). Although we cannot characterize this condition as intense bodily pain, loss of self in the case of Alzheimer's patients seems immediately agreeable from the point of view of the ontology of the self I describe in this chapter. This view in relation to the Alzheimer's disease is so prominent that resource books to caregivers of Alzheimer's disease from this perspective are now available (Cohen and Eisdorfer 2002). Herskovits argues that the thesis of the loss of self in Alzheimer's patients has also led to "the creation of a horrific and monstrous image of the person with Alzheimer's, which debased and erased the humanity of the individual" (1995, p. 159). But she does not offer a different and a more redeeming notion of the self, although she points out that the debates reflects "our very notion of what comprises the self and what constitutes subjective experience." The Alzheimer's patient is for her "a caricature or extreme version of the negative stereotype of the elderly" (1995, p. 160). But the problem of ill-treatment itself arises from essentializing being human as a self-substance and losing awareness of identity as losing a peripheral layer of the inner self. Whereas, from the stance of non-substance ontology, the self can be lost and regained, and so the aim of care here is to regain the lost self. It is also claimed that there is no total obliteration of the self in all Alzheimer's patients (Klein et al. 2003; Tappen et al. 1999), which is entirely possible. Capps (2008) also recognizes that Alzheimer's disease does not completely obliterate the self and advocates 'embracing of forgetfulness as an integral part of the self.'

The destroyed self, as Arendt contends, is an extreme form of selfhood, wherein the bare "I" alone is all that matters. The intolerability of the "I" makes that very "I" stark and naked. No other experience has any place in intense bodily pain. Biro points out that our usual self is social and we "literally face outward—our eyes, ears, nose, and tongue point us toward the people and objects in our environment... Our bodies as a whole continually push us into the world..." (2010, p. 25). Being-in-the-world is this self, the outward facing self, selfhood that is turned "inside out like a cloak" (Levinas 1998a, p. 48). It is this self that brings tears to our eyes in rejection and loneliness, and joy to our eyes in accepting company. Biro points out that this is the self, destroyed, suspended or diminished in intense bodily pain. If selfhood is exile from ipseity according to Levinas, intense bodily pain is exile from the world and the other. W.H. Auden's poem "Surgical Ward" speaks of the sufferer in the ward: "A bandage hides the place where each is living,/His knowledge of the world restricted to/The treatments that the instruments are giving.../Truth in their sense is how much they can bear..." (quoted in Biro 2010, p. 28). Biro notes that intense bodily pain and the consequent suspension of the world has driven sufferers to contemplate suicide and some have taken that route because what makes the self is meaningfully dealing with what is not the 'I' myself. The disengaged ego of metaphysical pretense, as Kierkegaard shows, is building castles in the air, is shadowboxing. It is a king without a real castle. Such a self is a riddle because "in the very moment when it seems that the self is closest to having the building completed, it can arbitrarily dissolve the whole thing into nothing" (Kierkegaard 1980, pp. 69–70). Hence, rather than thinking of the self as constructing the world of meaning, we must think of the self and world as inherently caught up in a mutual relation of entanglement.

The self of intense bodily pain is a destroyed self by virtue of its dissociation from the world and others. That the self can be recovered in most cases of intense bodily pain, or at least reconstituted, should salvage this conception from the accusation of inhumanity. Destruction of self in intense bodily pain does not make a human being something else, but rather speaks about the need of the human being in a specific situation—intense bodily pain. The accusation of inhumanity usually arises from the metaphysical notion of the self. The thesis of self-destruction is problematic in the eyes of the substance-ontologist, who is sometimes said to be caught up in what is called "the transcendental pretense" (see Solomon 1988, pp. 1–2). From that perspective, what is lost is the contingent and peripheral layers of the core self, which is above pain and pleasure. However, if we abandon the metaphysical pretense and understand ourselves in terms of contingent, finite, embodied, narrative being-in-the-world, we realize that the self can not only be lost as it can happen in intense bodily pain but also can be regained or recovered in many cases. I have not enough space in this chapter to dwell on self-recovery at length. However, a few remarks on it are in order.

3.4   The Self Recovered

The destroyable–recoverable way of being that the self is, rather than the inflexible, inalterable substance, makes possible the way for the broken, destroyed self in intense bodily pain to be whole again. Although some bodily pains are intense and terminal like that of Rilke, most pains are either acute and temporary or chronic and not terminal. Hence, the intensity of insufferable bodily pains could be made endurable or completely erased and the self can be thus made whole again. Pain is the aversive component of the tempestuous movement of life, and yet pain is also the individuating, rending open and differentiating integral element inherent to human existence as sensually open, embodied being-in-the-world. Because at the extremity of its intensity pain can destroy word, world and self, removal or reduction of human suffering is also inherent to all human striving. For the sake of simplicity, I now turn to elaborating meaningful human encounter with pain in two ways: (i) self-expression relating to all our making and creating of artifacts, and (ii) caring relation toward the suffering other.

For the first of these two, I shall refer to Elaine Scarry alone because perhaps the only thesis of *The Body in Pain* is: intense bodily pain denies both word and world, and all world-making artifices (self-expressive, creative, imaginative, cultural artifacts) are premised on the world-shattering, word-denying experience of pain. Scarry argues persuasively that relieving the suffering human body through material self-expression unites such divergent sets of writings as Judeo-Christian scriptures and Marxian revolutionary texts, both central to modern western culture. She puts on display the humaneness of materialism. If a chair were not imagined somehow as objectifying and thus negating the pain of managing one's body weight, it would not have become such an important cultural artifact that relieves pain. Similarly, all artifacts, right from the complex computer that relieves the calculating mind to the most humble wheel that relieves the porter and traveler, eliminates the limitations of the sentient body-being or magnifies its powers, thus making "sentience itself an artifact" (Scarry 1985, p. 255). In the Judeo-Christian scriptures and the texts of Marx, writes Scarry, "the material artifact is a surrogate or substitute for the human body, and the human body in turn becomes an artifact... the object is a displacement of sentient pain by a materialized clarification of creation" (257). The Scarry thesis is the following:

> All intentional states—physical, emotional, mental—take intentional objects: the more completely the object expresses and fulfills (objectifies) the state, the more it permits a *self-transformation* out of that embodied state; conversely, the more the state is deprived of an adequate object, the more it approaches the *condition of physical pain* (261; my emphasis).

That is, the job of the artifact is to eject the recoiling, private, inexpressible self, salvage it from destruction, give it the world back and let its reconstitution begin. By virtue of the artifact's morphology of being the objectification of an inexpressible human pain, it helps to relieve that pain in order to reconstitute the self. For Scarry, the teleology of culture and its products, whether it be the gods or the plough, have this sole purpose of figuratively and imaginatively entering the human body, feeling its pain and expressing what relieves that pain in objectifiable forms. Scarry argues that

> it is the benign, almost certainly heroic, and in any case absolute intention of all human making to distribute the facts of sentience outward onto the created realm of artifice, and it is only by doing so that men, and women are themselves relieved of the privacy and problems of that sentience (288).[4]

But, while the moralism of conceiving the artifact structurally as pain reliever is unwarranted, we may still say that if it is not primarily for encountering pain, our artifacts have no meaning. It is because the human is a constitutively sentient being-in-the-world that human artifacts can be sensually created to relieve aversive sentience (pain) and gratify desirable sentience (pleasure). For this reason, even if all technologies become superfluous and creative culture were to be detechnicized, medical technologies and techniques would be justifiable. Alluding to Heidegger's influential critique of technology, Levinas observes that "medicine as technique, and consequently the technology as a whole that it presupposes... does not derive solely from the so-called 'will to power'" (1998b, p. 94). Material making remakes the self destroyed by pain.

When we see all human pain as evil in itself, human making or the culture of the artifact is a good in itself. Scarry does not say so, nor does she allude to it, but the unproblematic tenor of her analysis of objectification and artificial making, laid out upon the background of the brutality of the intensely tortured body, might betray the narcissistic spirit of Enlightenment humanism in its triumphalist avatar. The valorization of the problem of pain and its solution—human making—has created what Arendt calls the 'perpetually labouring society', fashioned after the ideal of the *homo faber* and practised as the instrumental approach to things. Everything is thus reduced to a means for something else and its intrinsic or independent value is disparaged. Arendt remarks that it was due to this vulgar reductionism that the Greeks considered all productive enterprises as *banausic*, philistine or mundane. The Baconian search for knowledge that assists 'the relief of man's estate' is based upon the same ontology of the artifact. Relating the Kantian injunction that only human beings are outside the means-ends relationship to the saying attributed to Protagoras that the human being is the measure of all things, Arendt refers to Plato's criticism of Protagoras's statement:

---

[4]But I would hasten to suggest that the ontology of the artifact should begin with the notion of the pain-pleasure mélange that existence as a turbulent movement is composed of. Should pleasure only be conceived negatively as relief from pain so that every artifice takes the place of a reliever? This moralism appears to me unwarranted. The site of the artifact is the whole space of the movement of life, most of which is occupied by the mélange of pain-pleasure. The artifact relieves the human body-being from pain as well as gratifies her desire, but does so always as if by inhabiting the ontology of the body-being. Indeed, there is a moral imperative to direct our self-expressive powers primarily to relieving pain on account of its power to destroy the self. This moral critique, I think, needs to extend to contemporary material culture wherein the ceaseless production of the artifact seems to have become a sport by and for itself.

Plato knew quite well that the possibilities of producing use objects and of treating all things of nature as potential use objects are as limitless as the wants and talents of human beings. If one permits the standards of *homo faber* to rule the finished world as they must necessarily rule the coming into being of this world, then *homo faber* will eventually help himself to everything and consider everything that is as a mere means for himself. (1998, p. 158)

Arendt remarks that everything would thus become profane use-objects, and as Plato contends, the wind would no longer be considered as a natural force as such but as that which fulfills the human need for warmth and refreshment. The givenness of things would thus be eliminated from human experience.[5] On the one hand, inhuman pain cannot be justified under the pretext of the love of nature, and on the other, human pain cannot be the pretext for our reductionist technological culture, the limits and wrongs of which are already plain.

How do we come upon that tenuous balance between absolute reductionism and a reasonable approach to the problem of pain? Human condition cannot be fully pain-free and the fragility of existence cannot be fully overcome. This is why Heidegger repeatedly asserts that "[t]o be a human being means to be on the earth as a mortal. It means to dwell" (1971, p. 145). The human being alone is mortal because she/he is capable of death and she/he alone can die "indeed continually, as long as he remains on earth…" (1971, p. 148). Not that mortals are called upon to suffer pain stoically and wither away with the wind, but as language animals that express the meaning of all beings and as mortal dwellers on the earth, humans also take issue with or care for the being of entities they live among on the earth. "Mortals dwell in the way they preserve the fourfold in its essential being, its presencing" (Heidegger 1971, p. 148). It is as preservers of the world (fourfold) just as it reveals itself to us that we dwell or exist meaningfully upon the earth. The Scarrian ontology of the artifact has its authentic place within the sphere of existence only when fundamental human mortality, fragility and contingency are fully acknowledged and the problem of pain is situated within such an ontology of existence.[6]

From a Heideggerian point of view, Scarry's cultural artifacts are the handy or *zuhanden* things or tools that we imaginatively objectify with reference to the ontology of the body in pain. But Scarry—and Heidegger—has nothing to say about the second constitutive component of our being-in-the-world, which is not an artifact, indeed not handy at all. Levinas thinks of it as completely outside all handiness, all representational reduction. This is the other human being, the witness to our suffering and destruction of self. Does Levinas's argument that among all different sorts of affectednesses, the voice, sight and touch of another human being has an uncompromising predilection have any significance? Russon, while arguing

---

[5]We find a more celebrated version of this analysis of the humanly objectified and reduced world in Heidegger's writings on the technological understanding of all beings as the essence of modernity (see Heidegger 1977).

[6]See my article "Wellness in illness" (2011). Here, I give an existential analysis of the ill body and how one can exist well even in conditions of illness.

that "we are beings who are sensitive to our environments... [and] feel our placement within the world", places his emphasis clearly on the fact that "we care about how we stand with others, and our relations with others affect us... to have others already influencing, already *inside our experience*... it is as a bodily involvement with another that we are invaded, that we are satisfied, that we are embarrassed, and that we enchant" (2003, p. 22; my emphasis). While it is true that we are that "sort of open circuit that completes itself only in things, in others, in the encompassing earth" (Abram 1996, p. 62), our completing ourselves in other humans seems to have a very special meaning for us. True, we need to restrain this spontaneous 'affection' for the other human being in our speciesist, moralistic justification for cutting ourselves off from the 'encompassing earth' and exploiting nonhuman reality seen solely as raw material for human gratification, as Heidegger warns. Nevertheless, the unique meaning of the 'face of the other person' seems to be at the center of the 'humus' of the human, and, thus, to what drives the tumultuous, restive movement of our lives—the pain-pleasure mélange. If this is true, then Scarry's inflexible concentration on material making is at least lopsided. True, she concentrates single-mindedly on imaginative expression in material terms, so that the bodily being that the sufferer is, is relieved and reconstituted. But the being in pain is a being awake to the irreducible face of the other human person like no other; indeed, its selfhood is something constituted most significantly in relation to these others. The self is the 'other in the same.' There seems to be a reawakening of the self destroyed in pain by the touch, call and empathic presence of a dear one, something even the most skillfully constructed artifact cannot do.

Scarry suggests that western culture's humane approach to human suffering shifts the intensely felt character of pain from the human body to the body of the artifact with the purpose of releasing the human body from pain, and hence there is "an increased pressure toward material culture, or material self-expression" (1985, p. 14). She writes: "If western civilization is characterized by a long list of attributes, two that must occupy a central position in any list are first, its Judeo-Christian framework of belief, and second, its insistent thrust toward material self-expression" (1985, p. 179). I suggest that the problem of alienation, breakdown of community, technologization of the human and the disappearance of connection with the earth, which so many western scholars—from Karl Marx, Max Weber, Heidegger, Levinas, Derrida, Jean-Luc Nancy to Charles Taylor—have bemoaned, something that has become our global fate too, should also be connected derivatively to this list. What is happening in this pronouncedly humane emphasis on material self-expression is a forgetfulness and undermining of the concretely sensual and material (but different from the materiality of the artifact), relational aspects of the human comportment toward the suffering of the other person. Indeed, this emphasis on artifacts and the artificial to relieve suffering is in itself pregnant with humane potential. But isn't this emphasis also the subtext of the 'white man's burden' and the whole complex history of colonialism?

Both Biro and Scarry note the absence or severe inadequacy of verbal articulation of one's suffering to another. This inadequacy adds to the suffering. And, (alas!) if the significant other or dear other takes the lack of words for the lack of pain, a world indeed comes tumbling down. Such unempathic relation to the other in pain not only denies the other's pain but her *self* (Biro 2010, p. 33). Pain destroys self; nonrecognition of pain by the caregiver certifies and seals that destruction. As Hannah Arendt observes, our most intense feelings need to be expressed in order to make them palpably real and public; approval (and disapproval too!) creates truth. The artifact reconstitutes the self destroyed by pain by pain's relief, leading to the gradual reemergence of the self eclipsed by the onslaught of pain, but cannot affirm the other person's pain and make it verbally real. The Hegelian dialectics of the sense of the self as conditioned on the recognition of the self by the other is paramount here. The several layers of human affirmation of another human being is a sovereign activity of sentience, which alone has any effect on the reemergence of the self, for example, in terminal pain. The touch of life upon life has a totally different constitution to the touch of the artifact. If the artifact is imagined as entering the body in pain, empathic caring is standing 'inside' another in an attempt to be that self. Deep, self-reconstitutive care is possible because our selfhood is already 'the other in the same', already substituted for the other. Our body-being is of that kind which can be made whole *only with reference to the other*. While an artifact can be empathically created, empathic caring is more direct and cuts one step short in the creation of the artifact, for empathic caring is not empathic *creating for* the body in pain, but empathic *being toward* the body in pain. To privilege the artifact-aided relief of pain over human care is to privilege the historical meaning of the human as the "technologized animal" (Heidegger 2012, p. 78).

For an instantiation of the recovery of the self destroyed by pain through human caring and affirmation, I will now look at an episode in Amitav Ghosh's *Sea of Poppies* (2008). The scene is chapter fourteen: Neel Rattan Halder, the Raja of Rakshali, is imprisoned in Alipur Jail, falsely charged with forgery. The Raja's companion is a Chinese opium addict, Ah Fatt, in whose convulsive seizures "a fire would seem to come alight under his skin and he would begin to slap himself all over, as if to snuff out the spreading flames… [and gouge] into his flesh as if to rip off a coating of charred skin" (322). Gradually the Raja begins to feel that 'he was somehow implicated in his cell-mate's plight' and setting aside his repugnance, begins to clean the cell and Ah Fatt's body 'soaked in his own waste.' Neel was surprised with his accomplishment, and discovered that "the mere fact of using one's hands and investing one's attention in someone other than oneself, created a pride and tenderness that had nothing whatever to do with the response of the object of one's care" (326). For many days without success, the Raja made a ritual of asking his cell mate's name, as if to help him recover self. The response to the question, indeed the recovery of self, came on a gloomy night in Alipur jail during the Diwali festival season, the day before their ship would set sail for Mauritius. Neel was despondent, thinking of his son and wife celebrating a Diwali without him and the prospect of the looming departure. In the darkness of the night, an embrace awakes Neel, and the scene of recovery is signed with the utterance of the name, a determination of the self: "My name Lei Leong Fatt… People call Ah Fatt. Ah Fatt your friend" (342). Of course, Ghosh sets up the scene also to say that Ah Fatt's self-recovery was a gift of friendship to Neel, which has far-reaching consequences for the storyline even in the sequel, *River of Smoke* (2011). But as for the scene here, a voyage is about to begin with the sunrise, a new life of shared fates, the name of the body-being in self-destroying pain uttered by himself—all symbolizing, for me, the recovery of the self destroyed by excruciating pain.

I must also record here the personal memoir of isolation and pain while undergoing a bone marrow transplant for multiple myeloma in 2011. During a six-day bout of intense nausea, diarrhea, and delirious insomnia, what I recollect most vividly is an eagerness to be left alone untroubled, unprobed. Phone calls and probing by doctors and dear ones I averted. Intense nausea is weariness with body-being; one truly does not recognize one's self and its affectednesses. In such moments there is only the tiring, sickening sensation; there is no way of making meaning out of that experience in a simultaneous moment. This is what is meant by the loss of the self. But it was not really a desire to be *left alone* but left untroubled, left without having to respond; in short, without having to do anything. Is this surrender of agency equal to turning away from all presence and entering a state of worldlessness? This state could be compared to Levinas's *Il y a* or the 'there-is', his term for existence without existents/beings, the anonymous, dark, horrifying state of blank, non-intentional awareness. Isn't the blankness in pain an experience of the there-is, a terror of selfless existence? The terror of my aloneness in the isolation ward of the hospital seems to belie the angst of the loss of self and, with it, the anxious desire for the other to affirm self. The desire to be left alone arose from the inability of meaningfully comporting oneself toward one's being-in-the-world, and did not mean any consolidated entrapment in the self. The last phrase in Rilke's '*Komm du...*', "no one knows me" reminds me of the terror of being alone in pain. *Affirmation aids self-recovery*, even when caring affirmation cannot be reciprocated with a response by the sufferer.

Let me make a brief reference to deep, intense trauma. The fact that intensely traumatic experience can throw some sufferers into absolute collapse and even mental illness, fleetingly or more enduringly, suggests that trauma can also be self-destructive. Robert Stolorow, a practitioner of what he calls 'post-Cartesian psychoanalysis', makes this case with reference to his own experiences, both personal and clinical, and to Heidegger's philosophy. His autobiographical reference is to the traumatic loss of his wife Dede to cancer. He writes that "the loss of Dede shattered my world and permanently altered my sense of being" (2007, p. 24). Stolorow uses the term 'ontological unconsciousness' to refer to the loss of the sense of being, and his clinical practice and psychoanalytic approach is to help patients to regain their sense of being shattered by trauma. He emphasizes the difficulty of sharing intensely traumatic experiences and the difficulty of caregivers to feel with the sufferer as they could come to feel 'painfully erased' by the experience. And yet, Stolorow's stress is on affirmation. What is lost in trauma and any intense suffering is not a self-substance but a way of being that is based on our ability to bring about unity and significance to our existence in terms of what Heidegger calls 'the ecstatical unity of temporality' or our ability to project a future at each moment of the now and, thus, own up our past. "Thus, although the possibility of emotional trauma is ever present," observes Stolorow, "so too is the possibility of forming bonds of deep emotional attunement within which devastating emotional pain can be held, rendered more tolerable, and, hopefully, eventually integrated" (2011, pp. 64–65).

I want to reemphasize in conclusion that it is the self itself that is shattered in intense bodily pain—the self, understood as embodied, sensuous, affected, substituted, narratively structured, ecstatically temporal being-in-the-world—and not merely word and world. In the reconstitution of the self in pain, the centrality of human care needs to be reaffirmed in the face of the technological culture of the artifact. Rilke's final poem says that the self in pain is unrecognizable to oneself and unknown to others. Caring affirmation of the sufferer's self, I have argued, attempts to stamp that self with being and reality. Pain is self-destroying; human care is self-affirming. At the same time, we may also note that intense pain cannot be undone and the self in pain cannot be made whole by something like the opposite of pain—intense pleasure. It is also, therefore, clear that while intense pain is self-destroying, intense pleasure is not self-constituting in an unproblematic sense. Rather, often painful healing processes are required in order to recover and restore the self destroyed in intense bodily pain. Although intense, totally aversive, self-destructive pain is to be overcome, pain as such is not an evil per se, but an inherent part of our sensual, finite and constantly dying existence.

References

Abram, D. (1996). *The spell of the sensuous: Perception and language in a more-than-human world*. New York: Vintage.

Aho, K. (2009). *Heidegger's neglect of the body*. Albany, NY: State University of New York Press.

Arendt, H. (1998). *The human condition (1958)* (2nd ed.). Chicago, IL: University of Chicago Press.

Biro, D. (2010). *The language of pain: Finding words, compassion, and relief*. New York: W. W. Norton.

Burley, M. (2013). Retributive karma and the problem of blaming the victim. *International Journal for Philosophy of Religion, 74*(2), 149–165.

Capps, D. (2008). Alzheimer's disease and the loss of self. *Journal of Pastoral Care and Counseling, 62*(1–2), 19–28.

Charmaz, K. (1983). Loss of self: A fundamental form of suffering in the chronically ill. *Sociology of Health & Illness, 5*(2), 168–195.

Charmaz, K. (1991). *Good days, bad days: The self in chronic illness and time*. New Brunswick, NJ: Rutgers University Press.

Cohen, D., & Eisdorfer, C. (2002). *The loss of self: A family resource for the care of Alzheimer's disease and related disorders*. New York: W. W. Norton.

Derrida, J. (1983). Geschlecht: Sexual difference, ontological difference. *Research in Phenomenology, 13*(1), 65–83.

Fagenblat, M. (2010). *A covenant of creatures: Levinas's philosophy of Judaism*. Stanford, CA: Stanford University Press.

Frankl, V. E. (1985). *Man's search for meaning (1946)*. New York: Washington Square Press.

George, S. K. (2011). Wellness in illness. *Samyukta: A Journal of Women's Studies, XI*(2), 49–65.

Ghosh, A. (2008). *Sea of poppies*. New Delhi: Penguin-Viking.

Gotlib, A. (2013). On the borderlands: Chronic pain as crisis of identity. In L. F. Käll (Ed.) *Dimensions of pain: Humanities and social sciences perspectives* (pp. 41–59). Abingdon, UK: Routledge.

Heidegger, M. (1962). *Being and time* (1927). (J. Macquarrie & E. Robinson, Trans.). New York: Harper & Row.

Heidegger, M. (1971). Building dwelling thinking (1951). (A. Hofstadter, Trans.). In *Poetry, language, thought* (pp. 143–159). New York: Harper & Row.

Heidegger, M. (1977). The question concerning technology and other essays. W. Lovitt (Trans.). New York: Harper & Row.

Heidegger, M. (1984). *The metaphysical foundations of logic* (1928). (M. Heim, Trans.). Bloomington, IN: Indiana University Press.

Heidegger, M. (1987). *Zollikon seminars: Protocols—conversations—letters* (1959–71). (M. Boss, E.; F. Mayr & R. Askay, Trans.). Evanston, IL: Northwestern University Press.

Heidegger, M. (1988). *The basic problems of phenomenology* (1927). (A. Hofstadter, Trans.). Revised Edition. Bloomington, IN: Indiana University Press.

Heidegger, M. (1992). *The concept of time* (1924). (W. McNeill, Trans.). Oxford: Blackwell.

Heidegger, M. (2012). *Contributions to philosophy (of the event)*. (R. Rojcewicz & D. Vallega-Neu, Trans.). Bloomington, IN: Indiana University Press.

Herskovits, E. (1995). Struggling over subjectivity: Debates about the 'self' and Alzheimer's disease. *Medical Anthropology Quarterly, 9*(2), 146–164.

Hopkins, J. (1998). Death, sleep, and orgasm: Gateways to the mind of clear light. *Journal of Chinese Philosophy, 25*(2), 245–260.

Kierkegaard, S. (1980). *The sickness unto death: A Christian psychological exposition for upbuilding and awakening* (1849). (H. V. Hong & E. H. Hong, Trans., & Eds.). *Kierkegaard's Writings* (Vol. XIX). Princeton, NJ: Princeton University Press.

Klein, S. B., Cosmides, L., & Costabile, K. A. (2003). Preserved knowledge of self in a case of Alzheimer's dementia. *Social Cognition, 21*(2), 157–165.

Langer, L. (1991). *Holocaust testimonies: The ruins of memory*. New Haven, CT: Yale University Press.

Levinas, E. (1998a). *Otherwise than being, Or beyond essence* (1974). (A. Lingis, Trans.). Pittsburgh, PA: Duquesne University Press.

Levinas, E. (1998b). Useless suffering (1982). (M. B. Smith & B. Harshav, Trans.). In *Entre Nous: Thinking-of-the-Other* (pp. 91–101). New York: Columbia University Press.

Levinas, E. (2003). *On escape* (1935). (B. Bergo, Trans.). Stanford, CA: Stanford University Press.

Merleau-Ponty, M. (2012). *The Phenomenology of Perception* (1945). (D. A. Landes, Trans.). London: Routledge.

Morris, D. (2008). Diabetes, chronic illness and the bodily roots of ecstatic temporality. *Human Studies, 31*(4), 399–421.

Morris, D. B. (1991). *The culture of pain*. Berkeley, CA: University of California Press.

Ricoeur, P. (1992). *Oneself as another* (1985–86). (K. Blamey, Trans.). Chicago, IL: The University of Chicago Press.

Rilke, R. M. (2010). *Come, you…* (1926). (R. G. Stern, Trans.). In R. G. Stern, *Still on call* (p. 99). Ann Arbor, MI: The University of Michigan Press.

Russon, J. (2003). *Human experience: Philosophy, neurosis, and the elements of everyday life*. Albany, NY: State University of New York Press.

Scarry, E. (1985). *The body in pain: The making and unmaking of the world*. Oxford: Oxford University Press.

Smith, J. A., & Osborn, M. (2007). Pain as an assault on the self: An interpretative phenomenological analysis of the psychological impact of chronic benign low back pain. *Psychology and Health, 22*(5), 517–534.

Solomon, R. C. (1988). *Continental philosophy since 1750: The rise and fall of the self*. Series: A History of Western Philosophy (Vol. 7). Oxford: Oxford University Press.

Stolorow, R. D. (2007). *Trauma and human existence: Autobiographical, psychoanalytic, and philosophical reflections*. Series: Psychoanalytic Enquiry Book Series. New York: The Analytic Press, Taylor & Francis Group.

Stolorow, R. D. (2011). *World, affectivity, trauma: Heidegger and post-Cartesian psychoanalysis*. Series: Psychoanalytic Enquiry Book Series. New York: Routledge, Taylor & Francis Group.

Tappen, R. M., Williams, C., Fishman, S., & Touhy, T. (1999). Persistence of self in advanced Alzheimer's disease. *Journal of Nursing Scholarship, 31*(2), 121–125.

Taylor, C. (1989). *Sources of the self: The making of the modern identity*. Cambridge, MA: Harvard University Press.

Woolf, V. (2002). *On being ill (1926)*. Ashfield, MA: Paris Press.

Zbrorowski, M. (1969). *People in pain*. San Francisco: Jossey-Bass.

Chapter 4
Waiting to Speak: A Phenomenological Perspective on Our Silence Around Dying

Kirsten Jacobson

Abstract Drawing from existential and empirical accounts, I consider the pain that relates to our recognition of our own mortality, especially focusing on our contemporary silence around mortality and our tendencies to generalize and medicalize death. Examining Heidegger's distinction between "ontic" structures concealing death and the "ontological" significance underlying this concealing, I argue that, though this silence arises from our way of being-in-the-world, there are reasons for challenging institutional and social structures pushing us to cover over death and the existential suffering associated with it. I argue it is incumbent upon the medical community specifically, and ultimately all of us, to respond to silence surrounding dying by cultivating practices of listening, thereby opening possibilities for a more authentic relationship to our dying.

Keywords Martin Heidegger · Being-towards-death · Existential health · Anxiety · Dying · Medicalization

In this chapter, I use existential authors—Martin Heidegger, Rainer Maria Rilke, and J.H. van den Berg—as well as empirical discussions from medical practitioners and patients to consider the pain that relates to our recognition of our own mortality, focusing especially on ways in which contemporary silence around our mortality as well as our related tendencies to generalize and medicalize death often work toward covering over this pain. Drawing especially on Heidegger, and his distinction between the "ontic" or worldly structures that conceal the nature of our death and the "ontological" or existential significance underlying this concealing, I ultimately argue that, though this silence arises from the existential depths of our way of being-in-the-world, there are nonetheless reasons for addressing this by challenging the worldly institutional and social structures that push us toward this covering over of the experience of dying. I argue it is incumbent upon the medical community specifically, and all of us more broadly, to respond to this silence around dying by cultivating practices of *listening*, and thereby to open up possibilities for a more authentic relationship to our

K. Jacobson (✉)
University of Maine, Orono, USA
e-mail: kirsten.jacobson@maine.edu

© Springer India 2016   75
S.K. George and P.G. Jung (eds.), *Cultural Ontology*
of the Self in Pain, DOI 10.1007/978-81-322-2601-7_4

own dying and the pain we experience in facing our mortality. I begin, in Sect. 4.1, with a brief look at Heidegger's argument that it is in anxiety that we come face-to-face with our own nothingness, whereas in experiences of fear we are wrapped up in "worldly" concerns. In Sect. 4.2, I use this insight to analyze what lies behind contemporary examples of the silence and resistance we demonstrate toward dying. In Sect. 4.3, the focus of the chapter, I begin to articulate the demand upon us to break up such resistances in our own experience and in the healthcare arena, arguing that changes at the ontic level can open up ontologically significant realizations for us; specifically, I emphasize the value in *listening to the voices* of the dying. I conclude, finally, that resolute being-towards-death, far from being a "morbid" activity, in fact opens up sites for true intimacy within our ontic experience.

4.1   Fear, Anxiety, and the Disclosure of Care

Heidegger differentiates between fear and anxiety. He argues that something that is fearful to us—the threatening—has "detrimentality as its kind of involvement" and "comes from a definite region" (Heidegger 1962, H. 140, M/R. 179–180).[1] The fearful is something on which we can focus our attention, something that stands against us "out there" and that looms before us threatening to "attack" us. As such, the fearful must be something within the "world." Heidegger argues, however, that we are not beings set against a pre-formed "world." Rather, the way the world appears to us reflects our way of caring for our own Being, our way of "being-in-the-world."[2] The object of our fear, then, though it immediately seems to be something worldly—something "ontic," in Heidegger's language—more deeply reflects back to us something about ourselves—something "ontological" about our very nature as being-in-the world, as "*Dasein*"—even if we do not recognize it as such.[3]

Anxiety, in contrast to fear, is precisely the mood that urges us to shift from understanding the surrounding world as a fixed entity to realizing that the significance of the world arises through us and answers to the demands of our care.[4]

---

[1]Citations of Heidegger's *Being and Time* will begin with pagination from the 8th edition of the German text—e.g., "H. 187"—and conclude with page numbers from the Macquarrie and Robinson translation—e.g., M/R. 232.

[2]This is not to say that we simply "make up" the world we desire or need. There are, of course, factical realities that we encounter and to which we must respond; but, the way in which these "realities" are held together by us in a meaningful and oriented whole—in a world—is made possible only because we are beings for whom these things can matter.

[3]For core portions of Heidegger's analysis of "*Dasein*," see *Being and Time*, H. 11–15, M/R. 9–12 and H. 42–45, M/R. 39–42.

[4]Heidegger emphasizes that the awareness of our being-in-the-world that comes to us in anxiety is not a conceptual awareness or recognition. What we experience in the state of anxiety is less settled and definite than this; there is nothing for us to hold onto as there would be if we had a clearly articulated "cause" for the problem. For Heidegger's discussion of this point, see *Being and Time*, H. 187–188, M/R. 232–233.

Anxiety can bring about this shift insofar as the way in which it unsettles us is not through causing us to feel unsettled about any *thing* in particular, but rather pointedly about *nothing* (Heidegger 1962, H. 187, M/R. 232). Whereas our fear is of something specific in the world, we cannot pin our anxiety on our worldly affairs, on our worldly possessions or interests, on our involvements with and through other people, or on any other determinate feature of our lives. In fact, it is just these things that drop away and appear utterly insignificant when we are anxious.

The experience of anxiety thus invites the *revelation* that our state of being cannot be explained by these things, cannot be explained on the basis of the world.[5] As a result, we become aware of the world and ourselves as *being* essentially "nothing and nowhere" (Heidegger 1962, H. 343, M/R. 393; H. 188, M/R. 233), and we become aware of the fact that we are existentially *free* beings. Heidegger writes: "Anxiety makes manifest in *Dasein* its *Being towards* its ownmost potentiality-for-Being—that is, its *Being-free* for the freedom of choosing itself and taking hold of itself" (Heidegger 1962, H. 188, M/R. 232, emphasis in original). We come up against ourselves *as* being-in-the-world—that is the beings for whom there is a world, by whom there is a world, and who are, therefore, spread throughout the world and typically involved in understanding themselves in terms of the world. In short, then, anxiety leads us to encounter the existential nature of the world—not in a thematic way, but rather in a feeling of the utter emptiness of the daily world and in a corresponding sense of our way of being responsible for worldhood as such.

Though anxiety invites this authentic recognition of our existential nature and the attendant responsibility for rendering life meaningful, we most often evade this recognition. It is profoundly unsettling to our daily lives to feel the "nothingness" of our being, and there are countless diversions by which we can and do readily distract ourselves when we begin to feel anxious (Heidegger 1962, H. 189, M/R. 234). Even if we are not willfully distracting ourselves in such ways, our very way of having a world is essentially distracting. We are unavoidably wrapped up in the things (and people) of the world insofar as it is our way of existing to care for ourselves by means of our concern for these worldly things. Thus, for reasons both of evasion and of the very structure of our way of being, the "world" for the most part prevents us from noticing the freedom and responsibility that are announced through anxiety.

For each of us individually, death is the end of our care: our death is not the end of reality, but it is the end of that very capacity we have that lets the world matter, and so in addressing ourselves to our own death, we are addressing ourselves to that very freedom, that very responsibility for meaning, that we typically evade. Anxiety in the face of death, Heidegger argues, is what brings a person "face to face with itself as delivered over to that possibility which is not to be outstripped" (1962, H. 254, M/R. 298; H. 262, M/R. 306–307). And, to evade this recognition—a recognition, Heidegger argues, that catapults us into the "uncanny," into the feeling of ultimately "*not*-being-at-home" in the world—we typically concern ourselves with...

---

[5]For an extensive explanation of the theme of anxiety and authenticity in Heidegger's philosophy, see Russon (2008, pp. 99–103).

transforming this anxiety [in the face of the possibility of the measureless impossibility of existence] into fear in the face of an oncoming event. In addition, the anxiety which has been made ambiguous as fear, is passed off as a weakness with which no self-assured *Dasein* may have any acquaintance…. The cultivation of such a "superior" indifference *alienates Dasein* from its ownmost relational potentiality-for-Being (1962, H. 254, M/R. 298).[6]

In our fears around death, we see our evasion of anxiety and also the impossibility of escape from this very anxiety.

We will turn now, in Sect. 4.2, to consider more specifically this evasive character of our fears of death in the context of modern healthcare practice. In Sect. 4.3, we will examine the specific theme of *listening* to investigate how specific ontic practices of engaging with dying can offer us important resources for connecting us to the ontological issue at their root.

4.2   The Silence in Evading Death

In the opening pages of *The Notebooks of Malte Laurids Brigge*, Rilke's narrator laments the lack of people's "owning" of their deaths, and, in doing so, resonates at certain key points with Heidegger's discussion in *Being and Time* of the ways in which we regularly turn away from our own dying—at both ontological and ontical levels.[7] He wonders:

> Who cares anything today for a finely-finished death? No one. Even the rich, who could after all afford this luxury of dying in full detail, are beginning to be careless and indifferent; the wish to have a death of one's own is growing ever rarer. A while yet, and it will be just as rare as a life of one's own. Heavens, it's all there. One arrives, one finds a life, ready made, one has only to put it on. One wants to leave or one is compelled to: anyway, no effort: voilà votre mort, monsieur. One dies just as it comes; one dies the death that belongs to the disease one has (for since one has come to know all diseases, one knows, too, that the different lethal terminations belong to the diseases and not to the people; and the sick person has so to speak nothing to do) (Rilke 1949, pp. 17–18).

We are here described as beings who, so far from considering what death may mean for our own way of being, can only speak about death—and even the mere "facts" of death—in borrowed institutionalized and technical terms. We speak in the words of the "they-self" (*das Mann*), as Heidegger maintains, and, in doing so, keep death at a distance from ourselves.[8] We consider death as something that happens to some *one*, not to ourselves, and we focus on death in terms of a generic disease or

---

[6]For Heidegger's central discussion of the "uncanny" (*unheimlich*), see *Being and Time*, H. 188–189, M/R. 233).

[7]See especially *Being and Time*, Section 51. "Being-towards-death and the Everydayness of *Dasein*."

[8]For a discussion of the everyday way in which we evadingly "take up" death in terms of the "they-self," see Heidegger (1962, Sections 51 and 52).

accident of which we might die, or perhaps of the types of pain or incapacities that we might face depending on the biological form of the death.

As long as we are wrapped up in biological or factual terms, we are focusing, Heidegger argues, on our "demise"—the falling apart of our organic body, not on our death.[9] It can be important to take up the issues of our demise: pain and the fear of impending pain are significant concerns, and diseases put specific demands upon us if we are to deal with them well. Indeed, in attending to these demands, we are often responding quite rightly to the worldly realities of our ontic existence. Yet, Heidegger argues that such attention to the body's demise can and typically does overlook the ontological "problem" with which our own death confronts us.[10] Heidegger describes this turning away from death as a key marker of our "falling" into the "world." He writes: "As falling, everyday Being-towards-death is a constant *fleeing in the face of death*" (1962, H. 254, M/R. 298).

This fleeing is further supported by the contemporary sense that hospitals, clinics, and funeral homes provide the "experts" who will take care of business for us.[11] We hand our bodies—whether living or dead—over to the professionals of these institutions, and they will handle the problem. At the end, we will be discharged from their care, and, if anything, we may have to follow the directions given to us by the professionals.[12] As Rilke suggested above, we ourselves have nothing, so to speak, to do.

This covering over of the particularity of our dying and its meaning is also mirrored by the routinized and uniform character of many contemporary Western

---

[9]For Heidegger's distinction between our dying and our demise, see Heidegger (1962, Section 49).

[10]See Heidegger (1962, Sections 46–50). For interpretations of the ideas therein, see de Beistegui (2005, Chapter 2: "The Truth That Lies Beneath"); and, Lingis (2009).

[11]As an existential structure of *Dasein*, evasive approaches to death can and have taken different forms throughout history and across cultures. In Western history, we could interpret as such evasions the once general and resigned sense that young children were more likely to die than adults, the pre-modern emphasis on the afterlife, and the quite formalized process from the mid-sixteenth century until the medicalization of the twentieth century of having a "good death." For studies of different ontic approaches to death in Western culture, see Kellehear (2007, pp. 85–104 for a discussion of "the good death"), Ariès (1974, 1981), Illich (2002), Howarth (2007), Cassell (1986), and Walter (1996). Howarth (2007), following Illich (2002), argues that what distinguishes the contemporary approach to death is the replacement of a "natural" death with a "technological" death (116–123). Many have argued that this shift toward medicalization and a "managed death" has intensified our distance from death (see, for instance, Howarth (2007, pp. 123–125); Kellehear (2007, pp. 145–146); and Ariès (1974, 1981)), while others have suggested death has come to be more public and less concealed by these moves (Armstrong 1987). Heidegger's argument would suggest that regardless of whether death has become more discussed or studied, as long as it remains a discussion of our demise—that is, concerning the ontic possibility of our body's biological end—we are falling, and, thus, concealing from ourselves the ontological significance of our death.

[12]See Gatchel et al. (1989, pp. 163–165) for a brief, but illuminating discussion of "good patients" as those who comply readily and without question with the directions of hospital staff, and also of the increased likelihood of such patients (in contrast to "bad patients") to develop sometimes health-threatening traits of helplessness both during and after their hospital stay.

institutions and practices that deal with terminal illness and death.[13] Hospitals and clinics have white-washed walls, repetitive hallways, impersonal waiting rooms, and they often demand of one that one remove all private traces of clothing and ornamentation, and that one behave according to a strict procedure. By becoming generically clothed and well-behaved—and, thereby, becoming a mere "case"—patients arguably make it easier for their visitors, their caregivers, and even themselves to avoid altogether the sense that the dying being encountered will ever be a personal death, "our" death. The aspects of the body and its wastes that are off-putting to our polite sensibilities are whisked away quickly from our view and from our senses of scent and touch. J.H. van den Berg observes that, in contrast to pre-modern times when death and sickness were present in the heart of towns—for instance, in sick persons begging there, in centrally placed cemeteries, and in the tolling of church bells for the dead—nowadays,

> the sick are removed from our every-day life. They live in hospitals or institutions. A visitor to these centers of sickness usually notices very little of disease and death. There is singing and laughter; there is hardly any suffering to be seen. For serious patients are moved to private rooms; they are more or less sick in secret. ... And even for the patient himself, death has to be camouflaged. Morphine is administered to him—of course, only to remove the pain. But the universal secret wish that death should come to a patient while he is unconscious is gratified all the same (1966, pp. 47–48).[14]

Following a person's biological death, funeral homes and cemeteries have their own means of "cleaning up" and "quieting" the experience. The corpse is quite immediately covered and stored away from our ready view (Rosenberg 1987, pp. 292–293). The dead person has erased from her body the look that she has "gone through something"; instead, she looks merely like she has fallen asleep, and in many cases a gentle smile on the corpse's face suggests that it is an untroubled, sweet sleep.[15] In general, these institutions regularly seem to discourage reflection on ourselves and our situations as *particular*, encouraging us instead to see ourselves as one of many, as having replaceable, interchangeable experiences that, therefore, do not require us to attend to them as being specific to us. In other words, they announce themselves as places not for the intimacy and particularity of our ownmost situation, but rather as

---

[13]In *The Birth of the Clinic*, Foucault (1994, pp. 96–105) famously traces the historical movement beginning in the eighteenth century toward treating the body and an individual "not so much [as] a sick person [but rather] as the endlessly reproducible pathological fact to be found in all patients suffering in a similar way" (p. 97). See also Foucault (1995, pp. 184–194). See also Rosenberg (1987, Chapter 12: "Life on the Ward," and pp. 332–336).

[14]Van den Berg draws there on Huizinga (1999), especially the chapter "The Vision of Death," which discusses the significant presence of death in everyday life experience toward the end of the Middle Ages.

[15]For instance, in Ajmani's *Embalming: Principles and Legal Aspects*, the chapter "Cosmetics and Presentation" begins: "Care should be taken to maintain the pleasant appearance of the face. The eyelids should be gently closed to give an appearance of sleep" (1998, p. 179).

places for regularity and protocol, for the "they-self" and its generic forms of grasping onto—or, more to the point, of evading—that which is most individual.

Indeed even if a person wishes to speak of her dying or a terminal illness, she may find resistance. Following Erving Goffman, Havi Carel maintains that "being a good ill person, a good patient, is conforming to the expectations of the healthy, not to be offended or polluted by your illness" (2008, p. 56). After discovering she had a terminal illness, Carel found that many people, including close friends of hers, were resistant to speaking to her about her dying and in some cases to speaking to her at all. "And so my illness remains the elephant in the street, the café, the office. The elephant in the friendship" (Carel 2008, p. 56). Carel amplifies Rilke's and Heidegger's complaints about this *seeming* indifference to our death:

> Perhaps we would have all been better off if my illness did not present itself as a taboo, something arousing pity and terror, the emotional components of tragedy according to Aristotle. I sometimes think that what is tragic about being ill is this silence (2008, p. 56).

Perhaps more tragic than the mythic figure of Cassandra whose words of warning are unheeded until it is too late, Carel experiences her words about her own death as threatened by the possibility of never being heard, and this while she is surrounded by those who listen to her in many other arenas and who love and care for her deeply.

Here we see quite pointedly a significant problem of covering over and avoiding our personal experience of dying in favor of something generic or already understood. Carel feels she has become an object of pity and terror, some *thing* to be avoided (2008, p. 59). The public and even her friends have come to see her *as* a diagnosed illness with its unpleasantnesses that are to be stepped around and avoided. While she herself is the sort of being—*Dasein*—who is fundamentally "that-for-the-sake-of which," she is treated in this situation as a "worldly" entity. Her ontological status is itself denied. Understandably, then, for Carel, the silence that surrounds her in light of this is perhaps even more unbearable than the physical pain of her illness and the fact of her dying. She is being treated as a pariah, like a living dead person. She is being held apart from the communication that marks the experience of human life even around the most trivial things, and this is happening when she is facing one of the most significant experiences of human life. Moreover, insofar as she is not acknowledged as going through this experience, she misses out on the possibilities of "mutual recognition" that Hegel and others have argued are central to our experience of self-consciousness and identity: if everyone around her is turning away from something that is most fundamentally shaping her experience, there is a fundamental way in which she is denied the ability to feel that she is there.[16]

As evasive as many contemporary pathways for "dealing with" death may be, they are nonetheless our average, everyday way of being-towards-death. As we saw

---

[16]For discussion of recognition, see Hegel (1977, paragraphs 178–196); and, Russon (2003, Chapter 4). See also Laing (1969, Chapter 3, especially pp. 35–38) for a discussion of the importance of the other in helping us to establish "ontological security."

in our discussion of fear in Sect. 4.1, it is a regular structure of our way of being that we wrap ourselves up in "worldly" concerns, and in doing so cover over our underlying anxiety; nowhere more than when "facing" our dying do we "feel a need" to flee in this way. The ontic structures of our "world" that we have just been examining reflect this everyday evasive way of Being-towards-death: they *show* us —if we pay attention—our anxiety in the mode of being covered over by worldly concerns. Let us turn now to consider the demand for facing this anxiety, as well as the ontic character of the situations in which such authenticity surrounding our being-toward-death may arise or, alternatively, may continue to be especially thwarted.

4.3   The Imperative to Listen to Ourselves and to Death

Heidegger describes at length what it would take for us to enter into an authentic relationship with our being-towards-death.[17] Authentic being-towards-death is not a matter of "dwelling upon our end," but rather a move toward cultivating our anticipation of the possibility of the measureless impossibility of meaning that faces us in our death (Heidegger 1962, H. 261, M/R. 305). By anticipating our death in this way, we shatter the tenaciousness with which we otherwise would cling to and fall into this "world" (Heidegger 1962, H. 264, M/R. 308). The end of this does not, however, lead to an abandonment of meaning or of our responsibility for the creation of meaning, but rather allows us a freedom towards death that summons us out of "lostness" in the they-self and into authenticity (Heidegger 1962, H. 266, M/R. 311). At the center of this move toward authenticity is the move toward *Dasein* hearing itself, rather than "listening away" to the "they" (Heidegger 1962, H. 271, M/R. 316). And, at the core of this transformation away from living through the "they-self" is a need for *Dasein*, if *Dasein* is indeed to make the transformation *itself*, "to find itself as something which has failed to hear itself" (Heidegger 1962, H. 271, M/R. 315–316). The "listening-away [to the "they"] must get broken off; in other words, the possibility of another kind of hearing which will interrupt it, must be given by *Dasein* itself" (Heidegger 1962, H. 271, M/R. 316). This hearing responds, "not to what *Dasein* counts for, can do, or concerns itself with in being with one another publicly, not to what it has taken hold of, set about, or let itself be carried along with" (Heidegger 1962, H. 273, M/R. 317), but to "*Dasein* in its uncanniness," and the call is that of caring for *Dasein* as such (Heidegger 1962, H. 276–277, M/R. 321–322), and for doing so in a way that also allows others to "co-disclose" their ownmost potentiality-for-Being (Heidegger 1962, H. 298, M/R. 344–345). Let us consider three aspects of listening in empirical contexts of dying.

---

[17]See Sections 53–60 of *Being and Time* (Heidegger 1962).

a. *Listening to Our Own Voice*

In *The Notebooks of Malte Laurids Brigge,* Rilke's narrator offers an example of a man he takes to have had his "own" death, and to have done so in part through his embrace of the loudness and unavoidability of his own voice. The narrator describes a chamberlain, Chrisoph Detlev, in his dying weeks. The body of Detlev is large and literally getting larger with the effects of his illness. The servants are watching what Rilke describes as a "great darkening heap" in the middle of a room, and they wish that "it were nothing more than a large garment over some rotten thing" (Rilke 1949, p. 21).

> But it was something more. It was a voice, that voice which 7 weeks before no one had known yet: for it was not the voice of the chamberlain. It was not Christoph Detlev to whom this voice belonged, but Christoph Detlev's death. Christoph Detlev's death had been living at Ulsgaard for many, many days now and had spoken to everyone and demanded: demanded to be carried, demanded the blue room, demanded the little salon, demanded the large hall. Demanded the dogs, demanded that people should laugh, talk, play and be quiet and all at the same time. Demanded to see friends, women, and people who were dead, and demanded to die itself: demanded. Demanded and shouted (1949, p. 21).

We see a contrast here between Detlev's demanding voice and the silence described earlier by Havi Carel—the silence not only that her friends have toward her, but also the silence that she felt was expected of her in dealing with her illness. Carel felt she was being a "good sick person" when she faced her illness with a courageous silence and stoicism. Detlev, by contrast, lets go and shouts out his death, or as Rilke's narrator describes, his death simply and fully gives way to shouting and demanding to be heard. Detlev's death is heard throughout the surrounding fields and the nearby village, keeps workers awake and exhausted, threatens to send women prematurely into labor, scares even Detlev's most companionable dogs, and sends taunting, murderous nightmares to those desperately wishing for this death to complete its business and move on from the vicinity. In this story, people cannot get away from the calls of Detlev's death, whereas Carel finds there is no space even for the quietest utterances regarding her death.

Rilke's narrator identifies the particular loudness and demandingness of Detlev as he nears death as a mark of *his* way of having a death. He writes: "How the chamberlain would have looked at anyone who asked of him that he should die any other death than this. He was dying his own hard death" (1949, p. 23). It would be absurd to the chamberlain to consider the notion that he adjust himself and his death to the interests, the delicateness, or the politenesses of other people. According to this line of thought, Carel, who feels herself shaping her thoughts and conversations according to the pressures of others, is failing to have a death "of her own."

To bring out further the contrast between Detlev's taking up of his own death and the ways in which we may often feel pressured to live the "quiet" or prefabricated death that others expect or desire from us, let us turn to a passage in Rilke's *Notebooks* in which Rilke speaks not of death directly, but rather of the narrator's relationship to his own writing of dramas:

[W]hen I wrote my drama, how I went astray. Was I an imitator and a fool that I needed a third person to tell of the fate of two human beings who were making things hard for each other? How easily I fell into the trap. And I ought to have known that this third person who pervades all lives and literatures, this ghost of a third person who never was, has no significance and must be disavowed. He is one of the pretexts of Nature who is always endeavoring to divert the attention of men from her deepest secrets. He is the screen behind which a drama unfolds. He is the noise at the threshold of the voiceless silence of a real conflict (1949, p. 27).

Lamenting the way in which a third-person voice "pervades all lives and literatures," the narrator again draws our attention to ways we so commonly "lead" our lives according to the standard norms of the "they-self." We "decide" how we ought to do things because this is how such things "are done" by others. We see this in the often pre-set paths that people take toward such serious issues and actions as going to college, getting married, buying a house, taking a particular job, having children, and so on.[18] Decisions to embark on these paths are often less like actual *decisions* than they are akin to *societal habits* we pick up from the third-person narratives of our surrounding culture. Thus, rather than struggling with our "deepest secrets" and the "real conflicts," it is common for us to cover over these sites of authentic experience and struggle with the readymade answers of safe decisions, clichéd "insights," or diversions into more palatable topics.[19] In many situations where our choices are so strongly driven by societal norms, it is not even clear if there is a "screen behind which a drama unfolds." That is to say, those norms may be so pervasively and unreflectively carried out by us that we cut ourselves off from the very lifeblood of our personal existential drama, keeping the relevant issues from ever actually touching us, and behaving instead as "characters" of a third-person-driven life.

It is this squelching of *our* personal experience that Rilke's narrator, Carel's account, and Heidegger's discussion of death and the they-self seem to suggest occurs in the modern person's relationship to his or her death. The voice that might have screamed out as Detlev's did is so far suppressed that it is not easily audible even to its owner. The curtains are drawn over a person, so to speak, far before the moment of her actual demise, since she is, according to Rilke's narrator, not living the very life that is her own. That we would separate ourselves from *this* experience —our relationship to our own dying—is arguably the most problematic form of taking on third-person narratives instead of working out our own authentic engagement with this aspect of our existence. Heidegger argues that "death reveals itself as that *possibility which is one's ownmost, which is non-relational, and which is not to be outstripped*" (1962, H. 250–251, M/R. 294, emphasis in original). Dying is the epitome of what no other can do for us (Derrida 1995, pp. 41–44). It is

---

[18]See de Beauvoir (1948, pp. 45–52) for a relevant discussion of the "serious man." De Beauvoir contrasts this with the never-ending call for us to engage the ethical situations of life—whether they be "extraordinary" or daily—through the creation of "original solution" (p. 142).

[19]Compare the discussion of "second-order speech" by Merleau-Ponty (1962, point 1, Chapter 6: "The Body as Expression, and Speech").

integral to the unique experience of my *own*. It is thus quite significant and problematic that around this experience we would take on other people's narratives about how we should die or how we should think about our own dying. Other people may be with us as we struggle with something, might help support our own work on something, etc. Yet, no one can quite be there with us in our death. Indeed, there is a way in which we cannot even be there with ourselves. We cannot come back from death to reflect on it and share our insights with others, since "death is the possibility of no-longer-being-able-to-be-there" (Heidegger 1962, H. 250, M/R. 294). The "meaning" of death is precisely the *death of meaning*, the end of the very uniqueness that is *my* experience. Again, our being-towards-death is, as Heidegger says, a possibility "that is non-relational and not to be outstripped."

b. *Listening and its Lack Within the Institution of Healthcare*

In "Death in the First Person," a student nurse who is dying articulates this very tension in the face of her hospital caregivers who seem to deal with her experience as something generic, as something belonging to the anonymity of the third-person way: "Death may get to be a routine to you, but it is new to me. You may not see me as unique, but I have never died before. To me, once is pretty unique!" (Anonymous 1975, p. 26). This woman is only going to get to "do" this—her dying —once. Even if someone is in a marriage, and may desire for this to be the one and only marriage, it remains the case that marriage is something that can be undone and redone. This is true of all of our experiences in our lives, but such experience meets its limit in our death. The student nurse expresses this well: she has never done this before and she will never do it again. It is striking, then, that the institutions that care for people who are dying are ones that, as this student nurse suggests, become so inured to death that it may be extremely hard for persons working within these institutions to understand, feel, or recognize the freshness of *this* person's death, to face the momentousness of the fact that death is happening for the first time for a *you*, not for a *they*.

Moreover, not only might a caregiver's regular experience of people dying inure him or her to the existential significance of death; there may also be professional norms that limit what the caregiver is trained to "show" a patient even if the caregiver does retain a sensitivity to the uniqueness of death.[20] For instance, even if a nurse were "touched" by a person's illness or imminent death, it might not be condoned for the nurse to show that feeling to the patient. Yet, the student nurse again writes:

> If only we could be honest, both admit of our fears, touch one another. If you really care, would you lose so much of your valuable professionalism if you even cried with me? Just person to person? Then, it might not be so hard to die—in a hospital—with friends close by (Anonymous 1975, p. 28).

---

[20]See Todaro-Franceschi (July 2008); and, Ferell and others (2007). A further impediment to such conversations arises in the decrease in contact hours between nurses and patients owing both to shorter hospital stays and changes in the last two decades in nursing management that tend to diminish extended contact between any one nurse or caretaker with a particular patient. For a discussion of these issues, see Weinberg (2003, pp. 60–68 and 143–146).

As a student nurse, this woman has been trained in and understands various professional codes, but she is heavily aware of the tensions surrounding the professionally approved treatment of someone who is dying, and she questions why it would count as professional to cover over the significance of death. Her concern arises in direct response to the contemporary emphasis in the medical field to attend to death, illness, and the ill or dying person in strictly biological rather than existential terms. The professional keeps his or her eyes on the "relevant" issue, and in this realm that issue is the body, but the body not as the rich site of meaning that Merleau-Ponty, for example, reveals it to be, but rather the body as a discrete "physical" object that can be understood and treated in reductive biological terms (Merleau-Ponty 1962, Part I: "The Body," especially 128–130 and Chapter 4: "The Synthesis of One's Own Body").

In the medical approach, the body is x-rayed, poked with needles for injecting or extracting fluids, fed chemicals, manipulated, reshaped, bandaged, cut open, cut away, kept cool or kept warm, cleaned, measured, and recorded in quantifiable and generalizable terms. While all these approaches to the body are helpful and even necessary for the maintenance of life or "health," the *significance* of illness and dying is largely overlooked in such reductive treatments. Indeed, someone may be receiving successful life-prolonging treatment, but nonetheless find herself hindered or perhaps crippled by the emotional or even the practical issues arising around her dying: she may well be as incapable of carrying out her daily life—of living—as she would be without such treatments.[21] Bringing this issue to the fore, van den Berg questions:

> Is not the overemphasized medical interest in a longer and longer average life-span an incorrect over-accentuation of one of the many medical tasks? The very pleasing statistics prove much in favor of the effectiveness of medical management, but in some respects they do not prove anything. The duty of a doctor is to save the life of his patients, to aid health in its struggle against disease. But human life is misunderstood if there is only an interest in the number of years and if medical care only includes the condition of the body (van den Berg 1966, p. 57; see also Aho and Aho 2008, Chapter 9).

Terms of mere biology—terms that pointedly find the universal or the generic character of something—cannot address the "ownmost" character of death.

Perhaps, as the student nurse further suggests, it is not merely the medicalizing of health care institutions and practices that steer caregivers away from dealing with the existential significance of death; perhaps instead this narrowing of the professional's attention arises from the professional's fear of his or her own death. The student nurse writes:

> You slip in and out of my room, give me medications and check my blood pressure. Is it because I am a student nurse, myself, or just a human being, that I sense your fright? Why are you afraid? I am the one who is dying! (Anonymous 1975, p. 26).

---

[21]See van den Berg (1972, pp. 92–95) for a discussion of a medically "healed" patient who continues to be ill, because existential problems have still not been addressed in his case. See also Carel (2008, Chapter 3: "Illness as Dis-ability and Health Within Illness").

Even in a situation in which professional codes guide caregivers not to "touch" the existential issues of dying, this student nurse can sense her caregivers' own existential concerns seeping through in their care of her. In this case, then, there is not only a professional distance between her and those most entrusted to care for her as she is dying, but also an additional distance of fear that she believes leads her caregivers to turn away from her as something that reminds them of their own mortality.

Though there are certainly countless instances of existentially rich practices of caring for persons' dying by particular individuals and even by institutionally based organizations or protocols, such as the hospice movement, studies suggest nonetheless that the current emphasis within the medical community at large is significantly biological, to the near exclusion of dealing with existential concerns.[22] For instance, a recent study by the Carnegie Foundation for the Advancement of Teaching presents an analysis of the current state of nursing education, and notes a particular tension between the emphasis in nursing education on attention to facts and theories and attention to care and practice (Benner and others 2010). The study argues that not enough attention is paid to engaging students in the latter, and that even when attention is given to the existential and ethical issues that nurses will encounter, the mode of educating student nurses about these issues is often problematically abstracted from the lived situations in which these issues are most palpable and in which student nurses could begin to work practically on addressing them (Benner and others 2010, pp. 12–14, 23–24, 59–62, 64–70, 82–89, 143–153). This Carnegie study resonates with the insights of Elisabeth Kübler-Ross, whose work in the mid-1960s revealed widespread resistance within healthcare institutions to address the existential issues surrounding death. Kübler-Ross worked to bring these conversations into the open, providing, among other things, conversational interview-forums in hospital settings in which a person with terminal illness discussed his or her experiences in the face of their dying with nurses, therapists, doctors, chaplains, family members, and community members. Kübler-Ross reported significant opposition to these forums: many doctors and other

---

[22]Indeed, Groopman (2007), M.D., notes in *How Doctors Think* that "medical students and residents are being taught to follow preset algorithms and practice guidelines in the form of decision trees," and further that "a movement is afoot to base all treatment decisions strictly on statistically proven data" (2007, p. 5). "This so-called evidence-based medicine," he continues, "is rapidly becoming the canon in many hospitals" (2007, p. 5). Groopman gives the example of one such "orderly" approach to practicing medicine called Bayesian analysis on pp. 61–62, and criticisms of that approach on pp. 150–151. Critical at points of the human elements (such as social context, personal history, patients' comprehension of their bodies and their abilities or inabilities to communicate their experiences, etc.) that are left out by such reductive approaches, Groopman begins his book with an apropos epigraph by William James: "We carve out order by leaving the disorderly parts out" (2007, front matter). Physician Richard J. Baron (1992, 1985) makes a compelling case for the existential as well as the medical and ultimately financial reasons for integrating phenomenological analysis into the medical practice of physicians.

caregivers argued that these issues were too "sensitive" to ask a dying person to address or even consider.[23]

Both at the institutional and the personal levels, this avoidance of facing our death is existentially and morally problematic. To begin, as Heidegger argues, death is that which cannot be outstripped, so to "avoid" it is fundamentally to turn away from our existential situation, to live inauthentically (Heidegger 1962, Sections 50 and 52). Van den Berg argues in a similar vein: "However emphatically we may ban death from our lives, we actually never cease to communicate with it; it determines our way of life" (1972, p. 53). The arguments of both authors and of this chapter should be read to apply not merely to those who are pointedly close to their demise: we are *all* faced with our mortality, all always being-towards-death. The person who is terminally ill, chronically ill, or even acutely ill simply exists in an ontic situation that privileges the possibility for coming to ontological awareness. In spite of this "privileged" situation, as we have seen in so many ways in this chapter, such a person may in fact be the one most shielded from such an opening.

c. Ontic Results of Ontological Listening

With a view both to existential concerns and to the responsibilities and possibilities of healthcare, both Kübler-Ross and van den Berg argue that it is important for us— whether we are professionals or visitors in arenas of healthcare—to overcome our own hesitancies around facing death in order to allow those who are dying to have the room to discuss their own experiences of dying with us should they wish this (Kübler-Ross 1969: Chapter 3: "First Stage: Denial and Isolation"). Van den Berg makes a strong existential criticism of the doctor who refuses such conversation:

> The doctor who is convinced that his patient's sickbed will be his deathbed and who forbids himself and others to speak of these things, even if the patient emphatically asks for it, acts as if death were only significant at the time of its occurrence, as if death were a symptom of a disease rather than of life itself. But death is even a norm of life. Thus, the physician's silence is not right (1972, pp. 52–53).

While he distinguishes the responsibilities of the doctor from those of the visitor, Van den Berg's criticism extends at its core to us all:

> Many patients suffer because they cannot discuss the problems that really matter to them. It is the healthy person who is to blame for this. It is he who goes through life with a completely unjustifiable levity in these matters (1972, p. 45).[24]

Kübler-Ross speaks also of the importance of such communication for those who will remain living after someone close to them will have died. She reports that a high percentage of spouses who have not worked through such conversations prior to the death of their partners will later appear in physicians' offices showing somatic

---

[23]For a discussion of the "Death and Dying Seminars" and the resistances Kübler-Ross initially faced in organizing them, see Kübler-Ross (1975: "Preface: A Journey into the Realm of Death and Growth," and Kübler-Ross (1969, p. 36).

[24]For his distinction between the doctor and the visitor in such situations, see van den Berg (1972, Chapter 5: "The Patient and His Physician").

signs arising from unaddressed grief (Kübler-Ross 1969, p. 169 and Chapter 9: "The Patient's Family").

Kübler-Ross and van den Berg emphasize in compatible ways that what is required of us in discussions about dying does not depend upon any particularly special training or articulation, but rather that we be open to listening both to ourselves and others, and also to speaking genuinely rather than in prepackaged terms that fail to listen to this person's or to our own experience (van den Berg 1966, p. 116 and Chapter 2, especially pp. 78–79; Kübler-Ross 1969, pp. 19–23, 31–34). In describing her own experience of dying from a mortal illness, Carel notes her desire that more people would simply acknowledge her dying, without seeking anything highly insightful or reflective from people when they speak to her of her death (2008, pp. 54–60). Carel's personal sense and Kübler-Ross's and van den Berg's professional assessments underscore the importance of trying to be open to conversations about death with those who are dying—and also perhaps with others and ourselves even when death does not appear to be imminent. While such conversations are no doubt an "ontic" matter, the fundamental thrust of these authors' arguments suggests that it is precisely such conversations that can open a space in which people can indeed begin to face the ontological consideration of what it means to face the certain, yet impossible to grasp, possibility that our struggle to "deal with" "this" life will no longer matter, at all.

This form of talking and listening to one's own existential situation as being-towards-death can be a fundamental way of acknowledging a person's need —and ability—to work cooperatively to adopt a new, even if temporary, way of *living*. Carel emphasizes that certain forms of conversation can help to open up new possibilities for the terminally as well as the chronically ill person. She specifically notes the benefits of shifting away from the nearly exclusive contemporary emphasis by caregivers on either the many problems and limitations facing the patient or on the medical-based protocols for addressing these problems. She argues that such emphases miss the possibility for helping the patient to develop a form of "health within illness" (Carel 2008, pp. 77–80). Carel refers to studies that have indeed shown that many patients are not only able to find a localized sort of health within their illness, but also that some sick persons end up finding that their illnesses bring a greater sense of value to their lives than they had before they were ill. In such studies, it was found that "for some chronically ill people illness became a tool of self-discovery and a fundamental source of later self-development," and that chronically ill and disabled persons experienced and reported their situations as allowing for "honouring the self, creating opportunities, celebrating life and transcending the self" (Carel 2008, pp. 77, 79, respectively).[25] A person may be impelled by serious illness, for instance, to mend a relationship that was otherwise floundering, or may become more clear about or focused on what truly matters to him or her. Van den Berg has witnessed a similar shift in ill persons' comportment

---

[25]Carel is here referring significantly to Charmaz (1983) and Lindsey (1996). See also Carel (2007).

to life, noting that "the certainty of death makes life very much alive" (1966, p. 40). Indeed, he adds:

> Can it not be said that every intensification of our personal existence is the result of difficulties, sorrow, and affliction? No one becomes mature unless he undergoes the crisis of maturation. … A deeper insight into the wonder of our existence, a more human and consequently a more acute way of experiencing the paradoxes and controversies which characterize our existence is always the result of an uneasiness akin to despair, and the challenge of a pressing uncertainty. Death only becomes a friend after a fierce and painful duel. Therefore, it cannot be right to reduce difficulties and sorrow to a minimum artificiality (van den Berg 1966, p. 96).

In this way, a mortal or even a potentially mortal illness can and should be the impetus for us to "pop out of" the hold that the third-person narrative or the they-self often has on us, and encourage us to work on crafting for ourselves the character we would like our world to have. In other words, this can be a call to live authentically.

Whether possibilities for recovered health exist or whether there is a certainty that death is near, van den Berg's argument, reminiscent of Heidegger's charge to cease "listening away" to the they-self, emphasizes the importance of "tak[ing] care that our conversation with the patient is indeed *with* the patient," not prepackaged according to social norms or even according to what we might have planned ourselves before engaging directly with the patient him or herself (van den Berg 1966, p. 95). "For every patient begins his sickbed with his own past and with his own expectations of the future. Every patient makes his sickbed his own personal situation, which is after all unique" (van den Berg 1966, p. 135). Just as de Beauvoir argues there will always be a need to "create an original solution" in the ethical conflicts of life, so too is there a demand to recognize a need for an original taking up of death insofar as it is our "ownmost" experience—one that cannot be taken over or defined by anyone else, even if others may be essential in our coming to our own unique grappling with our dying (de Beauvoir 1948, p. 142). So, the "conversation" that allows one person to hear herself, to respond to her own self rather than the they-self, will likely look entirely different than what another will require. The challenge, then, for us and for healthcare—if we are to continue working toward fostering an authentic being-toward-death and, thus, the possibility for authentic being-in-the-world—is to allow for an openness, an "original solution," that will allow us to co-disclose our ownmost potentiality-for-Being.

4.4   Conclusion: The Intimacy in Being-Towards-Death

After someone close to us has died, returning to our lives can in many ways be an immeasurably difficult process: it is the process of coming to terms with the pain of the loss of a voice and of the loss of the possibilities of that voice. I cannot, for instance, call my grandmother up to ask her how the bread dough should feel at a particular stage in her recipe, nor can I continue our conversations about spirituality, about her history, about my aspirations, about silly things that indeed do not seem silly when you consider they are part of the fabric of a person's life, part of the things on which a person "spends" her breath. Coming to terms with the pain of losing these possibilities is important not only as a mourning of the loss of communicating with that voice, but as much, I would argue, as a way of opening or re-opening the importance of tending to those relationships that persist and in which we may fail or succeed at both being heard and hearing.[26]

If an important part of being human is to be heard and to hear another, and if facing one's own dying is facing the point at which *one will no longer have a voice* —when one will no longer be able to respond to another or to have another respond to oneself—then it seems that coming together with people to face the pain and fear arising around our no longer having the possibility of a voice is, in a way, coming together around the very issue that defines what intimacy is. Communicating about our being-towards-death—in whatever ontologically significant, but ontically diverse form that may take—is, then, communicating about our vulnerability around being heard and our fears of not being heard—of not being heard in this "world" and, ultimately, of not being heard ever again. As such, far from being a site of pain we should continue to cover over or attempt to amelioriate, facing our mortality with one another stands as a preeminent site for intimacy—with others and with our own selves.

References

Aho, J., & Aho, K. (2008). *Body matters: A phenomenology of sickness, disease, and illness.* Lanham, MD: Lexington Books.

Ajmani, M. L. (1998). *Embalming: Principles and legal aspects.* New Delhi: Jaypee Brothers Medical Pub.

Anonymous. (1975). Death in the first person. In E. Kübler-Ross (Ed.), *Death: The final stage of growth* (pp. 25–26). New York: Simon and Schuster.

Ariès, P. (1974). *Western attitudes toward death* (P. Ranum, Trans.). London: Johns Hopkins University Press.

Ariès, P. (1981). *The hour of our death.* (H. Weaver, Trans.). Harmondsworth: Penguin.

Armstrong, D. (1987). Silence and truth in death and dying. *Social Science and Medicine, 24*(8), 651–657.

Baron, R. J. (1985). An introduction to medical phenomenology: I can't hear you while I'm listening. *Annals of Internal Medicine, 103*(4), 606–611.

Baron, R. J. (1992). Why aren't more doctors phenomenologists? In D. Leder (Ed.), *The body in medical thought and practice* (pp. 37–47). Dordrecht: Kluwer Academic Publishers.

Benner, P., Sutphen, M., Leonard, V., & Day, L. (2010). *Educating nurses: A call for radical transformation.* San Francisco: Jossey-Bass.

Carel, H. (2007). Can I be ill and happy? *Philosophia, 35*(2), 95–110.

Carel, H. (2008). *Illness: The cry of the flesh.* Stocksfield Hall, Stocksfield: Acumen Press.

Cassell, E. J. (1986). The changing concept of the ideal physician. *Daedalus: Proceedings of the American Academy of Arts and Sciences, 115*(2), 185–208.

---

[26]For further discussion of the relationship between intimacy and discussions of dying, see Jacobson (2014).

Charmaz, K. (1983). Loss of self: A fundamental form of suffering in the chronically ill. *Sociology of Health & Illness, 5*(2), 168–195.

De Beauvoir, S. (1948). *The ethics of ambiguity.* (B. Frechtman, Trans.). New York: Citadel Press.

De Beistegui, M. (2005). *The new Heidegger.* New York: Continuum Books.

Derrida, J. (1995). *The gift of death.* (D. Wills, Trans.). Chicago: University of Chicago Press.

Ferell, B. R., Dahlin, C., Campbell, M. L., Paice, J. A., & Virani, R. (2007). End-of-life nursing education consortium (ELNEC) training program: Improving palliative care in critical care. *Critical Care Nursing Quarterly, 30*(3), 206–212.

Foucault, M. (1995). *Discipline and punish.* (A. Sheridan, Trans.). New York: Vintage Books.

Foucault, M. (1994). *The birth of the clinic: An archaeology of medical perception.* (A. SSheridan, Trans.). New York: Vintage Books.

Gatchel, R. J., Baum, A., & Krantz, D. S. (1989). *An introduction to health psychology* (2nd ed.). New York: Random House.

Groopman, J. (2007). *How doctors think.* New York: Houghton Mifflin.

Hegel, G. W. F. (1977). *Phenomenology of spirit.* (A. V. Miller, Trans.). Oxford: Oxford University Press.

Heidegger, M. (1962). *Being and time.* (J. Macquarrie & E. Robinson, Trans.). Oxford: Blackwell.

Howarth, G. (2007). *Death and dying: A sociological introduction.* Malden, MA: Polity Press.

Huizinga, J. (1999). *The waning of the middle ages.* Mineola, NY: Dover.

Illich, I. (2002). *Limits to medicine: Medical nemesis: The expropriation of health.* New York: Marion Boyars.

Jacobson, K. (2014). The temporality of intimacy: Promise, world, and death. *Emotion, Space and Society, 13,* 103–110.

Kellehear, A. (2007). *A social history of dying.* Cambridge: Cambridge University Press.

Kübler-Ross, E. (1969). *On death and dying.* New York: Scribner.

Kübler-Ross, E. (Ed.). (1975). *Death: The final stage of growth.* New York: Simon and Schuster.

Laing, R. D. (1969). *The divided self.* London: Penguin Books.

Lindsey, E. (1996). Health within illness: Experiences of chronically ill/disabled people. *Journal of Advanced Nursing, 24*(3), 465–472.

Lingis, A. (2009). Experiences of mortality: Phenomenology and anthropology. *The Pluralist, 4*(3), 69–75.

Merleau-Ponty, M. (1962). *Phenomenology of perception.* (C. Smith, Trans.). New York: Routledge and Kegan Paul.

Rilke, R. M. (1949). *The notebooks of Malte Laurids Brigge.* (M. D. H. Norton, Trans.). New York: W.W. Norton and Co.

Rosenberg, C. E. (1987). *The care of strangers: The rise of America's hospital system.* Baltimore, MD: Johns Hopkins University Press.

Russon, J. (2003). *Human experience: Philosophy, neurosis, and the elements of everyday life.* Albany, NY: SUNY Press.

Russon, J. (2008). The self as resolution: Heidegger, Derrida and the intimacy of the question of the meaning of being. *Research in Phenomenology, 38*(1), 90–110.

Todaro-Franceschi, V. (2008). Don't worry about caring for the dying: It isn't on the NCLEX. In International Proceedings (Ed.), *Centre for nursing ethics conference, nursing ethics and health care policy: Bridging local national and international perspectives.* Hartford, CT: Yale University.

Van den Berg, J. H. (1966). *Psychology of the sickbed.* Pittsburgh, PA: Duquesne University Press.

Van den Berg, J. H. (1972). *A different existence: Principles of phenomenological psychopathology.* Pittsburgh, PA: Duquesne University Press.

Walter, T. (1996). *The eclipse of eternity: A sociology of the afterlife.* New York: St. Martin's Press.

Weinberg, D. B. (2003). *Code green: Money-driven hospitals and the dismantling of nNursing.* Ithaca, NY: Cornell University Press.

Chapter 5
Pain and Catharsis in Art, Ritual and Therapy

Roman Meinhold

Abstract Catharsis in the context of healing rituals, psychotherapy and narratives often involves the (re-)experience of pain. Ideally, catharsis in these three domains is a medical homoeopathic discharge and 'Aufhebung' of negative emotions, experiences or 'personal aspects'. The approach taken in this investigation is transdisciplinary, utilizing research findings in fields such as comparative religion, anthropology, philosophy, art theory, humanistic psychology, ethnology and ethology. The chapter emphasizes the need to re-valuate medical 'western' mainstream treatments that attempt to eliminate or reduce pain and further research on ethno-medical, holistic, preventive, humanistic and 'eastern' alternative treatments in order to intensify the discourse on such matters.

Keywords Catharsis · Alternative pain treatment · Healing rituals · Homoeopathic discharge · "Aufheben" · Imitatio prominentis

5.1 Introduction

Certain healing processes involve painful experiences the result of which may be a catharsis, despite the fact that, in many cases, severe painful experiences are (potentially) traumatic. This chapter compares catharsis involving violence and the experience of pain in (I) traditional initiation and healing rituals, (II) therapy and (III) art, especially narratives (stories, films, etc.). One purpose of this chapter is to find out under which circumstances and in which context the (re-)experience of pain may result in catharsis. The chapter is divided into six sections. The first section brings catharsis and pain in context with Sect. 5.2 the issue of human negativity and Sect. 5.3 the therapeutic connotations of "aufheben". The second, third and fourth

R. Meinhold (✉)
Guna Chakra Research Center, Graduate School of Philosophy & Religion,
Assumption University, Bangkok, Thailand
e-mail: rmeinhold@au.edu

© Springer India 2016
S.K. George and P.G. Jung (eds.), *Cultural Ontology of the Self in Pain*, DOI 10.1007/978-81-322-2601-7_5

93

sections deal with manifestations of catharsis due to pain, fear, horror, terror and violence in (2) initiation/exorcism/healing rituals, (3) narratives, and (4) (psycho)'therapy'. The fifth section examines the relation of pain and catharsis in the aforementioned three spheres in order to highlight its three functional essential elements: Sect. 5.8 discharge, Sect. 5.9 homoeopathic treatment and Sect. 5.10 *imitatio prominentis*. The last Sect. 5.6 contains a plea for intensified discourses on alternative treatments that take the relation of pain and catharsis into consideration.

5.1.1   Human Negativity

One reason why humans sometimes need psychotherapeutic support is due to traumatic painful experiences. Quite often such problems are caused by what has in the philosophical tradition been called evil. An analytical distinction of the kinds of evils which might be the source of such problems provides us with three possible sources: (1) divine or spiritual evil, allegedly caused by a spiritual, divine or evil entity, which is by definition non-human or at least not completely human. Examples of such evils can be found in Asian and African animism, Greek myths or in the Bible and the Koran. (2) Natural evils—if we assume that neither a God nor another spiritual entity is responsible for an evil event—such as natural catastrophes (earthquakes, floods, volcano eruptions etc.) are the second category. (3) The third category of evil is human evil: evil caused by humans and most often inflicted on humans (evil originating from humans can also be inflicted on animals and the environment at large). Buddhist laymen and monks try to avoid violence and the infliction of pain; even more so Jain householders. But Jain nuns and monks need to avoid it by all possible means, which includes to protection of insects and microorganisms.

In some traditional indigenous societies, in cases in which it is believed that a spiritual entity is the trigger or mediator of a possession or a disease, quite often a human being is the one who wished something evil for another human with the spiritual help of sorcerers for example. When tracing this kind of evil back to its roots, we can see that this evil, which on the first glimpse seems to belong to the first category, is in fact an evil caused by humans in order to inflict pain on (other) humans.

However, the problem of evil in general is not my concern in this chapter. I hold —following the analytical nature and scope of this chapter—that evil does not exist beyond human categories, meaning all evil is in fact 'human inflicted evil'. From an atheistic point of view, the first category of evil cannot exist. Assuming that evil is generally related to morally negative attitudes, behaviour and conduct of human beings, the term evil cannot be applied to the first and the second categories. One must not necessarily agree with this kind of categorization and with its assumptions or conclusions. The important aspect here is that if I am going to employ the notion of evil in the following chapter, I will confine my inquiry into coping strategies, especially catharsis, for human psychic or psychosocial problems (e.g. due to inflictions of pain) which have been intended or unintended, caused or triggered by other humans. Some might argue that unintended infliction of pain might not be straightforwardly labelled evil, but if it involves ignorance, carelessness, stupidity it is, or comes close to, human (inflicted) evil. "All that is necessary for the triumph of evil is that good men do nothing", is an often quoted adage in this context.[1]

According to Sigmund Freud, human beings have an inborn drive of destruction, aggression and cruelty (cf. Hügli 1980, 700), and Carl Gustav Jung holds that we have to be aware about the evil in ourselves and have to acquire the capacity to deal with it (cf. Hügli 1980, 700). "We are all demons, we just pretend to be human" Slavoj Žižek stated his view of human negativity succinctly in an interview (Taylor 2005). But he is only partly correct with this statement. Of course, we are human(s), but, in particular circumstances, within seconds, we can be 'demons', especially if there exists a problematic personal, psychological, social or political history in relation to such a particular circumstance.

The Etiologist Konrad Lorenz holds that humans—unlike dangerous animals—have a low intrinsic intraspecific killing barrier on one hand, but due to the faculty of reason (and its utilization for developing sophisticated technology), we also have a high potential to kill, inflict pain and destroy in a superlative manner. This combination of a low intrinsic intraspecific killing barrier and the potential to develop and use sophisticated technology for destruction is responsible for what we call "evil". Lorenz proposes two kinds of strategies for coping with the so-called human evil, which for him is mainly aggression. He suggests two different forms of "Katharsis" or purgation: one is *sublimation* and the other *abreaction at substitutes* ["Abreaktion … am Ersatzobjekt"], which seems to be the most promising strategy for (Lorenz 1983, 247–248). As an example of *abreaction at substitutes*, he mentions sport (or—less eloquently—smashing one's fist on the table instead of smashing it into another's face); an example of *sublimation* is to write a well-argued letter, a paper, a story or a poem instead of inflicting physical pain. It goes without saying, but was not mentioned by Lorenz, that the content of artworks might be violent and potentially inflicting psychic pain too. This is very much in line with what Žižek writes about the evil things happening in our mind and in our dreams: we have to do something about it so that we do not get crazy. This simply means that aggressive thoughts, human evil, the infliction and experience of pain are part and parcel of human nature; we cannot abolish such phenomena, but we should try our best to cope.

5.1.2 Catharsis as a Form of 'Aufheben' in the Therapeutic Context

According to Aristotle's *peri poietikes* tragedy operates through "the arousal of pity and fear effecting the katharsis of such emotions" (Aristoteles 1993a, 1449b–1450).

---

[1]Usually attributed to the philosopher Edmund Burke (amongst others).

But what *katharsis*[2] is and how it works in practice are neither described in depth nor in detail in the entire *corpus aristotelicum*. Catharsis is—etymologically seen— a form of *discharge*, not recharge. It discharges painful experiences, or in general *distress,* and it seems that in most cases, catharsis in art, ritual and therapy follows a *homoeopathic* process by administering, repeating, imitating and symbolizing a phenomenon or substance of outstanding importance. Catharsis seems to be a more or less holistic experience related to pain and pleasure, not only affecting body, soul or mind but also the entire human being. Thus, a working definition could read as follows: Catharsis (occurring in the context of art, ritual and therapy) is a homo-eopathic distress discharge of the body–soul–mind–complex resulting in a relieving pleasure.

The German word "aufheben" (already explored by Hegel in its various con-notations)[3] reflects different stages of a therapeutic process: the word connotes (i) to 'pick up', (ii) to 'store', (iii) to 'eliminate' (catharsis) and (iv) to 'lift up to higher level' (meaning to re-evaluate or re-value). The variety of meanings of "aufheben" applied to therapeutic components or steps suggest that catharsis is just one—more or less essential—step in the therapeutic context, but not the therapeutic process itself. Depending on the particular underlying therapeutic theory and on the psy-chopathological problem, catharsis is neither an essential nor a sufficient step in psychotherapeutic treatments. But if it comes to the therapeutic treatment of pain infliction, catharsis seems to play a crucial role.

5.2 Pain and Catharsis in Southern African Rituals

Today's modern analytical distinction between healing and religious rituals is made from a Western-influenced perspective. Most often in today's world, distinct pro-fessions are dedicated to certain professional tasks in restricted and well-defined areas. In contrast, indigenous cultural rituals do not only cater to religious and spiritual needs, but also to therapeutic, social and artistic needs as well. The division of labour and a narrow professionalization is a standard in high-income milieus and cultures, while in lower income cultures, a more holistic view of person, envi-ronment and cosmos is more prevalent. Examples are Lana culture in Thailand and Koisan Bushmen culture in the southern African Kalahari desert.

Paintings and engravings of the Koisan show illustrations in which the so-called trance dance rituals are performed for the purpose of healing. In such rituals, shamans for example draw arrows—signifying sickness—out of the body of a

---

[2]Two different kinds of spelling of the word catharsis are used in this chapter: *catharsis* and *katharsis*. While *catharsis* refers to the more general usage of the word which includes temporary and ancient connotations *katharsis* plays tribute to its meaning in the ancient Greek and German context, mainly referring to the term katharsis used in the two Aristotelian texts (the *Poetics* and the *Politics*).
[3]Cf. Hegel (1973, 89, 94, 146, 150, and 476).

patient, where the arrows have been shot by malevolent shamans or sorcerers in an evil act (Lewis-Williams and Dowson 1998, 38–39). The process of drawing out arrows is a painful but cathartic process: a pain which was already experienced when the arrow entered the body is re-experienced and will be followed by the re-experience of pain and the consecutive healing of the disease. The process of drawing out the arrow symbolizes a homoeopathic cathartic discharge of a disease. In trance, the shaman sometimes suffers from nosebleeding, indicated on the paintings by lines dropping vertically from the nose; nasal blood signifies shamanic trance. Additionally, shamans sniff out (discharge) sickness from the nose. In general, the nose seems to be a place where power is located (Lewis-Williams and Dowson 1998, 40, 46). The sniffing out of the sickness can be interpreted as a cathartic process, since the negative aspects of sickness will be discharged.

In an initiation ritual performed by the Xhosa[4] and some traditional Basotho[5], several rites are performed which include the infliction of pain in terrifying and horrifying contexts. According to Basotho tradition, what happens during that initiation ritual of medicine men is a secret, and can only be communicated within the group of people who are gathered for that ritual in a remote place in the mountains. Nelson Mandela in one of the first chapters of his Autobiography *Long Walk to Freedom* describes the Xhosa initiation ritual as a very painful and even horrifying event (Mandela 1990, 25–31).

According to Manyeli, Basotho initiation rituals for girls and boys include a number of horrifying, terrifying and painful experiences, which should prepare them for future obstacles, suffering and pain, but also for life in marriage (Manyeli 1992, 68–79).[6] A minority of the traditional people in the mountains still perform the initiation rituals. The girls' initiation includes ritual performances in which the girls are whipped and beaten on several occasions at different stages of the ritual, they are narrated mythical stories about dangerous animals (wolves, snakes, lions) and they are confronted with a "mythical person", acted by "women wearing terrifying masks which gave them a horrible appearance" (Manyeli 1992, 75). This "mythical person" lashes the girls mercilessly. It must be noted that this infliction of pain is not to be understood only as symbolic but happens in fact as real physical violence. The boys' initiation involves similar elements of violence and in addition the rituals of wrestling with a bull and the performance of traditional circumcision. The penalties for runaways even include capital punishment and secret burying of an unsuccessful neophyte tobe.

Mircea Eliade interprets terrifying, horrifying and painful experiences in transition rituals—especially initiation rituals—as symbolic or ritual *death* which usually

---

[4]Southern African indigenous group with various (sub-)tribes belonging to the Bantu ethnic group (Nelson Mandela, Desmond Tutu, Thabo Mbeki are prominent Xhosa).

[5]The Basotho too belong to the Bantu ethnic group. The majority of Basotho live in the Republic of South Africa (RSA), but Lesotho, a Kingdom landlocked by the RSA, is the ethnically most homogenous country in Africa with a majority of 99.7 Basotho.

[6]An investigation comparing such traditional tribal imitation rituals and those of urban gangs would be a particularly interesting project.

is followed by a symbolic or ritual rebirth (Eliade 1988, 14). The symbolic death in such rituals is the process of leaving the former life behind. The former life is either the life (1) as a child, (2) as a profane human being, (3) or as a sick human being. In any of the three cases, negative elements will be discharged (sickness or painful experiences) or the ontological status of the human being will be changed (child-hood–adulthood transition; or transition from a profane to a holy status) (Eliade 1988, 104). However, I am mainly interested in the therapeutic meanings of such rituals: the discharge of negative aspects in such rituals has to be seen as a cathartic process.

Another example of a painful transition ritual of the Xhosa minority in Lesotho has been communicated by a Mosotho.[7] A few of the traditional Xhosa people still perform a painful ritual to harden the boys and to make them brave. When a boy is about the age of 4 months, a fire is prepared by the elders with branches of trees and green leaves so that thick smoke is created. One limb of one of the fingers of the child is cut (except the thumb and the forefinger, and among the other fingers which is to be cut depends on the tribe) and will be thrown into the fire or will be buried. After that the child is placed on a blanket or an animal skin and two elders hold the skin or the blanket with the child above the fire; after some seconds they take the child away from the fire and place he again over the fire. This ritual is performed for about thirty minutes with the performance of chants.

Applying the interpretation of Eliade's transition rituals to the Xhosa ritual, it can be said that a symbolic death occurs during the ritual. The cutting of the limb signifies a ritual death which is even emphasized or reinforced by holding the child over the smoke of the fire. The cut limb will be buried or burned, symbolizing the burial of the "un-hardened" child. The child, without the limb, has a new ontological status as a "hardened" brave boy, since he will face all future obstacles, risks and calamities with the new braveness and boldness he has acquired due to the infliction of pain in the ritual. On the other hand, the placing over the fire could also be interpreted as a symbolic rebirth, since fire—in the shamanistic context—is a symbol for power and energy (Eliade 1974, 470–477). The heat and the smoke could be a symbol for supernatural power exposed to a being which is born again with new powers.

It must be noted that the therapeutic implication is not one which implies healing of a sickness which had been acquired in the past in the strict sense, but a pre-ventive treatment which should keep future sickness, pain and harm away from the person. Nevertheless, I believe that this ritual contains cathartic elements as well. If the cut limb symbolizes possible weakness of the being, which will be discharged during the ritual, then the ritual involves that cathartic element of discharge. According to a different source, the cutting of the limb is performed not only for boys in that particular age of four months, but also for any patient and for all sorts of therapeutic purposes.[8]

---

[7]The reference here is to an informal interview with Ntate L., National University of Lesotho on 26th November 2007 in Roma.

[8]I am referring to an informal interview with David Ambrose, National University of Lesotho, 27th November 2007 in Roma.

5.3 Pain, Catharsis and Psychotherapy

According to Eliade, the "archaic mentality" (Eliade 1988, 16) is convinced that a condition cannot be changed ('aufheben' in the sense of 're-value') if it is not first eliminated ('aufheben' in the sense of 'eliminate'). In transition rituals, the status of a person can only be changed if the person dies a ritual or symbolic death and is symbolically or ritually reborn afterwards, but in healing rituals, the problem causing the sickness must be eliminated (e.g. drawing out arrows during the trance dance ritual) before the "patient" is cured. Thus according to theories of various forms of psychotherapy, certain psychopathological conditions cannot be changed until the problem itself is eliminated; otherwise, only symptom treatment is performed. In many variants of trauma therapy, a patient will be (re-)confronted—really or ritually symbolically—with the pain, the object, the subject or the event that caused the trauma in order to facilitate the healing process of the psychopathological problem.

For illustration, I am picking out one particular method of treatment in psychotherapy, namely, Victor Emil Frankl's *Logotherapy*. One of logotherapy's methods is the *Paradox Intention*. Paradox Intention is a method which tries to eliminate expectance anxiety, an anxiety which expects a personal psycho-physical worst-case scenario (excessive blushing, stammering, sweating, etc.) in a situation of personal weakness (Lukas 1996, 487–490). Someone who for example blushes in particular situations and is also afraid of blushing in such situations will with a very high likelihood really blush in such a situation. The same applies to stammering, sweating and other symptoms. The psychopathological problem is a kind of negative self-fulfilling prophecy. The Paradox Intention method utilizes the element of humour and combines it with a homoeopethic strategy in imagining worst-case scenarios. For therapeutic purposes, the therapist advises the patient *paradoxically* to strongly wish what s/he is so afraid of, for example, to 'blush more reddish than a ripe tomato', to 'sweat or to weep so intensively that a dry river can be filled', etc.

Two phenomena seem to contribute to a catharsis due to paradox intervention: one is the exact imagination of the event, situation or object, but in a ridiculously and horrifyingly exaggerated way; and the other is the element of humour. The wish to want such a ridiculously embarrassing situation or event is not only a paradox, but also funny and thus the humoristic aspect provides the distance between the client's real problem and the client. The imagination of the disaster is a kind of 'imitation of an outstanding problem', an (exaggerated) mimicking of a prominent issue referred to as 'imitatio prominentis' (Meinhold 2013, 48–50). Besides that, paradox intention follows a 'homoeotechnique' since it fights the problem with the imagination of the problem itself. According to Lukas, there is clinical empirical evidence that the method of paradox intervention cures such psychopathological problems as expectation anxiety or neurotic anxiety (Lukas 1996, 513).

I want to add here my experience with an (unintended) "experiment" repeatedly made with one of my daughters who at the time of the occurrence of it was about four years old and had developed a habit (since she was around two) to nearly and sometimes really lose consciousness for a few seconds. When this occurred, she fell down regardless if she was standing or sitting. Such a situation was triggered by excitement over something she did not get as she wanted to, for example an object she saw on the shelf or especially if her sister had teased her or if somebody had annoyed her. Various trials to calm her down usually did not calm her down but reinforced her anger, once she collapsed on a tiled floor and her forehead began to bleed. After this incident, I advised her—when she was developing the same pattern of getting annoyed or angry—to beat her head thoroughly against the floor so that blood would flow intensely. I even reinforced my advice by staging and showing what she should do. Every time—without exception—when I applied this method, she was so annoyed with me and about my suggestion that her annoyance disrupted her schema and she was shouting "nein!" (no!), and calmed down after a few minutes without falling unconscious.

It seems that my aping of her pervious and anticipated behaviour lead to a change of her actual behaviour. The method I used seems to follow a homoeopathic schema. The situation I imitated was a painful one, while the funny aspect of that procedure is more on the side of an observer.

5.4 Pain, Horror and Terror in Narratives: Distress Discharge Due to Ideal Distance

The attempt to answer the question "why do we watch horror?" and imagery of inflictions of pain has for some time entered the discussion at the intersection of ethics and aesthetics or art and morality. The approaches to answer the question are various. Epistemic motivations include for example curiosity since one wants to know who is the murderer or the monster. The benefit of enlightenment or knowledge is a general reason why we admire artworks, even if they are horrifying. Another argument is that we admire the skill of the artists involved in the creation of the artwork although the artwork displays horrifying elements such as humans in pain. Another reason often stated for enjoying horror and terror, or horrifying and terrifying news, is that of a pleasant feeling of being 'relatively better off' than those in pain. Some observers experience *Schadenfreude*, and some might even be sadists, enjoying others' experience of pain as their own pleasure; again others might be masochists who take pleasure by imagining themselves being in the position of the pain sufferer. One further important reason why we enjoy narratives and images of pain experience in art (and in reality) is the momentum of catharsis. Indulging in observation of violent narratives and images might be a strategy to cope with our own inner aggression potential.

My approach here is not to claim that everybody likes renditions of humans in pain, but I claim that nearly everybody likes stories (storytelling, literature or film) which implicitly or explicitly involve a certain degree of violence, horror or terror or at least likes stories that induce some kind of fear or suspense. German folktales by the Brothers Grimm which we tell or read to our children are sometimes so cruel and brutal that it is better not to imagine the calamities of such stories in vivid details. Little Red Riding Hood and her grandmother are eaten by a sarcastic wolf; a cannibalistic witch wants to fry and eat Hänsel, a small boy; malevolent queens are burnt alive; princes who cannot solve the magic riddle will be held captive and their heads pinned on upright standing spears. Such stories are full of painful experiences, terrifying and horrifying scenes and if such folktales would be transferred to realistic films with state-of-the-art special effects and acted by real actors, age restrictions would apply for audience. The same applies to some Ancient Greek myths like King Oedipus and passages of the Bible, e.g. the sacrifice of Isaac. Pain inflictions, violence, horror and terror as crucial components of narratives are not a contemporary phenomenon but a very old one. It is common place in Ancient tragedy and the philosophical reflection of the tragic begins with Gorgias and Aristotle. What is a *novum* in today's films is the explicitness and closeness in which violence is presented. Films, in which the plot is played by actors, presented on large screens and with modern sophisticated sound systems bring us even closer to reality. Not everybody enjoyed or even watched the realist horror movie *Saw* or Pier Paolo Pasolini's *Salo* (at least many may not admit it), but some more mainstream movie goers watched *The Passion of Christ* or cartoons such as *Tom and Jerry*. A person not knowing the cultural context and the entire plot of the *Passion of Christ*, watching only the last scenes, might categorize the film in the genre of realist horror or a sadomasochist subgenre. But what is the difference between *The Passion of Christ* and, for example, *The Life of Brian*? The element of humour makes violence more palatable. If *Tom and Jerry* were acted by real cats or mice, we might find the cartoon less funny and animal rights activists would protest against such a genre. The crucial credential in order to find something more funny, disturbing, involving or brutal is related to what Thomas Scheff calls [ideal] distance. Scheff in his book *Catharsis in Ritual and Drama* argues that the (re-)experience of properly distanced negative emotions leads to a distress discharge. According to Thomas Scheff, catharsis is a method to *discharge distress* for which an *ideal distance* which he calls "aesthetic distance" (Scheff 2001, 57) and a *double ontological status* of a person are necessary (Scheff 2001, 12). The ideal distance refers to a mean between two extreme opposites: *under* distance and *over* distance. The discharge of distress is only possible if a "person's attention is not taken up by the return of repressed emotion from past events" (Scheff 2001, 57). The person thus must be properly distanced but not under-distanced (emotionally too much involved). If a person is over-distanced, s/he is unmoved. The most exciting drama (or film) is of course one in which the audience is under-distanced and thus taken away by the story, so that "they forget where they are" (Scheff 2001, 57). From the artistic point of view, under distance of the audience might be most desirable, but this is not the therapist's aim. On the other hand, an over-distanced drama is just boring for the audience because emotions are not addressed sufficiently. The audience in a boring drama is just observer of the plot, but does not participate emotionally. In a therapeutic method like for example Moreno's psychodrama, but also in many indigenous (therapeutic) rituals, a patient is not merely a member of the audience, but *participant in* and *observer of* the ritual or the therapeutic process. In mourning or funeral rituals for example of religious societies, the religious person on one hand sees and thus knows that the person lying in the coffin is dead, but on the other hand—if s/he believes in an afterlife—s/he simultaneously disbeliefs that the dead person has departed forever. This "double vision, of both believing and not believing simultaneously" (Scheff 2001, 113) leads to a status which could be philosophically seen as 'double ontological' or 'janus ontological' status because a person is both *participant in* and *observer of* a certain incident. Scheff illustrates his theory, applying it to the peekaboo game.

> In the game of "peek-a-boo", the mother first hides her face with her hands; then she removes her hands, moving her smiling face toward the baby, and says "peek-a-boo!" This cycle is repeated over and over. If the mother's timing is right, the baby will begin to laugh each time she shows her face. If she hides too long, the game is spoiled; the baby may cry or become frightened. If she does not hide long enough, the baby will not be sufficiently aroused lo laugh. (Scheff 2001, 109)

The baby's distress in that game is evoked due to the mother's separation when she hides her face. It is discharged when the mother shows her face again: the baby laughs. "The baby knows that the mother is not really gone" (Scheff 2001, 109); it believes and disbeliefs that the mother had disappeared. If the mother hides her face too long, the baby will be under-distanced and frightened if she hides it not long enough it will be over-distanced. The distress will best be discharged at ideal distance. Distancing is "the balance between distress and security" (Scheff 2001, 12).

Applying his theory to mass entertainment, Scheff argues that in many cartoons, violence is distanced properly (due to the less-real characters) and therefore the viewing of such films results in catharsis. Violence and the rendition of pain experience in more realistic movies—*realist horror*[9] might be a suitable example—are under-distanced according to such an understanding.[10]

5.5 Common Elements of Catharsis in Art, Ritual and Therapy: Discharge, Aufhebung, Homoeotechnique and *Imitatio Prominentis*

5.5.1 Discharge—Recharge

It must be noted that discharge is only one of two basic possibilities of improving mental, psychic or physical health. Catharsis—seen from the etymological

---

[9]The term *realist horror* is used by Cynthia Freeland to distinguish realistic horror stories (e.g. slasher movies) which depict possible "monsters" like mass murders, from *art horror*, whose monsters are not real or are less real, like ghosts or creatures such as created by Frankenstein. For a philosophical inquiry on art horror, compare Carroll (2004).

[10]On the other hand, we do not have to forget that it could be argued that in the genre of *realist horror*, a sublime and unconscious expectation of catharsis and thus pleasure might attract audience despite under-distanced violence as argued elsewhere (Meinhold 2012).

standpoint[11]—seems to be primarily a certain kind of *discharge* process. Depending on the circumstances, catharsis might bear or necessitate elements of recharge since it could be argued that catharsis creates some kind of "vacuum" that needs to be filled. This human nature also needs some kind of "recharging" of "positive energy" might sound quite "esoteric". However, being familiar with Mircea Eliade's comparative phenomenology of religious phenomena—e.g. the descriptions and interpretations of transition rituals—one might argue that a symbolic rebirth is an example of such a "recharge". Some examples for discharge and "recharge", however, have to be given here in order to illustrate the differences and similarities in various spheres where catharsis occurs. A simple (maybe oversimplified) example can be given with the following thought experiment. Let us think of a bottle partly filled with water, the quality of which as drinking water is merely acceptable but not excellent. In this example, one can think of two basic possibilities for improving the water quality *in* the bottle. The quality of the water can be improved by adding very high-quality drinking water (although this is neither a very logical nor useful idea in practice). The other possibility is to clean the water for example by filtering. The first strategy improves an initial substance by adding or "importing" a superior substance, while the second strategy removes negative elements from the substance to be cleaned. In psychotherapeutic practice, however, we can observe therapeutic methods that use both strategies: ridding off negative aspects *and* (parallel or consequently) recharge or "import" positive aspects. The cathartic process is comparable to the one which primarily rids off or "exports" negative substances or aspects.

What is illustrated with the bottle example can be applied to transition rituals described by Mircea Eliade for the sake of detecting the phenomenon of catharsis in cultural rituals based on myths. Also, these rituals described by Eliade have two ameliorative effects which apparently are appreciated in therapy: discharge and recharge (export of negative and import of positive aspects). The myths of world creation in traditional religious societies for example are often used or can be interpreted as healing rituals (Eliade 1957, 62).[12] In many such rituals—according to Eliade—a symbolic death is followed by a symbolic rebirth. The symbolic death *discharges* negative aspects of health, while the symbolic rebirth *recharges* a person with new reservoirs of energy (Eliade 1957, 62). In such a way, a sick person will be cured, or at least her health condition will be improved. Similar processes happen in rituals of transition. The "first natural life" (for example that of a child) will be ended by a symbolic death and will be begun newly by a symbolic rebirth or recreation (Eliade 1957, 110). *Death*, for example, is symbolized by the *loneliness* of the neophyte-to-be in the bush lands, or by isolation in huts, caves or holes; but death can also be symbolized by the amputation of a finger, as in the aforementioned example, by burning, cutting, bleeding and so forth (Eliade 1957, 111–112).

---

[11]Katharsis: cleansing, purgation, equalization, discharge, atonement, expiation.

[12]Furthermore, compare also Nürnberger (1999).

In a particular Sri Lankan exorcism ritual, catharsis at the intersection of art, ritual and therapy can be illustrated very clearly.[13] A patient complaining about stomach problems, vomiting and flatulence is believed to be "possessed[14]" by a demon. In this, ritualistic context to get rid of the demon (symbolically[15]) means to get rid of the sickness (in practice). In this kind of healing ritual, an exorcist dances in front of the patient *imitating* the demon and *imitating* the symptoms of the disease are done. Both kinds of imitations are instances of *imitatio prominentis*, since outstanding phenomena (demon and disease symptoms) are imitated. The imitating of the symptoms is a homoeopathic treatment (compare next section), since the 'same' (Greek: *homoios*) symptoms are mirrored "or repeated". The patient shivers due to the performance of the exorcist who imitates the demon. Later on, at midnight, a cock will be held above the patient's head where the disease is believed to be located. The disease will be transferred (exported) from the head of the patient (imported) into the cock. This act is the "Aufhebung" (elimination) and catharsis of the disease since the patient is cleansed by transferring the negative elements responsible for the disease from the patient's head into the cock.

5.5.2 Catharsis as Homoeopathic Process

It will be argued that the meaning of catharsis (documented since Gorgias and Aristotle) is chiefly and basically a discharge of negative aspects of the body–soul–mind complex of the human being that follows a homoeopathic or more generally a 'homoeotechnical' strategy.[16] Aristotle's father and grandfather were successful medical practitioners—successful in the sense that they served as royal medical doctors at the court of the Macedonian Kings Phillip and Amyntas—thus we have to assume that Aristotle was familiar with the function and process of catharsis from a medical perspective. According to the medical terminology in the school of Hippocrates, *katharsis* meant purification and the removal of disturbing or painful elements and thus an elimination of alien matter (Butcher 1894, 253). The background and usage of pity and fear in the context of *katharsis* lead Jacob Bernays, S. H. Butcher, Wolfgang Schadewaldt and other scholars of ancient Greek studies to the conviction that *katharsis* as used by Aristotle is a medical/therapeutical term or at least has medical therapeutical connotations in the context of tragedy

---

[13]Compare Nürnberger (1999, 19–20).

[14]For a substantial criticism of the application of western medical terminology to indigenous ritual–religious–medical phenomena, see Nürnberger (1999, 14–17).

[15]The insertion of the word "symbolically" is done from a "western" perspective. From the indigenous non-western perspective, the ontological status of the demon is *real*.

[16]The distinction Homöotechik-Allotechnik has been previously used by the German philosopher Peter Sloterdijk (Sloterdijk and Hans-Jürgen 2001).

and music.[17] Thus from the chief meanings of the word katharsis, which has medical, religious and moral connotations, the medical meaning is the one which Aristotle must have had in mind in his *Poetics* and in the last chapter of his *Politics* (Butcher 1894, 245). Aristotle's definition of tragedy is the following: "Tragedy, then, is an imitation of action [...] through pity (eleos) and fear (phobos) effecting the proper purgation (katharsis) of these emotions" (Aristoteles 1993a, 1449b–1450). The katharsis mentioned in this passage of the *Poetics* seems to follow a homoeopathic or 'homoeotechnical' principle. Through the arousal of *pity* and *fear*, a purgation of similar or even "identical" emotions (pity and fear) is effected.[18] "Pity and fear, artificially stirred, expel the latent pity and fear which we bring with us from real life..." (Butcher 1894, 246).

According to Butcher, a passage on music in the Aristotelian *Politics* as well indicates a homoeopathic operation of catharsis (Butcher 1894, 248–49). Flutes or pipes, which are used in origiastic celebrations, have a clear defined end, namely *"working off emotions"* (Aristoteles 1993b, 1341a20–1341a25). Music is used besides other ends (educational, higher-aesthetic and intellectual pastime, relaxation or relief after tension) (Aristoteles 1993b, 1341b35–1342a1) for cathartic purposes (Aristoteles 1993b, 1341b40).

> It may arise out of religious music, and it is noticeable that when they have been listening to melodies that have an orgiastic effect they *are, as it were, set on their feet* (alternative translation [Butcher]: fall back into their normal state), as if they had undergone a curative and purifying treatment. And those who feel pity and fear or other emotions must be affected in just the same way to the extent that the emotion comes upon each. To them comes a pleasant feeling of purgation and relief. In the same way cathartic music brings men an elation which is not at all harmful (Aristoteles 1993b, 1342a5–15).[19]

Following Butcher's argumentation, feelings (in particular pity and fear) are quieted for a certain time and the human "system" falls back to its normal level (Butcher 1894, 245). He interprets the orgiastic effect and the wild, restless and

---

[17]Bernays (1880); Butcher (1894, 245–253); Schadewaldt (1991, 15–18). Lessing's moral interpretation of *eleos* and *phobos* (Mitleid und Furcht) is dismissed by these authors.

[18]An example for a homoeopathic catharsis transferred to the physical sphere of the body, a physical homoeopathic catharsis, is the following: Due to bad food, somebody has a stomach-ache; eating the very food once again would cure her/his stomach-ache because the person would vomit all of that food and thus get rid of it; from the medical point of view, this is one possible variety of homoeopathic methods (because the problem is fought with the same "substance" which created it), while an allopathic method would suggest to take a medicine *against* the ache for example to calm the stomach.

[19]The German translation reads: "Denn durch diese innere [internal] Bewegung [movement] sind auch gewissen Menschen zu fesseln, und wir sehen diese unter dem Einfluss der heiligen Lieder, wenn sie Lieder aufnehmen, die die Seele in Weihestimmung versetzen, sich beruhigen [calm down], so als erlangten sie eine Heiligung und Reinigung. Kurz, ganz dassebe machen die mit, die anfällig sind für das Jammern und Schaudern [pity and fear] und überhaupt für den Affekt, und auch all die übrigen, soweit ein jeder von derartigem betroffen wird und in allen entwickelt sich eine geweisse Reinigung, und sie fühlen eine angenehme Erleichterung. Und in gleicher Weise also verschaffen auch die reinigenden Lieder den Menschen ein schadlose Freude [harmless pleasure]".

tumultuous melodies and music as *movement* that cures/soothes *internal trouble* (movement). The strong "movement" of music removes or cures emotional movement—a homoeopathic strategy (Butcher 1894, 248–249). Thus the result of *kathartic* music is a harmless joy or pleasure (Aristoteles 1993b, 1342a15).

Drawing out the arrows of disease—as depicted in the Bushmen cave-wall paintings—seems to be a 'homoeotechnique' as well since one can assume that a similar pain will be experienced when the arrows of sickness are shot and penetrate the skin. In the above-described African and Asian healing, initiation or transition rituals, we have a homoeopathic treatment as well since the soon-to-be neophyte will be confronted with anticipated pain, challenges or calamities. Pain is treated with pain, but in a preventive way; in this case, the therapeutic strategy can be described as preventive homoeopathy. The therapeutic examples of paradox intention point into the past, but also into the future: a problem which has occurred in the past is anticipated and fought with an exaggerated imagination of the very problem (Greek homoios = same). If it comes to film, it is difficult to prove if the 'homeo technique' works. It cannot simply be claimed that fear, pain or violent outbreaks can be prevented or past experiences of that kind can be cured with the (re-)experienced emotions in art. It seems that the ideal distance—described by Scheff—is essential for a therapeutic process. This is the reason why we have age restrictions which apply to realist horror movies of the slasher genre, but the same plot can take place in a different genre, in the framework of a cartoon, for example. The audience is more distanced if a sponge with head, legs and arms kills another creature of that kind under the sea than if the same narrative is acted out by real actors in a more familiar environment.

5.5.3 *Homoeopathy as Medical* Imitatio Prominentis

In many religious rituals described by Mircea Eliade, priests are 'imitating' certain rituals according to the myth that had been performed in "primordial times" by gods. The imitation of world creation is one example of such an *imitatio dei*. Also some imitations of Jesus' acts are performed by priests in Christian churches. The braking and distribution of bread during the Holy Communion or the remission of sins are acts of imitatio dei in the Catholic Church.

Potential, aim and ability to imitate is *inherent* in human nature; it can be recognized by observing small children and it is mentioned in Aristotle's, Friedrich Schiller's and Immanuel Kant's anthropologies.[20] But mere imitation alone seems not to cover the phenomenon of childrens' imitation of adults and young people's

---

[20]Aristotle (1993a: 1448b4-1449); Schiller (1983, 178); Kant (1998, 184). According to Aristotle, imitation is responsible for the genesis of poetry (Aristoteles 1993a, 1448b4–1449).

imitation of clothing styles and habitus of celebrities in media and art. The other component as discovered by Kant in his Anthropology is the factor that *important, distinguished, imminent* or *prominent* figures—those of supposedly higher status— are imitated, not those of lower status (Kant 1998, 184). This phenomenon which can be detected clearly in the domain of fashion and the consumers sphere in general, described by the term *imitatio prominentis* (Meinhold 2005, 40–49), is the more general phenomenon under which the more specific phenomenon *imitatio dei* described by Eliade can be subsumed. *Imitatio dei* is a specific form of *imitatio prominentis*.[21] In the rituals and examples for catharsis described above, such an imitation of something outstanding can be discovered.

In the example of the Sri Lankan exorcism, the exorcist (or therapist) imitates not only the demon (someone outstanding) but also the patient's health problems (flatulence, vomiting) in his dance. Although the exorcist imitates something negative (illness symptoms), he imitates something of outstanding importance (the demon, but also the symptoms). The homoeopathic principle—involved in these rituals—appears to be a medical form of *imitatio prominentis* or a repetition of something outstanding; if the problem was not outstanding in a certain way, we would not bother about it and getting rid of it would not be necessary. In order to get rid of an outstanding problem, it is essential to repeat or imitate the outstanding phenomenon or its symbol—the demon, the negative symptoms (pain or vomiting) and emotions (pity and fear).

In drama, the spectator *identifies* with the hero who is—in the Aristotelian conception of tragedy—neither a character of average nor flawless perfection, nor one of a rich and full humanity and as such outstanding (Butcher 1894, 261). In Scheff's terminology, an average character would be under-distanced, one of flawless perfection over-distanced. Thus the ideal tragic heroic character provides an *ideal distance* of the spectator which again is ideal to discharge negative emotions. Scheff in his book on catharsis argues that "[b]oth dramatic and psychotherapeutic theories involve the *re*experiencing of past emotional crises in a context of complete security: in the safety of the theatre or in the therapist's office" (Scheff 2001, 22). According to Moreno, the *repetition* of an *experience* in theatre-therapeutical context releases and purges its original experience, and the re-experience in the more secure setting effects a catharsis.[22]

---

[21] *Imitatio prominents* can not only be found in discharge but also in recharge imitation of media celebrities....

[22] Cf. Scheff (2001, 158ff); Moreno's Psychodrama is not only concentrated on elimination of distress (catharsis) but also on development of the personality, which could be interpreted as 'recharge' (Scheff 2001, 159–160).

5.6 Conclusion: A Plea for Intensified Discourses on Alternative (Pain) Treatments

Most cathartic processes at the intersection of Art, Ritual and Therapy follow a homoeopathic structure. One (unsuccessful) example of an allopathic treatment can be ascribed to Oscar Wilde's hero Dorian Gray who tries—according to the advice of his "teacher" Lord Henry—to cure the pain of his soul with the help of the senses (Wilde 2010, 181). But the text implies that this kind of allopathic pain treatment under the given circumstance is unsuccessful, with opium Gray's sins and their pains could not be cured. Also, Huysmans Hero Des Esseintes—admired by Dorian Gray—cannot cure his painful contempt and disgust of human beings with his luxury in loneliness.

I do not want to dismiss allopathic methods in the context of pain treatment as useless; I rather think that the circumstances prescribe which form of therapeutic treatment is most helpful. Drinking sage tea for curing a sore throat is a natural, but allopathic and not homoeopathic symptom treatment. It is quite effective, but it does not eliminate the cause of the sore throat. Using palliatives in medical pain care context is symptom treatment as well. Eliminating ('aufheben') pain in severe circumstances is an ethical necessity in order to prevent or shield (Latin *palliare*) severe suffering.

A hypothesis, which cannot be proved in this chapter, because the evidence of it requires a separate inquiry, is that in many cases, especially psychological issues such as phobias, a careful 'homoeopathic' method is effective and sustainable. Comparing the psychological sphere with the physical sphere, it could be argued for example that a manifested iterating headache cannot be cured simply by treating the symptoms, but only by elimination of the source of the headache (for example wrong posture, noise, air pollution, etc.). Allopathic methods may be most effective and suitable for treatments in severe emergencies. It is not my aim here to give medical advice, but I am convinced that the concepts of 'modern' 'western' medicine—according to which everybody has to be 'cured'—have to be re-evaluated (see Meinhold 2011). The torrent of complaints related to medical services in Germany in May 2014 as well as the current discourse on cancer 'overtreatment' in 'western' medical contexts are evidences for a need of re-evaluation from a more holistic perspective. Many alternative pain treatments are provided by ethno-medical and eastern medical concepts (such as Ayurveda, Chinese or Thai traditional medical systems) and by humanistic psychology with its positive health concept. It is high time to widen the outlook and intensify the discourses on this matter.[23]

---

[23]I would like to thank Siby George and Pravesh Jung Golay (both IIT Bombay, India), Taylor Hargrave (Assumption University, Thailand) and Chris Dunton (National University, Lesotho) for their insightful and critical–constructive comments on this chapter.

References

Aristoteles. (1993a). *Poetik*. Stuttgart: RUB.
Aristoteles. (1993b). *Politik*. Stuttgart: RUB.
Bernays, J. (1880). *Zwei Abhandlungen über die aristotelische Theorie des Drama*. Berlin: VWH.
Butcher, S. H. (1894). *Aristotle's theory of poetry and fine art, with a critical text and a translation of the poetics*. London: Macmillan.
Carroll, N. (2004). The philosophy of horror. In Carolyn Korsmeyer (Ed.), *Aesthetics: The big questions* (pp. 274–282). Malden, MA: Blackwell.
Eliade, M. (1957). *Das Heilige und das Profane: Vom Wesen der Religion*. Hamburg: Fischer.
Eliade, M. (1974). *Shamanism: Archaic Techniques of Ecstasy*. Princeton, NJ: University Press.
Eliade, M. (1988). *Das Mysterium der Wiedergeburt*. Frankfurt: Insel.
Hegel, G. W. F. (1973). *Phänomenologie des Geistes*. Frankfurt: Suhrkamp.
Hügli, A. "Malum". (1980). In J. Ritter et al. (Eds.), *Historisches Wörterbuch der Philosophie [HWdP]*, Vol. 5. Basel: Schwabe: 700.
Kant, I. (1998). *Anthropologie in pragmatischer Hinsicht*. Stuttgart: RUB.
Lewis-Williams, D., & Dowson, T. (1998). *Images of Power: Understanding Rock Art*. Johannesburg: Southern Book Publishers.
Lorenz, K. (1983). *Das Sogenannte Böse (oder: Über die Aggression)*. München: DTV/C.H. Beck/Robugen.
Lukas, E. (1996). Auf der Suche nach Sinn. Logotherapie. In *Wege zum Menschen: Methoden und Persönlichkeiten moderner Psychotherapie. Ein Handbuch*, edited by Hilarion Petzold. Band I. Paderborn: Junfermann.
Mandela, N. R. (1990). *Long Walk to Freedom*. Falmouth: Abacus.
Manyeli, T. L. (1992). *Religious Symbols of the Basotho*. Mazenod: Printing Works.
Meinhold, R. (2005). *Der Mode-Mythos: Lifestyle als Lebenskunst. Philosophisch-anthropologische Implikationen der Mode*. Würzburg: Koenigshausen & Neumann.
Meinhold, R. (2011). Comparative melioration and pathological pathogenization in viagra marketing. In Botz-Bornstein, T. (Ed.) *The Philosophy of Viagra: Bioethical Responses to the Viagrification of the Modern World*, 179–190. Value Inquiry Series. New York: Rodopi.
Meinhold, R. (2012). Catharsis and violence: Terrorism and the fascination for superlative destruction. *Boleswa Journal of Philosophy, Theology and Religion, 3*(3), 172–184.
Meinhold, R. (2013). *Fashion myths: A cultural critique*. Bielefeld: Transcript.
Nürnberger, M. (1999). Trance, Besessenheit und Hypnose in den Tanzriten Sri Lankas. *Ethnopsychologische Mitteilungen, 8*(1), 14–31.
Schadewaldt, W. (1991). Die griechische Tragödie. Tübinger Vorlesungen Bd. 4. Frankfurt: STW.
Scheff, T. J. (2001). *Catharsis in Ritual and Drama*. Lincoln: iUniverse.com.
Schiller, F. (1983). *Dramen und Dramentheorie*. Stuttgart: RUB.
Sloterdijk, P., & Hans-Jürgen, H. (2001). *Die Sonne und der Tod*. Suhrkamp: Dialogische Untersuchungen. Frankfurt am Main.
Taylor, A. (director). (2005). *Žižek!* The Documentary Campaign: Zeitgeistvideo.
Wilde, O. (2010). *The Picture of Dorian Gray*. Oxford: Oxford University Press.

Chapter 6
Traditional Philosophies and Gandhi's Approach to the Self in Pain

Douglas Allen

Abstract Traditional dominant Western philosophical approaches tend not to focus on the self in pain, regarding such concerns as prephilosophical or non-philosophical and as secondary to objective rational analysis. Traditional dominant Indian philosophical approaches often focus on the self in pain, but this *karmic* experience is viewed negatively, as based on illusion and ignorance and as an obstacle to the goal of *moksha* and *nirvana*. Gandhi formulates a new, creative, challenging, contextually informed and controversial philosophical approach to the self in pain. In his philosophical focus on *satya* and *ahimsa*, Gandhi provides a philosophical approach to relative truth, absolute truth, nonviolence and ontology in understanding and transforming the self in pain. After providing a formulation of Gandhi's diverse and sometimes contradictory approaches to the self and self-other relations that shape his analysis of the self in pain and its transformation, we conclude with a suggested approach to the self in pain as a constituted given.

Keywords Gandhi · Self · Pain · Ontology · Truth · Nonviolence

The experience of the self in pain is universal and it is sometimes claimed, constitutive of what makes us human. Indeed, in certain philosophical and mystical approaches found throughout the world, transcending the self's experience of pain is tantamount to transcending the human condition; transcending our human mode of being in the world and what makes us human. As will be seen, Advaita Vedanta, the best-known system of Hindu philosophy and other influential Indian philosophical approaches illustrate such an approach to the self in pain.

In analyzing the experience of the self in pain, there has been a wide range of contradictory positions in the history of philosophy that have attempted to analyse the complex nature of the self (or whether there is such a thing as "the self"), the nature and status of the self in pain, and how this self in pain analysis relates to reality. And yet, perhaps surprisingly, for thousands of years, much of philosophy has ignored

D. Allen (✉)
University of Maine, Orono, USA
e-mail: Douglas_Allen@umit.maine.edu

or devalued the analysis of the self's experience of pain as prephilosophical, nonphilosophical, unworthy of philosophical investigation or as having little onto-logical status or relation to reality.

6.1 Dominant Western Philosophical Approaches

Some of the reason for the philosophical undervaluing of the experience of the self in pain can be found in the dominant Greek ontology that so shapes later Western phi-losophy. It is important to acknowledge that what follows is typical but not invariable. The dominant, Greek, essentialized view of the self was of the human being as a rational animal. Although philosophers debated the nature of rationality, they tended to accept that the more rational we become, the more in touch we are with reality.

How does pain fit in with this dominant view of human rationality and the rational structure and nature of reality? Pain was often analysed as something subjective and sometimes as something we share with "lower" nonhuman animals. It is a prephilosophical and nonphilosophical concern that is not the focus of philosophy proper with its conceptual rational analysis. Of course, the self's experience of pain was not ignored in some of Greek philosophy and later Western philosophy, as seen clearly in philosophical hedonism, some stoicism, and Bentham's utilitarianism. However, the usual philosophical approach was to pro-vide a rational analysis of such experiences, as seen in the rational calculus of the principle of utility. In short, in most Western philosophy, the self's experience of pain is not what makes us distinctively human, what defines the highest levels of human development and what expresses the philosophical ontology.

This dominant Western philosophical approach, with its many variations and contradictory formulations, is evident in key conceptual distinctions in modern philosophy, in rationalism and in empiricism, and in later developments in for-mulations of the scientific method, logical positivism and recent formulations shaped by cognitive science and other scientific approaches. This is evident in post-Medieval, modern formulations of the distinction between primary and sec-ondary qualities. Primary qualities, such as the number of objects or the shape of an object extended in space, were viewed as more universal, more reliable, more objective and more open to intersubjective verification. The experience of pain, while certainly part of human experience, was typically classified as a secondary quality. It was more subjective, qualitative, shaped by emotions and feelings, and resisted quantifiable criteria of intersubjective verification necessary for knowledge. In short, the experience of the self in pain was typically devalued as having little or nothing to do with objective knowledge and the objective understanding of reality.

Of course, there have been numerous diverse philosophical approaches that have attempted to include sensations, emotional states and the self's experiences of taste, colour and pain and other "subjective" experiences in their philosophical formu-lations of knowledge and of reality. This is evident in various twentieth century approaches in analytic philosophy, with formulations of *qualia* and various formulations of physicalism claiming to explain (or explain away) the self in pain in terms of more rational, objective, scientific accounts. Such philosophical approaches, including many recent formulations in cognitive science and other scientific accounts, may be viewed as variations of extreme or more modest reductionism. However, as has been repeatedly noted, there is usually some sense of the mysterious or enigmatic nature of the self in pain and similar qualitative experiences that is not exhausted by or fully grasped by the reductive formulations. And this is not to mention the additional claim, often asserted in hermeneutical and phenomenological philosophy, that providing a causal or other explanatory account of an experience, say, of pain, is not tantamount to or a substitute for the philosophical task of the interpretation of the meaning of the experience.

In short, most of dominant Western philosophy has made a sharp dichotomy between reason, which allows for knowledge and comprehending reality, and emotions, feelings, including the experience of pain, which are part of our human existence but which are not essential for, and are usually viewed as an obstacle to, realizing the universal, objective, rational nature of knowledge and reality. Philosophers do not deny feelings of pain, but such nonrational and irrational subjective feelings must be controlled and suppressed in developing our philosophical analysis.

Of course, there are Western philosophers, for thousands of years, who reject this dominant approach. This becomes especially strong in many developments in Continental philosophy, including diverse formulations of existentialism, hermeneutical philosophy and phenomenology. For example, philosophical approaches that emphasize the subjectivity of truth, the prereflective and the nonreflective, and the need to empathize with and describe the real-lived experiences of the other have radically different approaches to the self in pain.

6.2 Dominant Indian Philosophical Approaches

Dominant Indian philosophical approaches, including both Orthodox Hindu and Heterodox Jain and Buddhist philosophies, share many of the characteristics of the dominant Western philosophical approaches, although they also incorporate significant differences in analyzing the self in pain. After providing a brief general formulation of the dominant Indian philosophical orientation, we will consider the innovative philosophical contributions of Mohandas K. Gandhi with regard to the self's experience of pain.

In the dominant Indian philosophical orientation, the experience of pain is viewed in negative terms. It is an integral part of the causal world of *karma* with cycles of birth and rebirth that imprison us in ignorance and suffering. It is an integral part of the world of *maya*, the mysterious cosmic process of human existence that generates and traps us in illusion and is removed from reality and liberation. *Moksha* and *Nirvana* point us to the teleological goal and transcending experience of freedom, liberation, salvation and enlightenment that are experiential realizations of a knowledge and realty beyond the self in pain.

Far from ignoring or marginalizing the human experience of pain, as illusory and separated from reality, dominant Indian philosophical approaches often focus on the self in pain. One cannot transcend illusion without understanding illusion. One cannot transcend the phenomenal world of pain without understanding, analyzing and transforming how we construct, maintain and become identified with the self in pain.

This is most evident in the philosophical foundations of Buddhism, as seen in the key teachings of the Buddha that are codified in the Pali Canon. In the Four Noble Truths, the first truth is that "life is *dukkha*," normally translated as suffering with the usual focus on pain and misery. The philosophical meaning and significance of *dukkha* is much deeper and broader than common interpretations of overt pain and suffering. *Dukkha* includes the sense that the experience of the (illusory) self in pain, as a universal feature of our spatial, temporal, historical, conditioned, ordinary human condition and mode of existence in the world, is separated from reality and involves friction and stress, discontent, alienation and lack of well being.

According to the Buddha's foundational teaching of *anicca*, everything in this phenomenal world is transitory and impermanent. This includes the foundational teaching of *anatta* or no-self in which there is no permanent ego, self, or individual being. Therefore, our normal human experiences of "happiness" are also identified with *dukkha* or suffering. Driven by our ego desires and attachments, we attempt to make permanent our impermanent experiences of happiness, and this leads to suffering.

In even broader and deeper philosophical terms, the Buddha teaches that what we construct and name as an ego or self as a unified mind–body individual or being is itself *dukkha*. In other words, our worldly phenomenal functioning as a human being is based on ignorance, separated from reality, and is *dukkha*.

Using the language of the self in pain, the Buddha's philosophical teachings point us beyond the ordinary meaning of physical and other overt manifestations of pain. Our usual ways of experiencing, denying and defending ourselves against impermanence are painful. And our dominant ways of constructing what it is to be a self and to be human are painful. According to the Buddha, the construction of the self always involves the construction of the self in pain.

The Hindu philosophical system of Advaita ("nonduality") Vedanta dramatically illustrates this dominant Indian philosophical approach to the self in pain. Indeed, there is a common view, really a misconception, that all of Hindu philosophy expresses the extreme nondualistic monism of Advaita Vedanta as formulated by its founder, the philosopher Shankara. In such a stereotypical misconception, all dominant Indian philosophy and religion is life denying and world denying, and grants no reality to our illusory worldly human experiences, including the self in pain.

It is true that of Orthodox Hindu philosophical systems, Shankara's Advaita Vedanta is at one end of the spectrum in classifying views of the status of this-worldly existence. One can submit that it most strongly analyses and devalues this world and human existence, including the self in pain, as *maya* or illusion. After all, Advaita's essential "definition" of *Brahman*, the Absolute Reality, as *satcitananda* describes *Brahman* as pure being (*sat*), pure consciousness (*cit*) and pure bliss (*ananda*). The *ananda* approach emphasizes that the Absolute Reality is free from all pain and suffering.

However, even Advaita's influential theory of illusion is more subtle and complex than the stereotypical views of its position as simply rejecting this human existence as unreal. Indeed, as evident in the name of Advaita's theory of illusion, *anirvachanyakhyati*, the object of illusion, including the self's experience of pain, is "indescribable" or "indeterminate" as either real or unreal.

In Shankara's theory of illusion, the illusory object (say, of the self in pain) is not completely unreal (*asat*, nonbeing or nonexistence). It is something that appears as real, and it is something that is finally "sublated" and overcome. However, the illusory object is also not completely real (*sat*, being or permanent existence). It is not real because it is sublated and removed by right knowledge. The self in pain, in particular, and the entire world of *maya* of our worldly human mode of being, in general, have this rather mysterious, complex, intermediate status in which they are indescribable as completely real or unreal. The illusory self in pain has epistemic status but no ultimate ontological status in reality.

Unlike the Buddha's teaching, Shankara clearly upholds the ontological status of the permanent, unchanging, spiritual Self, the *Atman*, but this is not the self in pain. In Advaita's theory of the illusory self, one finds such images as the white shell perceived as yellow because the perceiver has jaundice or is looking through yellow glasses. Unlike other worldly illusory objects, such as the illusory snake that is removed when we realize that is a rope, the shell is real but not as yellow. The Self is not sublated or removed but only the false characteristics we attribute to it. The true Self is real but not as conditioned, impermanent, *karmic* self in pain.

As was seen in the Buddha's teaching, Shankara's Vedanta takes very seriously the self in pain as an integral part of our human illusory world of *maya*. We need to understand *maya* in order to get beyond *maya*. We need to become mindful of the self in pain, so that we can understand its causes, nature and how it is fuelled and maintained as integral to being imprisoned in our human world of illusion. Without such philosophical analysis and appropriate transformative practice, we can never transcend the self in pain.

In terms of transformative practices, India has a long tradition of providing methods and techniques for developing a major focus on experiences of pain. One thinks of yoga and meditation. Pain may be a negative experience that needs to be transcended, but we must become mindful of it if we are to understand, transform and finally overcome it. Various yogic and meditational practices emphasize that the self in pain and other *karmic* phenomena function on all levels of human consciousness, not only conscious awareness, but also include the prereflective, the unconscious, emotions and feelings, and the imagination. Yoga and meditation offer methods and techniques for expanding consciousness of pain by bringing to conscious awareness painful phenomena that have been experienced as prereflective, nonreflective, subconscious, etc.

In this regard, Indian philosophies often emphasize the initial need to suspend ego-attached, contextually conditioned, "normal" assumptions and value judgments, such as the normative position that pain is something negative and needs to be avoided. This allows one to expand and deepen conscious awareness and to understand clearly how pain is experienced and expresses the functioning of the self in our human mode of being in the world. This is often similar to the insistence on the phenomenological *epoché* in much of philosophical phenomenology in allowing phenomena to appear and be described as phenomena.

In the dominant Indian philosophical approach, as illustrated by Advaita Vedanta and the Buddha's philosophical teachings, the basic problem in understanding and transforming the self in pain is ignorance. In the construction and functioning of the illusory world, including the self in pain, the basic defect is cognitive. In a wide variety of ways, as formulated by different Indian philosophical systems, we misapprehend, noncognize and live under illusion, separated from reality, and we then experience pain. Pain may be a symptom and consequence of ignorance, but it is not a root cause of the philosophical problem of our disconnection from reality.

This philosophical orientation, in which the major problem is cognitive and the root cause is ignorance, is expressed in the Buddha's foundational philosophical teaching, the Doctrine of Dependent Origination or Conditioned Genesis (*pratityasamutpada*). All worldly phenomena, including our experiences of pain and our constructions of a self that experiences pain, are causally and relatively interconnected. Nothing in our normal human experience is absolute, independent, or unconditioned. Each interconnected link is caused and conditioned and in turn becomes a causal and conditioning force that keeps us trapped in the illusory phenomenal world of pain and suffering. The basic problem is ignorance and the solution is overcoming ignorance, enlightenment, *Nirvana*. Overcoming ignorance, experiencing knowledge of reality, is the transformative process for transcending pain and other forms of suffering.

The dominant Hindu, Buddhist, and Jain philosophical approaches emphasize renunciation in relating to the self in pain and other *karmic* phenomena. The emphasis is on renunciation of ego desires and ego attachments that cause, condition and maintain our false and illusory self and world marked by so much pain. Although there are notable exceptions, as seen in "engaged Buddhism" and various activist Vedantic formulations, the strongest tendency has been to emphasize renunciation of active involvement in the world of *samsara* and *maya*. The usual exemplary contemplative model of the more enlightened and liberated spiritual being is of one who has transcended the self in pain by letting go and renouncing active involvement in the world, including the goal of actively transforming the spatial, temporal, historical world of so much pain and suffering. Among notable exceptions to this dominant traditional philosophical orientation is Mohandas Karamchand Gandhi, the best-known and most influential twentieth-century Indian proponent of truthful, nonviolent, action-oriented, this-worldly transformation of the self and the world in pain.

6.3   Gandhi's Philosophical Approach and Traditional Philosophy

As M.K. Gandhi sometimes writes, he is not a "philosopher" in any academic or scholarly way in the tradition of Shankara and other classical Indian philosophers or the Advaitin S. Radhakrishnan and other twentieth-century philosophers. His major focus is not on rigorous conceptual analysis, formulating rational arguments and refutations of alternative philosophical approaches and providing a rationally coherent philosophical system within which to understand the self in pain. And yet, as I have submitted in previous writings, Gandhi is far more philosophically significant than what is being done in most "academic" philosophy, East and West, and can serve as a catalyst for rethinking our approaches to the self in pain and other philosophical concerns.

In his moral, epistemological, and ontological approach to the self and the self in pain, Gandhi is influenced by many sources, mainly Indian but also Western. As is well known, he is indebted in his identification with certain Western scriptural sources, such as the Sermon on the Mount, and the writings of Leo Tolstoy, John Ruskin, and others expressing the dissident "other West" with which he feels most sympathetic. However, he is also influenced by dominant, post-Enlightenment, modern influences, such as the focus on the autonomous self with individual rights, while at the same time presenting a radical critique of such "Modern Civilization" and significantly reformulating and transforming its positive contributions. This includes his rejection of the dominant view that the ends justify the means and his view that individual rights must be grounded in social and moral duty (*dharma*).

Having acknowledged Gandhi's inclusiveness and indebtedness to Western influences, it is important to emphasize that the dominant influences on his approach to the self and the self in pain are Indian, especially Hindu and to a considerable extent Jain and also Buddhist. As Gandhi often answers, when asked about his religion or religious philosophy, he is a Hindu, although he sometimes answers that he is also a Christian, a Muslim and many other things. Nevertheless, in his innovative approach to the self in pain and other philosophical concerns, Gandhi is not a traditional Hindu or Indian, and he is extremely critical of much of the traditional ontological views and approaches to reality.

This is clear in Gandhi's approach to the Hindu sacred scripture, the *Bhagavad-Gita*, his favourite text, the strongest influence on his philosophy, and his practical guide to truthful moral living. Embracing the previously mentioned Indian focus on renunciation, Gandhi most identifies with the Gita's action-oriented philosophy and approach of *karma yoga*: act, based on knowledge of one's *karma* and one's duties or *dharma*, with an attitude of complete renunciation of all ego-attachment to the results of one's action.

In other words, as contrasted with the dominant Indian philosophical approach of renunciation of the world of action, including the self in pain, the Gita's *karma yoga* emphasizes renunciation in action, renunciation while acting. Thus, in traditional interpretations, Lord Krishna is instructing the warrior Arjuna to act according to his duty without attachment to results, such as killing or nonkilling or winning or losing the war. Refocusing his attitude and approach from his earlier doubts and indecisiveness, Arjuna should now free himself from any ego-attached focus on whether his renunciation in action in fighting will increase the *karmic* suffering of other selves.

Gandhi provides a remarkable interpretation of the highest moral and spiritual meaning of the renunciatory *karma yoga* philosophy, radically different from the numerous commentaries on the Gita by Shankara and other Hindu philosophers, mystics and political leaders over the centuries. As will be seen, Gandhi interprets renunciation in action as not devaluing the status or significance of the world of selves in pain. Just the opposite: he views the *Bhagavad Gita* as a gospel of selfless service with the major emphasis on meeting the needs of the most disadvantaged, the least free and the selves in greatest pain.

Even more remarkably, Gandhi, unlike the influential philosophical commentaries and the views of the hundred of millions of Indian devotees, interprets the seemingly violent Gita as a gospel of nonviolence (*ahimsa*). Obviously, this shapes his approach to the self in pain. As is well known, Gandhi is claiming that one should not read and interpret the Gita literally, as portraying an actual battlefield with the two armed forces about to inflict killing and great pain. For Gandhi, the profound message should be interpreted symbolically, allegorically, as, for example, expressing the conflicts and struggles with forces of violence and evil that we experience within and are obstacles to our moral and spiritual progress.

Even more significantly, in my view, Gandhi suggests a profound hermeneutical move in the reading of texts and the interpretation of meaning. As integral to the dynamic self-relations involved in the formulations of meaning, texts must be contextualized, disclosing social, cultural, economic, historical and other situated variables and structures. We are engaged in a complex, contested, hermeneutical project in which every reading is a rereading and every interpretation is a reinterpretation, textually and contextually related to the past, but also potentially creative and innovative.

Therefore, Gandhi can acknowledge that earlier Indian societies, religious expressions, and creators and receivers of the Gita often use violent language, uphold oppressive values and hegemonic teachings, and embrace hierarchical relations and institutional structures not adequately addressing selves in pain. However, texts are not static but are part of an ongoing, dynamic project. We today, reflecting on the profound moral and spiritual insights of the Gita, can purify and develop our reformulations and reinterpretations of meaning in ways that are more moral, truthful and nonviolent and that speak to our contemporary world of so much untruth, violence and the experience of so many selves in physical, psychological and other expressions of pain.

What is Gandhi's philosophy that allows him to understand such selves in pain? In this regard, Gandhi repeatedly asserts that he upholds two basic philosophical, moral and spiritual postulates and principles: *Satya* or Truth and *Ahimsa* or Nonviolence.

6.4 Gandhi's Philosophical Approach to Relative Truth, Absolute Truth and Ontology

Usually noted is that Gandhi is primarily a moralist, concerned with human beings living virtuous lives with character, and that his emphasis is on the primacy of moral practice, not conceptual analysis and systemic philosophical formulations. He experiences a great diversity of situations in which he as a self is in pain and, as integral to his self-realization, other selves are in great pain. To use the title of his *Autobiography*, he is engaged in practical "experiments with truth" in which he relates to and attempts to lessen the suffering of selves in pain. He frequently writes of his failed experiments with truth based on testing his assumptions, values, concepts, actions, *Satyagraha* campaigns of nonviolent resistance and implementation of his "Constructive Programme", including Hindu-Muslim harmonious relations, in terms of new contextualized practices. His experiments are failures when they fail to lesson the economic, political, psychological, cultural and other sufferings of selves in pain; fail to empower the suffering others; and fail to lead to their moral and spiritual development.

With this emphasis on practice, what is usually ignored or devalued is the key insight that Gandhi embraces a profound theory or philosophy of reality grounded in his formulations of truth and nonviolence and their integral relations. Such a moral and ontological philosophy shapes Gandhi's methodology and provides the interpretative framework in which he understands specific phenomena of selves in pain, why he engages in particular practices to overcome or lessen pain, and why he assesses his experimental practices as successes or failures.

In his approach to the self and the self in pain, Gandhi embraces a moral and ontological view of reality most often formulated in terms of his understanding of *satya* (truth, which he uses interchangeably with God, self, soul) and which has an integral relation and is sometimes used interchangeably with *ahimsa* (nonviolence, avoiding harm or injury, which he uses interchangeably with love). Similar to the dominant tradition of Hindu philosophy, Gandhi understands *satya* (upholding and sustaining truth, truth-force, reality, being) in terms of *sat* (truth, what is real, pure being, the true essence of existence, the self-existent or universal spirit, often presented as *Brahman*, the Absolute Reality).

In this philosophical approach to being and reality, through the process of self-realization, one gradually conflates or lessens the frequent philosophical distinction between the epistemological and the ontological: Knowing the truth is experientially realizing the truth; one comes to know the reality of the self (*Atman*) by realizing that one is *Atman*; one comes to know the reality of the Absolute (*Brahman*) by realizing that one is and has always been *Brahman*.

In many passages, Gandhi presents this approach to truth, being and what is real in language similar to influential passages in the scriptural *Upanishads*. He formulates *satya* as a spiritual force or power that reveals the underlying nature of realty, usually obstructed by our false assumptions, values, and views of untruth and violence. This truth-force of *satya* (often used interchangeably with soul-force,

God-force, love-force) is what is permanent and everlasting underlying the phenomenal experiences of impermanence and temporal existence. It is the force that brings the phenomena of our normal, untruthful, immoral, violent world of selves in pain into truthful, moral, nonviolent, loving and compassionate, meaningful relations and structures through which we can realize what is true and real. As Gandhi repeatedly asserts, such an experience of *satya* is radically different from normal sensations and perceptions, it can never be expressed adequately through language and conceptual formulations, and it defies all proof. But Gandhi is absolutely certain that *satya* exists and reveals to him what is true and real. How can he be so sure?

Gandhi is sure that *satya* exists as what is True, what is Real, because he experiences It. However, as will be seen in his key distinction between Absolute Truth and relative truth and its application to the self in pain, this is a very complex and controversial claim to the experiential verification of truth.

There are many Gandhi *satya* formulations in which it is tempting simply to identify his approach with a coherence theory of truth. Gandhi upholds an ontological view of the interconnectedness of all of life. Truth is that force which brings together untruthful and violent phenomena, such as those expressing relations of exploitation and hate, into meaningful, interconnected, truthful and loving relations that provide the understanding and means for relating to the self and lessening its pain.

There are even more Gandhi *satya* formulations in which it is tempting simply to identify his approach with a pragmatic theory of truth. This emphasizes the primacy of specific contextual practice in understanding and transforming the situatedness of the self in pain. Gandhi repeatedly affirms that one step is enough for him, and one step in actually alleviating the suffering of the self in pain is more important, truthful and real than any appeals to some coherent philosophical theory of truth.

In addition, Gandhi accepts moral philosophy as first philosophy, and there are numerous passages focusing on the self in pain in which it is tempting to identify Gandhi's ethical approach to truth and reality as that of a deontologist. This is especially the case when he so emphasizes the primacy of motives, intentions, acting with a pure will and doing what is truthful without any attachment to consequences. However, there are numerous other passages in which Gandhi is clearly a consequentialist, even if he specifically rejects Bentham's utilitarianism. This is repeatedly evident when Gandhi tests his truth formulations in practice and claims that even when he has moral intentions, if his action does not lesson the suffering of selves in pain, then this is a failed experiment with truth, and he needs to learn from his failure. And there are numerous passages in which it is tempting to identify Gandhi with a formulation of virtue ethics, especially with his emphasis on developing selves with moral character who embrace truth and nonviolence in acting morally.

The above reflections point to Gandhi's eclecticism, pluralism and openness to diverse experiences of selves in pain so that it is impossible to comprehend his overall approach and ontological theory by identifying them with a traditional philosophical category or system. To critics, this shows that Gandhi is muddleheaded, inconsistent and not a rigorous, systematic thinking. To sympathizers, this shows that Gandhi is extremely significant for contemporary philosophy and our world of selves in pain with his situated open-endedness, flexibility, contextualized pluralism and reluctance to imposed, violent, hegemonic theorizing on diverse others.

At the same time, Gandhi, while emphasizing the relativity of truth and pluralistic relative approaches to reality, wants to avoid a fashionable, unlimited and facile relativism. And while emphasizing differences and the diversity of other selves in pain, he endorses an ontological view of interconnected unity, a primary unity with a respect for diversity.

Gandhi's distinction between relative truth and Absolute Truth (which I'll capitalize in much of what follows) is invaluable for understanding how he approaches the self in pain. This distinction may seem to express the same dichotomy that Nagarjuna's Madhyamika Buddhism, Shankara's Advaita Vedanta and other traditional philosophers have made in distinguishing the world of relative truth, with the self in pain with its false views and illusions, from the enlightened and liberatory world of Absolute Truth that is free from selves in pain. Although Gandhi shares some of this traditional dichotomized approach, his distinction is much more complex in its relations, and he grants much more truth and reality to relative truth.

From passages in his *Autobiography* and other writings, many regard Gandhi as a rigid, often dogmatic absolutist. He uncompromisingly insists that we live according to the moral and ontological absolutes of Absolute Truth and Absolute Nonviolence. Nevertheless, if one examines thousands of pages of Gandhi's writings, along with how he actually lived his life in pursuing his experiments with truth, one realizes that this rigid absolutist interpretation is an abstracted oversimplification and serious misinterpretation of Gandhi's approach to selves in pain and his other existential concerns.

It is true that Gandhi affirms the reality of Absolute Truth. He claims an experiential basis for this philosophical view of what is True, Being, Self, Reality. Often, in times of crisis and despair, he expresses his faith commitment to such a view of Reality that gives him hope.

What is sometimes overlooked is Gandhi's repeated assertion that he, as an embodied, imperfect, situated self, at most has temporary, limited "glimpses" of Absolute Truth, Absolute Nonviolence and Absolute Reality. Gandhi's assertion can be related to the famous Indian fable and parable of the Blind Men and the Elephant found in Jainism, Buddhism, Hinduism and Sufism, and diffused widely. More specifically, just as Gandhi is deeply influenced by the Jaina key doctrine of *ahimsa* (nonviolence), he is here influenced by the Jaina key doctrine of *anekantava* (or *anekantava–syadvada*). *Anekantava* ('No-one-perspective-ism", "non-absolutism" and "manifoldness") is the theory of manifold predications, the manifold nature of truth. Often used interchangeably with *anekantava*, *syadvada* is the theory of conditioned predication, so that all of our judgments of truth are conditional.

It would be egotistic, arrogant and false for human beings to claim that they fully experience the Absolute. If one fully realizes the Absolute Truth, then differing views of other selves in pain would necessarily be false. This false view is the cause of much untruth, violence and pain in the world. Not only does such an orientation distinguish Gandhi from traditional Hindu and other Indian philosophers with their claims to experience Absolute Truth, the Absolute Self (or Absolute Void of No-Self) with the absolute realization of *moksha* or *nirvana*, but it also helps us to understand Gandhi's emphasis on pluralism with many legitimate relative paths to Truth. Such a Gandhi approach emphasizes the need for tolerance and mutual respect, including the view that the self can learn truths from other selves, since no self fully realizes the Absolute Truth. Such an encounter with other selves also serves as a catalyst for us to deepen our own moral and spiritual self and progress from untruth to greater relative truth.

As was seen, most of traditional Indian philosophy acknowledges that we must understand the conditioned, relative, illusory world of the self in pain in order to free ourselves from that world of ignorance, illusion and suffering, and realize the nonsocial, nonhistorical, noncontextualized Ultimate Reality. While Gandhi shares some of this traditional philosophical orientation, his approach to the self in pain, his values, and the emphasis in his philosophy and practice are radically different. As selves situated in our existential human mode of being in the world of relative truth, our philosophical project consists in the ongoing process of experiments with truth in which we attempt to move morally and spiritually from one relative truth to greater relative truth, closer to our imperfect glimpses and perspectival ideals of Absolute Truth.

What this means for Gandhi's focus on selves in pain is that philosophy must take the reality of relative truth very seriously with its social, historical, economic, political, psychological and other this-worldly self-relations, structures and conditionings. This means resisting the traditional renunciatory emphasis on devaluing, marginalizing and negating the world of relative truth with selves in pain as lacking ontological status. In granting moral, spiritual and ontological status to the world of relative truth, Gandhi is strikingly unlike most traditional Indian philosophy in his primary focus on this-worldly untruths and violence, with his highest priority of acting to transform this world of selves in pain so as to realize greater relative truth and nonviolence.

Probably, the most significant observation for distinguishing Gandhi's remarkably different approach to the self in pain in terms of the relative truth-Absolute Truth dichotomy is the following claim. Gandhi does agree that our relative, conditioned, *karmic* world is structured by relations expressing untruths and violence that are obstacles to the moral and spiritual realization of Truth and Reality and to understanding and transforming a world characterized by selves in pain. Nevertheless, relative truths are not inherently obstacles for our moral and spiritual development, for our truthful and nonviolent relating to selves in pain, and for our greater, not perfect, realizations of Absolute Truth, Absolute Being, Absolute Self and Absolute Reality. Indeed, in most dramatic terms, as contrasted with the emphasis on negating the relative to realize what is Real, Gandhi claims that relative truth is invaluable and is usually our only way for accessing Absolute Truth. In place of a traditional, essentialized, nonsocial ontology, Gandhi embraces a more open-ended, dynamic, relational and social ontology.

Three striking illustrations may bring out Gandhi's remarkable approach to relative truth and the self in pain. First, in contrast to most traditional moralists and exemplary spiritual figures, Gandhi's writings reveal his primary focus on economic, political and other this-worldly relations. For example, Gandhi criticizes traditional Hindu and other Indian philosophers for devaluing or ignoring worldly political concerns as expressing the world of illusion and unrelated to Ultimate Reality. Gandhi submits that just as the political must be grounded in moral and spiritual values and relations, the religious, if it is truly moral and spiritual, must be integrally related to the political. By this, he means that the only religious positions that are worthwhile and relevant to our existential concerns of selves in pain are those that emphasize the need to overcome poverty, class exploitation, caste and gender and other forms of oppression, violent and militaristic values and policies, colonial and imperialist and other forms of domination, and the lack of freedom, self-determinism and equality. To address such concerns of selves in pain is necessarily "political," although not reductionistically political in not reducing all of life and reality to some political perspective.

Second, in dramatic passages, Gandhi advises religious believers not to look for God or the sacred reality in some otherworldly supernatural realm of Absolute Reality. He is well aware of how Hinduism and other religions have traditionally used such supernatural faith appeals to justify or fail to address this world of selves in pain. Instead, Gandhi advises believers to take an existential approach focusing on those who are the most disadvantaged, the least free and the most in pain. When one identifies with other selves in pain and acts with them to overcome their suffering, then God, the Absolute Truth, will partially, imperfectly, but really appear in your life of greater relative truth.

Third and especially significant for our focus on selves in pain, Gandhi, in his primary focus on relative truth, does not evaluate pain as something inherently or always negative or as always disclosing untruth. Gandhi makes a basic distinction between voluntary suffering and involuntary suffering. He repeatedly emphasizes how involuntary pain and suffering—resulting from humanly caused and maintained poverty, hunger, exploitation, oppression and injustice—always reveal relations of untruth. However, voluntary pain and suffering—as seen in Gandhi's detailed accounts of his imprisonments, life-threatening fasting, acts of noncooperation and civil disobedience and other ordeals—reveal relations of truth to the self in voluntary pain and to other selves. Gandhi describes the experience of such voluntary pain as morally, economically, politically and spiritually transformative, as self-transformative and world-transformative, and even as joyful.

The distinction of Absolute Truth and relative truth does not remove all difficulties in Gandhi's approach to the self in pain. For example, if Gandhi has, at most, limited, imperfect, temporary glimpses of *Satya*, how can he justify the foundational lofty claims he makes about the universal, unifying, moral and ontological status of Absolute Truth? With his emphasis on diverse, perspectival, contextualized relative truth, how can Gandhi justify any key moral and ontological claims about the integral relations between the relative and Absolute Truth? As seen repeatedly in Gandhi's difficulties in justifying his philosophical and religious formulations with other philosophical and religious approaches, how can Gandhi relate to other approaches that reject his social ontology? For example, certain Christians and Muslims reject Gandhi's relative–Absolute approach to selves in pain, since they claim to possess the exclusive Absolute Truth. They claim that Gandhi's relative truths express ways of untruth, and they will never overcome the pain or allow the self in pain to realize Absolute Truth.

Gandhi's philosophy and practice express a variety of different responses to the above questions, expressing his views as to how he knows *Satya*, the ontological status of Absolute Truth, the integral relation between relative truth and Absolute Truth, etc. Some of his responses, in my view, are mutually exclusive and sometimes inconsistent. Nevertheless, the following is how I interpret and reformulate his philosophical approach to most adequately respond to these questions and understand selves in pain.

In responding to his own self and other selves in pain, Gandhi focuses on the conditioned phenomena and causal relations of untruth and relative truth. He also embraces an ontological view of *Satya*, but he only has limited, fleeting, imperfect glimpses of Absolute Truth. Now Gandhi reflects on his limited, worldly experiences of untruth and relative truth, and he also reflects on the occasional breakthroughs and disclosures of imperfect realizations of Absolute Truth. Such partial and limited realizations are only possible through self-sacrifice and transcending the ego, voluntary suffering that purifies the self, and other methods for moral and spiritual development. Then, through an ontological move involving a bold imaginative construction, Gandhi attempts to formulate the Absolute Ideal, Truth, Being, God and Self, what is ultimately Real. The limited realization of the Absolute Truth can serve as a regulative ideal, providing us with moral and spiritual values, guidance for our actions and hope in difficult times in which untruths expressed through selves in pain can be overwhelming.

Gandhi does not intend this dynamic, creative, ontological move to be some fantastic flight of imagination, some detached abstract utopian vision, or some theoretical substitute for real-lived experiences of the self in pain in the world of relative truths. This also is not some Gandhi recipe or mechanical formula in which one can apply the pure, nonsocial, ontological essences to the world of relative truth in order to experience Absolute Truth and Nonviolence.

In his relative–Absolute distinction and relations and his social ontological move relevant to selves in pain, Gandhi emphasizes complex, dynamic, open-ended, engaged encounters and struggles with the contextualized structures and situated relations of selves in pain. We can only know to what extent we have experienced or not experienced the Absolute Truth and whether we have realized dynamic integral relations holding between the relative and the Absolute through our failed or successful experiments in truth. This means evaluating the extent to which our experience-based and imaginatively constructed ideals allow us to explain the enigmatic and complex phenomena of selves in pain and engage in action-oriented transformative practice allowing us to move from one level of relative truth of selves in pain to a more developed moral and spiritual level of relative truth closer to the ideal of Truth, Nonviolence, Being, God and Self.

We end this section by emphasizing the ontological claim in Gandhi's approach to Truth/truth: There exists some deeper, permanent spiritual power or force that allows us to experience the meaningful interrelatedness and unity of all reality. Gandhi presents an inclusive, organic, holistic philosophical approach with presuppositions and principles that affirm the essential unity and interrelatedness of all existence, the indivisibility of truth that is manifested in diverse relative ways and the integral relation of truth and nonviolence. We now consider Gandhi's philosophical approach to nonviolence.

6.5   Gandhi's Philosophical Approach to Nonviolence and Ontology

Gandhi, best known for his philosophy and practice of nonviolence, greatly broadens and deepens our understanding of violence and nonviolence. Everyone easily grants that violence is a force, but Gandhi rejects the usual view of nonviolence as passive, as simply refraining from violence, as seen in *ahimsa* meaning not-harming. For Gandhi, nonviolence is an active force, our most powerful moral and spiritual force, more powerful than violence. Violence is often approached in rather overt and simple terms, as expressed in terrorist acts of setting off explosive devices or brutal acts of rape, but in Gandhi's approach, violence is usually viewed as complex and often hidden, camouflaged, and in need of our hermeneutical uncovering and deciphering.

Just as Gandhi made the key distinction between Absolute Truth and relative truth, he distinguishes between Absolute Nonviolence and relative nonviolence. He has limited imperfect experiential realizations of *Ahimsa*, while recognizing that all human beings, in their conditioned, situated human mode of being in the world, are necessarily violent. Even Gandhi's careful acts, with his self-disciplined reduced needs of simple living, such as acts involving walking, breathing, practicing hygiene or maintaining his vegetarian diet, involve some taking of life and other violence. Gandhi's action-oriented philosophical project is to become aware of, and eliminate as much as possible, our humanly caused and controlled voluntary violence. We do this by actively engaging in more nonviolent and truthful, interconnected relations with other selves in pain so that we move from one level of nonviolence to a more moral and spiritual level of nonviolence closer to the ideal of Absolute Nonviolence.

Gandhi greatly broadens and deepens our understanding of violence and nonviolence. We normally restrict our meaning of violence to overt, usually physical, expressions of pain and suffering (killings, assaults, torture, rape, domestic abuse, overt bullying, etc.). For Gandhi, this is significant, but it includes only a small part of the violence of selves in pain. In my research, I have introduced two key concepts: the multidimensionality of violence and the structural violence of the status quo.

In Gandhi's philosophy and practice, violence is multidimensional and includes inner psychological violence (often identified with hatred), economic violence (usually equated with exploitation with asymmetrical relations of economic domination), linguistic violence, social and cultural violence, political violence, religious violence, environmental violence and educational violence. We are contextually situated and socialized in ways so that all of these dimensions of violence interact, mutually condition and reinforce each other, leading to our violent assumptions and views of our self and other selves in pain.

Gandhi also focuses on the structural violence of the status quo. This is business as usual. Indeed, when the dominant economic, political and other violent systemic structures are functioning smoothly, without active nonviolent and truthful resistance and disruption, we usually consider the situation nonviolent and peaceful. But for Gandhi, the usual structural situation of selves in pain—suffering passively, feeling insecure and powerless, adopting religious and ideological justifications for their pain, not disrupting the structural violence of the status quo—is extremely violent and needs to be resisted and transformed through active nonviolent force.

Gandhi develops this approach to violence and nonviolence, focusing on overt and multidimensional and structural violence and nonviolence, through his famous means-ends analysis. Gandhi provides a radical critique of our dominant, violent and untruthful "Modern Civilization" with its view that the ends justify the means. For Gandhi, means and ends are integrally related and mutually reinforce each other. We cannot use impure, violent, untruthful means to achieve noble ends. In this regard, Gandhi usually presents nonviolence as the means to the realization of truth as the end, but he also says that *satya* and *ahimsa* are convertible or interchangeable as means and ends. Nonviolence is the means for realizing truth, but truth is also the means for realizing the goal of becoming more loving and nonviolent.

As interpreters easily note, Gandhi is providing a means-ends ethical analysis: immoral means lead to immoral ends, and moral means are the only way to realize moral ends. We cannot use hate to overcome hate, terrorism to overcome terrorism, injustice to overcome injustice, exploitation and domination to achieve freedom and equality, etc. The only way to break this vicious causal cycle of violence, greed, hatred, domination, inequality and injustice is to decondition and transform those immoral relative causes and structural conditions of selves in pain by embracing nonviolent moral ends and primarily focusing on integrally related nonviolent moral means.

What interpreters usually fail to note is that Gandhi's primary moral analysis is grounded in his means-ends ontological formulation of Reality, Truth, Being, God or Self. He is making a major ontological claim in relating *ahimsa* and *satya*. Violence is a force that maximizes ontological separateness and divisiveness. It is based on the fundamental view and orientation that the other self, the other self in pain—whether individual, class, caste, gendered, racial, religious, ethnic, or national target of my hatred, fear and violence—is essentially different from my self and our selves in pain.

By the way of extreme contrast, *ahimsa* is the most powerful moral and spiritual unifying force. Grounded in the basic view that what unites us as humans is more fundamental than what divides us, it brings selves in pain together in caring, loving, compassionate, cooperative relations that allow us to experience and act consistently with the interconnectedness and unity of all of life.

In other words, violence (hatred, exploitation, imperialism, sexism, homophobia, racism, religious persecution) is not only immoral, resulting in so much humanly caused pain and suffering, but it is also inconsistent with and an obstacle toward realizing the ontological nature of Truth and Reality. By the way of contrast, the active force of nonviolence, the activated love-force, is not only moral, expressing moral means-ends relations and consequences in relating to selves in pain. By unifying us in meaningful moral relations, by recognizing the basic interconnectedness and unity of life, a basic unity with a respect for differences, nonviolence is consistent with and the means for realizing the ontological nature of Truth and Reality.

6.6 Gandhi's Philosophical Approach to the Self and Ontology

Any adequate account of Gandhi's philosophical approach to the self in pain requires lengthy exposition of his pluralistic, eclectic, at times contradictory, and often confusing formulations of the self. Philosophers and other interpreters examine Gandhi's writings, privilege specific passages and formulations, and present differing views of Gandhi's philosophy of the self and self-realization. Our account is necessarily brief and inadequate, but presents what, in my view, is most insightful in Gandhi's philosophy and practice relating to selves in pain.

What is clear is Gandhi's major target for understanding our dominant false view of the self, at the basis of so much violence and untruth, and why this false view results in the self and other selves in so much pain. Gandhi's project involves the need to decondition and overcome such a false view of self in order to realize greater relative truth and nonviolence and develop the self in pain closer to what is the Absolute, Self, what is Real.

Throughout his writings, Gandhi focuses on the dominant false view of the self as the separate, autonomous, conditioned, relative, I-me, ego-driven and ego-attached self that is at the heart of our modern economic, political, educational, environmental and other systemic thinking and practices. This false view of self is a primary cause of so much pain in our lives and our world. Gandhi repeatedly claims that this ego-self, socially and contextually constituted, is the false self, the self of untruth and violence. This ego-self separates itself from other selves, other sentient beings and nature; from the unifying truth-force and love-force of *satya* and *ahimsa*; and from the social, ontologically grounded, unifying interconnectedness of the Self, Truth and Reality. Gandhi repeatedly expresses his philosophical project, his ongoing experiments with truth and nonviolence, as transformative with the ideal of reducing the ego-self, with its desires and attachments, to a "cipher" or to "zero". Only when we attempt to reduce our ego-self to zero, through nonattached renunciation and selfless action, can we experience greater relative truth, nonviolence, and the moral and spiritual Self that is an ontological expression of Reality.

In a wide variety of self-formulations, Gandhi frequently distinguishes the false, illusory, violent self from the true moral and spiritual self/Self. In his pluralistic and inclusivistic approach to self and selves in pain, in which Gandhi is attentive to personal and contextual differences and advises others to follow their own experiments with truth, Gandhi presents a wide variety of formulations of self and self-other relations. These differing formulations are often complementary, but they also express ambiguities, tensions, contradictions and unresolved philosophical problems and issues.

What cannot be developed here is my interpretation that Gandhi has at least three major formulations of Self (as used interchangeably with Soul, Truth, God, what is Real). First, Gandhi often affirms the true moral and spiritual self in terms of an inner individual essence, sometimes expressed as "the inner voice", conscience, or the God within each of us. This individual essence is often presented as nonsocial. We are advised to be true to our own inner voice, even in opposing the social. This is the moral and spiritual individual self and should not be confused with the modern Western separate individual. Gandhi often writes that his purified and disclosed individual inner voice, speaking to him in times of crisis and providing him with moral guidance, is used interchangeably with conscience, what is moral, Truth, God and Self. It is often not clear to me how Gandhi can justify some of his individual-essence self-formulations epistemologically, morally and ontologically.

Second, Gandhi sometimes expresses his personal preference for the impersonal, universal, unifying, pure Absolute Self or Soul that can be identified with the Hindu Advaita (nondualistic) Vedantic *Atman*. As was seen in our treatment of Absolute Truth, this is consistent with the Upanishadic monistic identification of *Brahman* (Being, Reality) with *Atman*, the Self that frees us from the illusory self in pain. A major difficulty in providing a coherent systematic formulation of Gandhi approaches arises from the fact that he not only rejects much of the traditional pure monism, with his primary emphasis on relative truth and selves in pain, but he also claims to believe in *dvaita* or dualistic approaches. In thousands of passages, he formulates a non-monistic approach, often in *bhakti* devotional contexts, in which he affirms his belief in a transcendent God or deities, and in which self/Self is realized through its moral and spiritual relation to the divine Absolute Reality.

Third, Gandhi usually expresses his philosophical approach to the self and self in pain by affirming the self as social and relational. His focus on moral philosophy as first philosophy and his understanding of the Hindu concept of *dharma* as ethical and social duty and obligation shape this approach to the self. For Gandhi, I am self only in relation to the other; the relational other is an essential part of my self-identity and dynamic open-ended process of self-development.

Sometimes Gandhi expresses his approach to the social and relational self by emphasizing the Hindu concept of *swabhava* (*svabhava*, one's essence or self-nature), our individual, unique, physical, mental and social nature and contextual situatedness. This is a dynamic approach in which we are born into this world with our own nature, not some universal static view of human nature, and we then develop and realize our individual self-nature through our social interactions and relations with others.

Gandhi's primary focus on an open-ended, social, contextualized approach to self and selves in pain is consistent with his approach to the complex relative–absolute relations informed by his truthful and nonviolent social ontological moves. Recognizing that the relational other is an integral part of my open-ended and contextualized self-identity and process of self-development is consistent with his ontological formulations of the interconnectedness of all of life. Situated and contextualized selves in pain—experiencing poverty, exploitation, hatred, fear and insecurity, lacking economic, political, spiritual freedom, etc.—make a moral demand on me, oblige me to act, as integral to my moral and spiritual self-nature and transformative development as a self in pain.

This is clearly expressed in most of Gandhi's experiments with truth, nonviolent and truthful actions, struggles and campaigns. It is most clearly expressed in his famous "Talisman" advising the confused and lost self in pain how to act morally and spiritually: Think of the other self in pain you may have experienced with the greatest suffering and least freedom, ask which of your possible actions will do the most to alleviate that person's pain and contribute to that person's self-determining freedom, and then your doubts will melt away. Responding to the needs of the other situated self in pain, as integral to your own self-nature, is Gandhi's major social relational response for moral and spiritual development and greater realization of Self, Truth, Nonviolence and Love, and God.

Our formulations of Gandhi's philosophical approach to the self, in terms of his approach to truth/Truth, nonviolence/Nonviolence and self/Self, do not resolve all philosophical difficulties in his philosophy and practices relating to the self and selves in pain. Consider one serious challenge to the above dynamic social relational formulation. Granted, one can use Gandhi's analysis to make considerable sense of relative untruths, causing and perpetuating selves in pain, when I do not embrace the relational other as integral to my self-nature and moral and spiritual development. I then act in ways that violate the social, ontological, interconnected and unified nature of Reality. As seen in the above formulation, illustrated by Gandhi's Talisman, one can also use this open-ended, contextualized, social relational approach to make sense of the moral and spiritual process for lessening the pain of situated selves and for the greater realization of relative truth and relative nonviolence, acting in ways consistent with Gandhi's social ontology.

But how does one adequately justify the key claim that there is an integral relation between the social relational self and the Self (Truth, Being, God, what is ontologically Real)? When we formulated Gandhi's approach to relative truth and Absolute Truth and their integral relation, we noted this same kind of serious challenge, along with some of Gandhi's possible responses.

Illustrations of this challenge to Gandhi's social self–Self relation can be seen throughout Gandhi's life and writings. As consistent with Gandhi's epistemological, moral and ontological emphasis on a basic interconnected unity with a respect for differences, he attempts to empathize with and show respect for the diverse situated views and practices of other selves in pain. He advises other selves in pain to follow their own inner voices, their own paths to truth/Truth, commensurate with their own personalities and cultural, religious and other contextualized structures, traditions, and developing situatedness.

However, this Gandhi approach does not express some unlimited facile relativism in which Gandhi accepts that selves are simply formulating their own differing narratives about self, Self and self–Self-relations with no larger criteria for evaluating their positions. For all of his pluralistic tolerance, respect for other approaches and views that I should be open to other truths for deepening my own understanding, Gandhi knows that other selves in pain claim to hear inner voices and divine voices that are violent and are voices of untruth; these social relational views of self are often responsible for so much untruth and violence. Therefore, how does Gandhi relate to other selves in pain that reject his approach to self, to Self and to his integral self–Self-relations?

Gandhi struggles with such relations with Hindu, Muslim, Christian, *Dalit* ("Untouchables," the downtrodden), women, British and other selves in pain. With his primary focus on practice and moral living, this challenge is never merely intellectual in refuting false views of self. He believes in the need for the organic, harmonious, integrated self as mind-body-heart (or soul) unity, and he formulates many innovative techniques and actions for relating to and transforming selves in pain expressing violent and untruthful values and actions. As seen earlier, he often goes beyond rational arguments and embraces other means, such as voluntary suffering that aims at touching the heart of the other and moving the other toward greater truth/Truth and nonviolence/Nonviolence. He promotes nonviolent noncooperation and resistance that aim at exposing and preventing the continuation of the untruth and violence, and he promotes his Constructive Programme that aims at providing nonviolent and truthful alternatives.

6.7 Concluding Suggestion: The Self in Pain as Constituted Given

We conclude this essay by merely suggesting a philosophical approach to self and self in pain as a constituted given. This may serve as a catalyst for developing our earlier formulations.

It is tempting to approach the self in pain in ways similar to modern empiricism and other recent approaches. We start with the basic experiential data of the self in pain as foundational and as a given. In our human mode of being in the world, Shankara, Bentham, Gandhi, and I experience our selves in pain. There are basic genetic, biological, environmental and other scientific "facts". If I place my hand in the fire, I feel pain; if I go into the freezing Atlantic Ocean waters during a Maine winter, I will soon experience painful life-threatening hypothermia; if I have certain allergies and eat certain foods, I will experience painful migraine headaches.

These experiential givens of the self in pain also include all kinds of contextualized structures and variables. Consider the typical situation of a social relational self that is socialized into a given status quo structured world, in which family, community and other social bonds have been destroyed, and in which one is bombarded by endless nonsocial and antisocial ego-driven rewards and punishments. Such a social relational self, situated and objectified in a given world one has not constituted, typically experiences an alienated, untruthful and violent self in pain.

Now it is tempting to formulate true and false views of self in pain as constructed from such experienced givens that then need to be analysed, interpreted and developed. Such an approach to self in pain is oversimplified and inadequate.

A more adequate philosophical approach to self focus on the self in pain as a constituted given. There is a phenomenological givenness revealed in our situated experiences of pain. But even at the experiential level of the self in pain, this experienced givenness is usually dynamic, perspectival, complex, hidden and overt, prereflective as well as conscious and shaped by all kinds of presuppositions and dominant structures and variables. This givenness, largely constituted for us by others, is both limiting and also enabling in our relating to the self and other selves in pain.

Therefore, it is necessary for our philosophical approach to examine how we filter through a dynamic, open-ended, relational, contextualized, social ontology our experience of a complex phenomenological sense of givenness, which is given to us without closure and always requires that we constitute its meaning and significance. It is in terms of the self and other selves in pain as constituted givens that we can develop our understanding of the situated social relational self, the idealized Self as experientially based and involving an imaginative, idealized construction and the self–Self-relations that can lessen the pain and allow for greater moral development and self-realization.

Part II
Culture, Politics and Ethics of Pain

Hurt

Daniel M. Becker

Email: DMB2Y@hscmail.mcc.virginia.edu

She hurts *here, and here, and here,* she's tender everywhere
except where I want her to be tender,
where the resident said she was tender.

It's a 4 hour drive to get here she says, *plus an hour to park,*
in her own defense for being an hour late.
We offer her a shot where it hurts the most. *Numbing medicine.*

She counter-offers: *something to get me through the night.*
I show her the print out with dates, locations and numbers of pills
where someone with her first, middle, and last names,

someone with her date of birth, had received three times
last month a one month supply of what she's asking for now.
She says *the nights are the worst.*

Then she blinks and begins to weep. She's right about the night.
The resident looks at me, I look around for the *Kleenex.*
It's 50:50 they're there when you need them.

I make a drawing of pain going up and pain coming down
and different pains not bumping into one another.
The X's are where the Rx's work, roadblocks

to redirect the traffic. Maybe it's worth sharing
a little neuroscience: *the MRI of pain looks different*
than the MRI of suffering, sunrise versus sunset different;

some kitchen table wisdom too—*loss needs grief*;
no—from the look on her face—*we're not saying it's all in the head,*
even though it mostly is, up there between the sounds,

behind the sights, above each whiff, but also where
and what we touch, what touches us, how in and in between
each breath, each gasp, there's a fear of drowning;

finally, getting to causes and effects, *post hoc*—
after getting rear-ended for instance—
doesn't mean it's *proctor hoc*. Not all of it. Not the part

that never sleeps. Meanwhile, there still isn't any *Kleenex.*
If I were on the *JCAHCO* inspection team,
Joint National Commission for the Accreditation

of Health Care Organizations, pronounced *Jake-O*,
I'd put facial tissue on the checklist.
But it's not just timely gestures we can't always offer.

The patients try to be patient with me, and the residents
act as if they listen, but the teaching evaluations don't lie,
nor the patient satisfaction surveys that manage

to equate good care with how easy it is to park.
It has not escaped our attention how many flat tires occur
on the way to being late again at clinic.

I'm surprised there aren't more.
If, as Pasteur said, *chance favors the prepared mind,*
then misfortune shadows the helpless.

Pain attracts pain. The pain it paineth every day.
Stroke it and it tingles, burns, and bristles.
It hurts to stand, to sit, to squat, to lie, to get out of bed,

to think about getting out of the bed.
Morphine receptors stop receiving, numbing medicine
won't numb, more meds make it worse

and no meds make it worse. Addicts get pain too,
they get cancer, bones get cancer. On rounds we ask,
as required by JCAHCO, *on a pain scale of 1 to 10*

what number would be you? The patient curls up in a ball.
He shuts his eyes. He's teaching himself to disappear.
He clutches a button that leads to morphine,

a button shaped like a joystick. No offense to JCAHCO
but there are only three sizes of pain, like the three bears.
The large size takes up all the space in the room,

it ignores time—a minute takes a minute and a half—
but it's never late. He opens an eye and shakes his head *no.*
His wife complains that's all he ever talks about.

It wouldn't hurt to change the subject? As if something else
could matter. Not in this world.
Someone's mother tucked into a death bed

surrounded by statues of saints? She's paying dues,
paying ahead, keeping a large balance, a down payment
just in case for getting out of limbo. Her son complains

she will not take the Percocet. He rattles the bottle.
In the documentary a man smiles at the camera
while ironing. No irony intended. He's teaching us how

to learn from adversity. On a scale of 1 to 10
he's smooth as silk. You'd trust him with your shirts.
Ironing, a mind-body practice that happens not to be

an ancient form of self-defense, takes his mind off
all those pins and needles. Recall that pain
is different from suffering. Our clinic patient is here

to share her pain. Everyone in range feels her pain.
Her family, her neighbors, the scary guy who brought her,
the guy with knuckles tattooed 1 through 10.

He's right about the gothic font. He gives us the look,
the look that includes our parents and our children,
our fancy schools, our knowledge and experience,

the limits of our knowledge and experience,
our sad white coats, our haunted white coats.
The robot in *The Day the Earth Stood Still* look,

its visor about to open, its beam about to melt everything
in the straight line it travels. I thank him for changing her tire.
If I had to drive 4 hours to see a doctor whose body language

wishes the spare was flat too, my look, a curious look
with skeptical syntax, would delete the parking garage
and type in valet parking. It would look up in wonder

and ask no one in particular: *it wouldn't hurt to wash the windows?*
It would look down and notice weeks of what the pigeons left
then mention such in the after visit survey.

My look would take a picture, make a slide, put together
a PowerPoint presentation that includes statistics
of prescription drug abuse and accidental overdose.

The residents come and listen, there's free lunch
and to give them credit, they're curious to learn
how people who hurt for a living hurt.

Chapter 7
The Infinite Faces of Pain: Narrative, *Eros*, and Ethics

David B. Morris

> *No moral theory can be adequate if it does not take into account the narrative character of our experience.*
> —Mark Johnson, *Moral Imagination* (1993: 11)[*].

Abstract This chapter begins by affirming the medical distinction between acute pain and chronic pain. It then discusses pain within a theoretical framework that divides illness between two large forces: *medical eros* and *medical logos*. While *medical logos* incorporates the familiar reason-based scientific molecular gaze of contemporary biomedicine, *medical eros* is an unfamiliar term that refers to the various ways that desire is expressed in the context of medicine, health, and illness. The chapter builds an argument holding that eros (or desire) and narrative have a crucial, connected role to play in the medical understanding and treatment of pain. This role is especially important for ethics. Bioethics is traditionally a discipline in which principles are the main focus. In an extended discussion of the 1944 film *The Great Moment*—which dramatizes the discovery of surgical anesthesia—the chapter concludes with an argument, based on the work of philosopher Emanuel Levinas, in which pain becomes a key test case for an ethics that sees in "the face" an image or metaphor for the infinite otherness of the other person. *Medical eros* thus serves to promote an ethics of pain opposed to the engineered and incidental facelessness of much contemporary medicine—and life.

Keywords Pain · Ethics · Bioethics · Eros · Emotion · The face

[*]My thanks for the invitation to revisit, to revise, and to rethink writing published in various sources over a dozen years. See especially *The Culture of Pain* (1991) and "Narrative, ethics, and pain: Thinking *with* stories" (2002).

D.B. Morris (✉)
University of Virginia, Charlottesville, USA
e-mail: dbmkirk@me.com

© Springer India 2016
S.K. George and P.G. Jung (eds.), *Cultural Ontology of the Self in Pain*, DOI 10.1007/978-81-322-2601-7_7

Medicine is the professional discipline to which modern cultures have formally or informally assigned the knowledge and treatment of pain, and in recent years have seen the creation of an entire subspecialty called pain medicine. For better or worse, pain is now enfolded securely within a medical frame regardless of its importance across the spectrum of contemporary culture, from law enforcement to cinema. Much of the writing about pain today, however, especially when it emerges from the social sciences or humanities, takes no account of the crucial medical distinction between acute pain and chronic pain. It may be true that a rose is a rose is a rose, but there are more than one hundred species of roses, and the distinction between acute pain and chronic pain is extremely important, outside as well as inside medicine. It matters enormously whether your model for pain is the hyperintense, almost blinding and world-obliterating acute pain of torture, with its political subtexts, or the unremitting low-level intractable ache of nonspecific low back pain. Psychological as well as physiological effects will differ too in ways that make the medical context crucial for the current discussion. It is now clear that protracted chronic pain produces measurable changes in the brain. In addition, as merely one example, low back pain patients in primary care—according to a study conducted in the western United States—develop their own beliefs about their back pain, about what it means for them, and such beliefs remained "very stable" over the 6-month period studied (Foster et al. 2008). "Common chronic pain conditions affect at least 166 million U.S. adults at a cost of $560–635 billion annually in direct medical treatment costs and lost productivity": so says a report from the prestigious Institute of Medicine (2011). The report calls for nothing short of a "cultural transformation" in how medical professionals understand and treat pain (2011, p. 1).

Medicine, meaning health-care in all its ramifications, accounts for a major global expenditure, and its cultural prominence alone suggests the need to take a medical perspective on pain into account. The World Bank estimates that, as a percentage of GDP, in 2012 total annual health expenditure (the sum of public and private services) ran at 17.9 % in the United States, 9.4 % in the United Kingdom, and 4.0 % in India. Even on purely economic or cultural grounds, it is important to consider a medical perspective on pain. Medicine, however, has been notably ineffective in dealing with the near epidemic of chronic pain—an epidemic especially noticeable in the developed world—so the timing is auspicious for a dialogue of medical and nonmedical voices. The Institute of Medicine, for example, in its call for a "cultural transformation" in the understanding and treatment of pain includes among its primary recommendations to healthcare specialists something like a game-changing proposal: to "promote and enable self-management of pain." In effect, the representatives of Western biomedicine (which I call *medical logos*) are saying explicitly that doctors must help patients *to manage their own pain*. Such self-management of pain might well find limited but crucial assistance in the everyday resources and neglected powers of what I describe—here and in a forthcoming book provisionally entitled *Eros and Illness*—as *medical eros*.

Medical eros, or erotic desire as expressed in a medical context, is certainly an unfamiliar concept, and it thus requires an extended discussion both to clarify what is unfamiliar and to confront the real and implicit dangers. At the onset it is enough to consider *medical eros* as simply referring to the numerous occasions, from the emotions surrounding childbirth to deathbed reconciliations and impassioned memorial services, when desire, feeling, affection, and their emotional surrogates accompany and even interpenetrate the experience of pain and illness. There is strategic value in a concept, however vaguely defined, that as yet has no official standing in medicine and whose meaning is still open to negotiation. Medicine after all specializes in a lexicon that remains opaque to outsiders. *Medical eros* reverses this process by opening up both medicine and everyday understanding to a concept that embraces nonrational, emotional, and sociocultural aspects (Morris 2010). Eros as it impinges upon illness certainly takes forms that are sometimes hazardous: a good reason to account for it. Western biomedicine, however, proves almost entirely unwilling to take it into account at all, doubtless in part because eros carries us beyond what many cultures regard as rational, sensible, measurable, and ultimately knowable. Eros notoriously traffics with the irrational, the nonsensical, the immeasurable, and the uncontainable, the unknown—carrying us away often despite our better judgment. Scientific biomedicine has every right to insist on operating within its chosen limits as defined by evidence, reason, and logic. Trial lawyers wait to pounce if it does not. Here I want to open up the understanding of pain to forces that lie just beyond or, like blind spots, concealed within the purview of *medical logos*. Pain, from this perspective, leads us less toward psychology than toward ethics.

7.1   *Medical Eros*: Pain and *La vie intérieure*

"A threshold has been crossed," writes sociologist Nikolas Rose, Director of the BIOS Centre for the Study of Bioscience, Biomedicine, Biotechnology and Society at the London School of Economics and Political Science, and the particular threshold is what he calls "a molecular vision of life" (2007, pp. 7, 4). Biomedicine places us if not exactly in a new world order—we have grown accustomed to medical near-miracles —at least well into a future when *medical logos* (as the institutional practice of a molecular vision of life) holds power over human affairs comparable to the role of theology in the Middle Ages. Unprecedented advances in technology, including biotechnology, now enmesh humans with computerized machines and with altered forms of life, ranging from genetically modified foods to clones and cyborgs, propelling us rapidly into an uncharted era that some are already calling *post-human* (Sharon 2014). Eros too has changed in the new age of biotechnology, as befits a born shape-shifter, beginning in 1954 (to be exact) with human experiments using oral progesterone—leading directly to The Pill, as the early female contraceptive was known, and to the sexual revolution of the 1960s. Eros adapts with seeming ease to ever-new technologies, from drugs to treat erectile dysfunction to hard-core porn at the click of a mouse. Sexuality, while clearly relevant to a study of pain, is not, however, what limits or defines the broad field of experience that we call erotic.

Eros is simply not identical with sex or sexuality, despite their many areas of correlation or overlap. "Sexual reproductive activity is common to sexual animals and men," writes Georges Bataille, the chief modern theorist of eros, "but only men appear to have turned their sexual activity into erotic activity" (1986, p. 11). Although this basic distinction requires extensive discussion, Bataille nonetheless accurately locates a bedrock for all subsequent analysis when he distinguishes eroticism from sex. Eros, as Bataille indicates, shares common ground with sexual activity, but erotic life also extends to distant and indirect psychological inflections of desire. A sonnet sequence, emails, a certain smile, breast-feeding, the way a man or woman crosses the room, even a lullaby under the right circumstances can be erotic. Consciousness matters for eros as much as erogenous zones, while the free play of mind provides an indispensable, and even self-sufficient erotic experience. "Human eroticism," as Bataille nails down the crucial point, "differs from animal sexuality precisely in this, that it calls inner life [*la vie intérieure*] into play" (1986, p. 29).

A diagram risks obvious self-parody, of course, in offering geometric patterns to clarify an inherently disorderly force, but as a simplified descriptive schema—like weather maps—even a self-parodic diagram can help to provide a basic alignment while also suggesting why a brief definition cannot avoid misrepresentation. Think of eros, then, as a libidinal energy in humans that (played out in consciousness or inner life) suffuses, in degrees, such disparate states as lust, love, empathy, and violence (Fig. 7.1).

The diagram—since it cannot appear in three dimensions spinning like a pinwheel—should embed a poison pill or kill switch for use when the explanatory apparatus grows too clear. It nonetheless recognizes that eros, in certain extreme states, dissolves into or makes contact with energies that also circulate entirely *outside* eros. Violence can be wholly unerotic, of course, but it is hard to explain the history of warfare, human sacrifice, and ritual cruelty without positing an erotic pleasure within at least certain violent cultural behaviors. The vicious philosophical sexuality in Sade belongs to eros, for example, while mindless brutality loses all

Fig. 7.1 Logos in (doomed) quest to make sense of eros

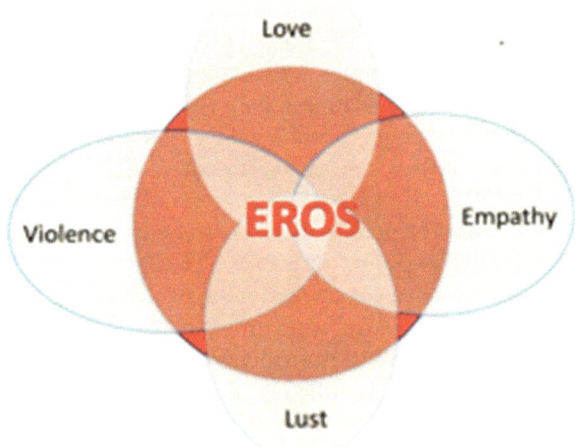

contact with the inner life. Such iffy distinctions and gradations, however, indicate how far *logos* simply falls short of fully *comprehending* eros. Eros, by definition, resists definition. It embraces the *in-definite*, *a-logical*, and *in-comprehensible*. My clock-face diagram allows for at least 56 additional shades of erotic practice, most unnameable and many unpleasant. *Medical eros* needs to maintain vigilance on behalf of patient safety. Nonetheless, pain too, especially chronic pain, often eludes the objective instruments of *medical logos* because, like eros, it remains so hard to disentangle from the vagaries of human consciousness and from the subjectivity of an inner life.

7.2   An Integrative Model of Pain: Narrative, Ethics, and Eros

Medical eros looks at pain in ways that differ from the perspectiveof researchers and clinicians dedicated solely or primarily to a molecular gaze. Pain and everyday trauma, for example, are inseparable from what, in Rose's phrase, "it is to be a biological organism" (2007, p. 17). Acute pain is not necessarily pathological even though it hurts, since the hurt may represent optimum biological function: a message from your nervous system saying *step away from the stove*! Medical reformers have recently rebranded pain as the *fifth vital sign*: equivalent in status to pulse or respiration, which means that hospitals, in order to retain accreditation, must now "chart" (or record) each patient's daily levels of pain. Chronic pain, however, by definition approaches pathological status—often nonstop misery with no redeeming biological function or clear biological cause. Such chronic pain entails possibly permanent neurological damage, as it alters brain pathways, and even constitutes a risk for suicide. In this difficult situation, the challenge for *medical eros* is to understand pain as something more than a vital sign or a technical problem in neurobiology. It is thus worth considering two paramedical resources that, while not incompatible with a molecular gaze, generally fail outside the purview of *medical logos*: narrative and ethics. *Medical eros*, in ways that potentially complement the efforts of *medical logos*, offers an incentive to focus on the particular *stories* we tell about pain and on what pain leads us *to do* or—equally important for ethics—*not do*.

We need to understand what we mean by pain before exploring its relations to narrative and ethics, and it is thus important to recognize that the best authorities in medicine now reject a strictly molecular understanding of pain. The International Association for the Study of Pain (IASP)—the authoritative scientific and medical organization worldwide—defines pain as an "unpleasant sensory and emotional experience associated with actual or potential tissue damage, or described in terms of such damage" (Merskey and Bogduk 1994, p. 210).[1] A quiet revolution is at work within this apparently bland account. The IASP invokes the traditional

---

[1]The IASP definition was first published in 1979.

molecular one-to-one link between pain and tissue damage—described as "noci-ception," or the transmission of neural impulses—only to reconfigure it as a loose network of possibilities. Tissue damage alone is no longer a prerequisite for pain. Expectation alone can suffice. In a study by Bayer et al. (1991), volunteers attached to a stimulator were told that the electrical current might possibly produce a head-ache, but they weren't told that the stimulator was set to produce nothing beyond a low humming sound. The result? Fully half of the volunteers—experiencing no more than the sound of a dull hum—reported pain.

The most important and counterintuitive implication of the new thinking about pain is that there is no longer a sound basis for dividing so-called *mental* pain from *physical* pain. This distinction, which seems to make good common sense, is really a legacy of the erroneous Cartesian split between bodies and minds that most scholars now reject and that cannot survive even a remote brush with eros. (Is sexual attraction *mental* or *physical*?) Pain, like eros, belongs to the conjunction of body and mind. The IASP definition describes pain not only as a sensory phe-nomenon but also, in an historic shift, as an emotional experience. Emotion, as pain specialist Mark D. Sullivan (1996) contends, is intrinsic to pain and not merely a response or a wholly separable add-on. Finally, for die-hards who cling to the distinction between mental and physical pain, which sometimes looks like pure common sense, the IASP adds a note to its *Classification of Chronic Pain* insisting that pain is "always subjective" and "always a psychological state" (Merskey and Bogduk 1994, p. 210). The object of study, if you are studying human pain, is not strictly an objective cellular process—say, a measurable electrochemical signal transmitted from the peripheral nervous system to the brain—but an event of consciousness. "The brain," as neurosurgeon and internationally respected pain specialist John D. Loeser puts it, "is the organ responsible for all pain." "All sensory phenomena," he adds, "including nociception, can be altered by conscious and unconscious mental activity" (1991, pp. 215, 216).

This new vision of pain—with its center in human consciousness—ultimately requires a new integrative model that seeks to combine a micro-level molecular understanding with macro-level psychological and sociocultural explanations. Here is one view—unfortunately static—of what such an integrative model might look like (Fig. 7.2).

The two levels of analysis are not in conflict. From a center of consciousness, the focus moves both inward and outward: inward toward the micro-level processes of cell biology and outward toward the macro-level sociocultural environments: families, nations, religions, media, international foundations and multinational corporations.

Two distinguished pain specialists (Carr and Bradshaw 2014) have argued recently that patients will be better served if medical students focus initially on macro-level sociocultural explanations. Over the last 50 years it has grown ever clearer that chronic pain often responds less well to drugs, surgery, and biomedical treatment than to psychosocial therapies. Many centers now favor a mix of cog-nitive and behavioral approaches. Clearly it represents an advance to understand gout at a micro-level molecular process triggered by high levels of uric acid—not,

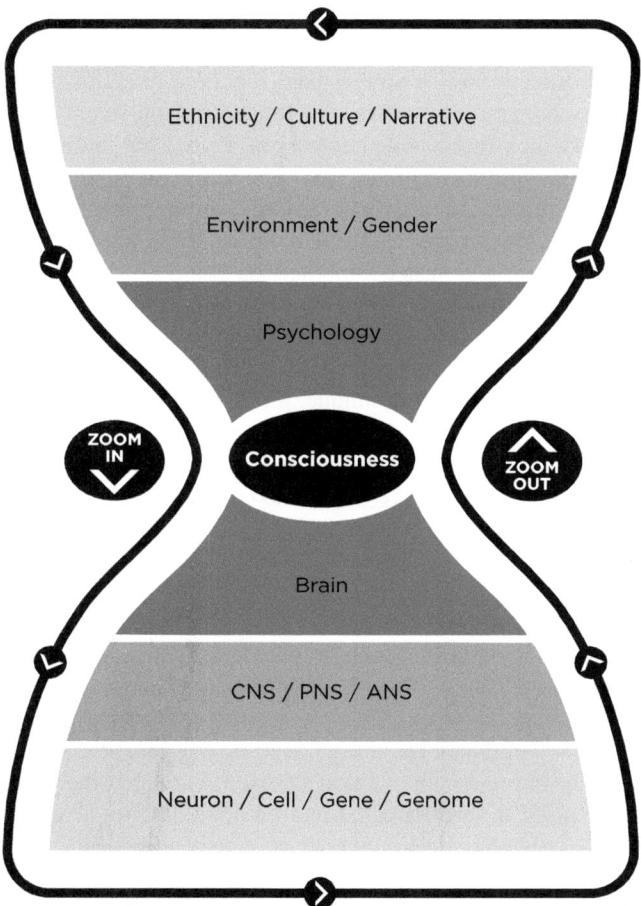

Fig. 7.2 An integrative model of pain. *CNS* Central nervous system. *PNS* Peripheral nervous system. *ANS* Autonomic nervous system

as in the nineteenth century, a moral affliction visited upon the rich idle upper class. Diet, however, is a macro-level sociocultural fact (indirectly dependent on wealth) that directly affects serum uric acid. The intense chronic pain of gout, moreover, especially when at times it accompanies other illnesses, such as life-threatening leukemia, is impossible to disconnect from psychological stresses and fears.

Pain moreover is almost impossible—outside a laboratory or textbook setting—to separate from emotion. Emotion, we might say, is the forgotten or neglected partner in the biocultural construction of pain. Its evident aversiveness does not exhaust the constitutive role of emotion in pain. The brain as the organ responsible for all pain communicates with complex neural networks that include the limbic system and its innumerable varieties of affect. The cultural and personal semantics of pain, then, which includes the deviously unnoticed ways in which pain absorbs

ad hoc or prefabricated meanings, could not achieve its crucial place within individual lives without this intrinsic link with emotion. *The Culture of Pain*, if I might
be allowed a retrospective self-critique, paid too little attention to how emotion
suffuses the experience of pain—not as an extraneous supplement to meaning or to
neurobiology but as their inseparable companion. Pain, even in our stoic denials, is
in effect shot through with feelings that may well linger on the far side of meaning,
pain's inescapable shadow, outside any shared language that might identify the
more subtle or subterranean shades of emotion, as when primary colors dissolve
into countless gradations and pastel combinations that have no name. The emotion
implicit in any semantics of pain—always individualized according to our personal
histories, fears, and desires—is what makes pain far more than just another aversive
event. Pain confronts us with and entangles us in meanings that carry an emotional
charge, explicit or hidden, shared or unique, multiple or singular. It is an emotional
charge absent from an abstract semantics—as in the statement *pain signifies death*
—but constitutive of a personal, embodied, urgent encounter with intense or
chronic pain, bone-deep, perhaps pre-linguistic or post-linguistic in a resonance that
meanings alone cannot adequately encompass: *I feel like I have no place here, I feel
too exhausted to speak, I feel crushed by an overwhelming weight impossible to
bear, I feel like I'm about to die....*

"Our concepts of pain, impairment, and disability," writes pain specialist
Wilbert E. Fordyce, "must consider environmental factors as well as the person"
(1995, p. 4). How might an environmentally sensitive integrative model work in
practice? We know that different cellular processes, for example, cause the stabbing
pain of post-herpetic neuralgia, the queasy pain of migraine, the dull ache of deep
muscle pain, and the burning pain of a skin abrasion. Similarly, the pain of childbirth
generally evokes quite different mental and emotional states than do the intense
facial paroxysms of trigeminal neuralgia, which a noise or breeze can trigger. Anger
and sadness increase pain reports in women, according to a 2010 study by Henriët
van Middendorp et al. Stigma, guilt, and blame affect the long undertreated pain of
people with HIV/AIDS (Breitbart et al. 1996). Undertreatment for pain is a cultural,
not biological, fact: it has nothing to do with the molecular gaze, unless we consider
what that gaze leaves out. Ethnicity, race, and gender influence pain, as a review of
the clinical and experimental literature confirms (Fillingim et al. 2009). In Japan,
chronic low back pain patients are less impaired—in psychological, social, voca-
tional, and avocational function—than similar patients in America (Brena et al.
1990). Pain, in short, is multicausal, with its molecular level open to the combined
influences of culture and of personal belief—as well as to our habits and noncon-
scious lives, from dreams to neuroses. It is irreversibly porous, open to the hubbub of
human social and psychic life, unlike the simple, direct neural mechanism that
Descartes compared to a rope that, when pulled, rings a bell at the other end, as if
pain were no more than a response triggered directly by a stimulus.

A full knowledge of consciousness is not necessary to an understanding that
consciousness establishes a "necessary condition" for human pain. If we turn off
consciousness—as happens under anesthesia, in sleep, or with drugs—there is no
pain to account for. Even in an illness with such a clear biological cause as gout,

consciousness links pain to beliefs, to cultural patterns, to social practices, and to modes of feeling that bring us back ultimately to *medical eros*. Although pleasure and pain at first appear diametrically opposed, pain in a new integrative model remains open to an intersection not only with sociocultural sources of distress but also with unexpected resources of pleasure. An integrative model thus offers an opportunity to explore how *medical eros*—in its attention to inner life—offers new ways to understand the complex interrelations among pain, narrative, and ethics.

7.3 Pain and Erotics of Narrative

Every child knows that stories give pleasure—filmmakers depend on the adult pleasures of narrative to fill cinemas—but it turns out that the brain will produce stories on its own, independently, even in the absence of pleasure. Taylor (2006), a brain neuroanatomist, suffered a massive left-hemispheric stroke that impaired the language processing areas of her brain. As her function gradually returned, she observed that her left brain "enthusiastically manufactured stories that it promoted as the truth." Taylor somewhat fondly refers to her left brain as "my storyteller." She recognized its power to lead her astray: "I learned that I need to be very wary of my storyteller's potential for stirring up drama and trauma" (Taylor 2006, p. 151). *Confabulation* is the term for pathological versions of this unwilled and unreliable narrative stream. As William Hirstein observes, "[t]here is also a clear connection here to the human gift for storytelling" (2005, p. 5). Paralyzed patients after a stroke, for example, sometimes deny their paralysis and confabulate bogus stories to account for their limitations. ("Why can't you lift your left arm?" asks the doctor. Reply: "I've got arthritis in my shoulder.") Such patients are not lying. Narrative simply appears to be a standard function of the human brain when we need an explanation: stories are what our brains *can't help* producing. In an integrative model, then, narrative is not an irrelevant, free-floating fiction, unrelated to human pain, but rather pain and narrative both triangulate through human consciousness, both inextricably somatic and cultural. Moreover, the reception of narrative is as mysteriously biocultural as its coproduction. If we *invent* and *tell* stories much in the way that birds build nests, as an evolutionary function of our brains, why are we also drawn to *hearing* and to *reading* stories? The allure of stories may belong to their primal role in social bonding, like myths for early humans who depended on groups for survival, but we are also doubtless drawn to stories by the same power that draws us to hear a joke or to see a film: an expectation of pleasure. Such pleasure matters especially because narrative holds the power to modify or to intensify pain.

Pleasure for*medicaleros* is hardly a frivolous experience. Eros is built on the desire for pleasure, which is why pain medicine needs to oppose the professional attitude that dismisses pleasure as inherently frivolous, uninteresting, and far less significant than, say, knowledge. Charon (2001), for example, in a ground-breaking article articulates the role of stories in medicine as offering "narrative knowledge." Her subtitle, it is important to note, also highlights the role of narrative in creating empathy and trust, but her cogent defense of narrative does not go so far as to defend pleasure. For an article published in JAMA, the corporate headquarters of *medical logos*, it makes strategic good sense to emphasize knowledge. Eros, on the other hand, makes no excuses for pleasure, which needs no defense. Pleasure may be hard to justify to funding agencies as a legitimate research agenda. It surely offers at times merely private rewards and fragmentary insights, as well as opportunities to run completely off the tracks. Isn't that why fundamentalists too so often warn against the dangers of pleasure? Pleasure, however, remains a primary force both in human action and in our taste for stories. French theorist Roland Barthes in *The Pleasure of the Text* (1973) characterizes the two main kinds of literary response as *plaisir* and *jouissance*. *Plaisir* (or garden-variety reading pleasure) he describes as the emotional response to texts that follow conventional patterns of syntax and meaning, like a newspaper or a fable. These texts he calls "readerly." The most intense and worthiest enjoyment, however, Barthes reserves for code-breaking, unconventional, indeterminate, so-called "writerly" texts that scramble syntax and resist clear meanings. The term that he applies to such heady pleasures—*jouissance*—covers in French both general bliss and sexual orgasm.

Thinking *with* stories, a crucial concept that I borrow from sociologist Arthur W. Frank, does not qualify as orgasmic, but it identifies a pleasure-based process very different from the operations of analytical reason (2013, pp. 23–25). Stories, from our earliest years, are little engines of pleasure. Yes, they are the product of mental operations with a complex underlying brain science (Herman 2013). From fairy-tale giants and elves to grown-up *cinéma vérité*, however, we are drawn to stories not from duty—not even a social obligation to stay up-to-date—but from off-duty desires for enjoyment. While thinking *with* stories, then, clearly involves reason in the process of cognition, it also involves a pleasurable collaboration with feeling often absent when narrative is identified as an object of study. Research clearly shows that the ancient Western binary habit that puts reason and emotion into opposing categories is a neurological mistake, with crucial implications both for narrative and for ethics (Damasio 1994). Work in cognitive neuroscience and brain imaging indicates how reason and emotion *collaborate*, so that the concept of thinking *with* stories (as a process involving both reason and feeling) in effect challenges the institutionalized academic practice of thinking or reasoning *about* stories, in which stories are both objectified and also artificially cleansed of their emotional power—since emotion and pleasure have been already automatically marginalized as that which keeps us from thinking straight. Thinking *with* stories, by contrast, is a zigzag, combinatorial, or sideways process less alien to medicine that many think. Clinical professor of psychiatry and best-selling author Kramer (2013) asks why doctors need stories, and he proposes that stories serve as corrective to the narrowed focus on *medical logos*. "Beyond its roles as illustration, affirmation, hypothesis-builder and low-level guidance for practice," he writes in a *New York Times* opinion piece, "storytelling can act as a modest counterbalance to a straitened understanding of evidence." Hunter (1991) has written at book length about the narrative structure of medical knowledge. Equally important, however, thinking *with* stories is a process in which we, as thinkers, do not so much work on narrative as, almost in a return to childhood experience, take a radical step back and allow narrative to work on *us*. The step back—a philosophical move with major significance for Heidegger—has particularlyimportant implications for bioethics as a discipline where, traditionally, reason and analysis rule. Is it just possible, following the path of*medicaleros*, that ethical action might depend less on principles, reason, analytics, evidence, and objectivity than on responding to a dilemma with the emotion-rich cognition that thinking *with* stories might engage?

7.4 Pain and Narrative Ethics: Three Probes

A young contemporary male Apache interviewedby anthropologist Keith H. Basso offers a refreshingly nonacademic and a-theoretical view of how stories can affect us, even in an ethical dimension. "That story is working on you now," he tells Basso. "You keep thinking about it. That story is changing you now, making you want to live right. That story is making you want to replace yourself" (1996, p. 59). Basso's purpose is to show how the Apache people today in the American southwest still inhabit a local world where the landscape is richly endowed with narrative meaning. Even a passing or oblique reference to specific places (such as Line-of-White-Rocks or Red-Ridge-with-Alder-Trees) instantly evokes tales of what supposedly happened there. As Basso demonstrates, in Navajo culture, where custom dictates an avoidance of direct rebuke for misconduct, these narratives provide unobtrusive but steady moral guidance. Family members might indirectly correct a child with an oblique reference to a specific place—a place that evokes the stories embedded there, including their implicit moral content. Such stories have almost literally gotten under your skin if they make you want to act better or "to replace yourself." Narrative and pleasure collaborate here in the service of ethics.

The stunning concept of stories that make you want to replace yourself might underwrite an entire ethics of narrative. Stories from this perspective are not casual entertainment, fictions, an escape into fantasy but rather—as Jean-François Lyotard and Jean-Loup Thébaud claim concerning the Cashinahua Indians of the upper Amazon—they are experiences that incur an obligation (1985, pp. 32–35). Such stories exert on the listener a kind of "call.' The moral "call of stories"—in the phrase used by psychologist Coles (1990)—is hardly restricted to indigenous peoples in remote locations. Coles describes how stories exercise a moral force among patients and students living in contemporary Cambridge. A few philosophers from Aristotle to Iris Murdoch and Mark Johnson have staked a serious claim for stories in engaging what we might call the moral imagination. There is even an emerging scholarly literature devoted to a so-called "narrative ethics."[2] Ample

---

[2]See, for example, Ellos (1994), Newton (1995), Lindemann (1997), Chambers (1999), Charon and Montelllo (2002) and Montello (2014).

precedent thus exists for challenging the still dominant approach that regards stories and narrative as either trivial products of the entertainment industry or as artifacts so complex, self-contradictory, and indeterminate that they require extended scholarly analysis. *Medical eros*, in a zigzag contribution to bioethics, might ask instead how narrative and its pleasures engage the always more than strictly rational processes by which stories work on us.

"Once upon a time," write physician Howard Brody and scholar Mark Clark, creating their own metanarrative about stories, "medicine dismissed narrative as unimportant and uninteresting" (2014: S7). Their own "state of the field" report accurately describes an increasing recent medical interest in narrativebioethics. The momentum owes much, as I have indicated, to the ground-breaking inquiries of University of Calgary sociologist Arthur Frank, as well as to the work of Rita Charon, as founding director of the program in Narrative Medicine at the Columbia University College of Physicians and Surgeons for which she is founding director. The new interest in narrative also involves a growing recognition that the dominant approach in medical ethics—known as principlism, or the four-principle approach —cannot provide a system of universally binding moral standards. Autonomy, beneficence, non-maleficence, and justice are certainly fine concepts, but they mean different things in different cultures, and, in particular instances, they may well enter into mutual conflict. Do they contain the power to make you want to replace yourself?

Principlism and its four pillars are still invoked with scriptural authority as the moral absolutes applicable to any medical dilemma, but they have also coincided with a long period marked by the widespread, systemic medical undertreatment for pain (Rich 1997). Fine principles do not necessarily lead to the ethical treatment of pain. Of course, it is hard to imagine any ethics surviving in a complete absence of principle. Mark Johnson from a perspective of cognitive semantics, argues that principles are best understood not as the products of pure reason but as "crystallizations of the insights that emerge out of a people's ongoing experience" (1993, p. 105). Tom L. Beauchamp and James F. Childress, coauthors of the bible of principlism, *Principles of Biomedical Ethics*, in effect agree, stating in the (1994) fourth edition: "These principles initially derive from considered judgments in the common morality and medical tradition…" (p. 37). The claims of pure reason, then, are increasingly difficult to uphold today, while scholars and theorists are now building a respected place for narrative ethics not as a replacement for principles but as a complementary, supplemental, or corrective discourse. The issues at stake for patients and families, however, might be translated into a very pragmatic question. How can narrativebioethics and *medical eros* help us understand and treat pain?

The process of thinking *with* stories might well begin, like lunar explorations, with a probe: two story probes, in fact. Recently I attended a medical school symposium on pain and ethics. I won't tell the whole story, but the procession of speakers concluded with the chair of anesthesiology. He spoke gravely about the burdensome demands on his budget and staff, citing multiple troubles that included university cutbacks in funding and state directives about mandatory care for the poor. His measured tones and visible integrity left me unprepared for his sweeping conclusion. When it comes to the treatment of pain in his department, he stated as an absolute deadpan matter of fact, "it is no longer possible to do the right thing."

This probe offers a revealing glimpse into the ethics of postmodernpain. The dilemma is distinctively postmodern not in embracing doubt, irony, contingent plural truths, or unresolvable indeterminacy. The speaker assumes, with an old-fashioned nonrelativist certainty, that he knows exactly what *the right thing* to do is, and he knows with equal certainty that doing the right thing is now impossible. What makes the dilemma distinctively postmodern is that reason, principle, and traditional moral agency all seem at an impasse. The speaker's impersonal construction ("it is no longer possible") suggests that this particular quandary does not concern the failure of specific moral agents—anesthesiologists or university administrators—but, on the contrary, it concerns the insignificance of individual moral agency and the irrelevance of personal choice. The problem lies instead with inflexible institutions and impersonal systems. An ethics responsive to such a distinctively postmodern dilemma may require tools as unfamiliar to biomedicine and to *medical logos* as inquiries into narrative point of view or into the dialogics of values-based decision-making. The chair of anesthesiology in effect identifies a point where ethics involves more than reasoning clearly about fixed principles: it also involves, in complex ways that his blunt one-line story encapsulates, the stories we tell and how they affect us.

Probe two concerns a story in the *New York Times* about a California Medicaid patient, Mrs. Ozzie Chavez. The necessary backstory, however, requires a brief comment on medical insurance and narrative patterns. Narrative, that is, especially in structuralist analysis, can often be reduced to a basic pattern: for example, boy meets girl, boy loses girl, boy gets girl. (The names and details are fungible.) Pain, moreover, is now often connected with medical insurance. This complicated social system as it applies to disability insurance could be reduced, at a structural level, to a mini-narrative: you have insurance, you get hurt, you get paid. Like most developed nations, Scandinavian countries face rapidly mounting claims for pain associated with automobile accidents. In Lithuania, however, where drivers had recourse to no such mini-narrative, studies showed no significant difference between accident victims and a control group in reports of headache and neck pain (Schrader and Obelieniene 1996). Chronic whiplash syndrome, it appears, is at least partly the artifact of social narratives about accident insurance. In the United States, a prestigious taskforce studied fast-rising workers' compensation payments for chronic pain. Chronic pain *in the absence of an organic lesion*, it concluded, should not be classified as a medical disability eligible for compensation but instead should be reclassified as "activity intolerance" (Fordyce 1995, p. xiii). *Activity intolerance* is clearly not a diagnosis but a slightly tone-deaf counter-narrative constructed in opposition to the dominant social narrative that offers disability status, cash payments, and freedom from work in exchange for medically certified chronic pain.

Narrative bioethicsmay demonstrate its value precisely in illuminating the conflicts native to every local world where moral action is no longer a choice of virtue or right action but rather concerns the shifting points of contact where powerful social narratives intersect with personal narrative identities or life stories.

The social narrative of disability not only entails large economic costs, often questionable, but also impedes medical treatment if the cash becomes an incentive for patients to retain pain (Mendelson 1992; Teasell 2001). Today, the personal narratives that we live out increasingly come into conflict with powerful social narratives—beyond the control or even the knowledge of individuals—that establish trajectories for patients as damaging as the ethically obtuse, nineteenth century narratives of hysteria.

Mrs. Ozzie Chavez—to return to probe two—met the income threshold at which obstetrical expenses were covered under the Medicaid program. Whatever medical circumstances attended the process of childbirth thus belonged to a familiar, predictable social narrative. The dilemma: Mrs. Chavez was refused a fairly standard form of anesthesia in labor because she did not pay an additional (and illegal) fee demanded in advance by the anesthesiologist. "I'm not a wimp when it comes to pain...," she told the *Times* reporter afterwards. "But it was a very painful delivery" (Pear 1999). Such demands for additional payment were not uncommon because of California's well-known substandard Medicaid reimbursement policies, so this encounter is more than simply a medical "horror story" about greedy doctors—a recognizable narrative subgenre—but the experience of Mrs. Chavez also offers a snapshot of under-medication for pain well-documented across various healthcare systems. "The anesthesiologist wouldn't even come into the room until she got her money," Mrs. Chavez is reported as saying. "I was lying there having contractions, and they wouldn't give me an epidural. I felt like an animal."

Narrative bioethics will not get to the bottom of this event—expose the bedrock truth about what really happened in Mrs. Chavez's room—but it helps to illuminate the conflicting narratives, personal and social, that define her experience. Bioethicist Tod Chambers reminds us that every narrative is "constructed": there is no such thing as a transparent narration that gives us all the facts and nothing but the facts. As Chambers explains:

> Every telling of a story—real or imagined—encompasses a series of choices about what will be revealed, what will be privileged, and what will be concealed; there are no artless narrations. All stories are shaped by a particular teller for a particular purpose, for all narratives are infected by their situatedness (1996, p. 25).

Narrative bioethics reminds us that all our responses to Mrs. Chavez' plight also partake of this *situatedness*. The American Society of Anesthesiologists ran an account about Mrs. Chavez in its newsletter that elicited one response from a member, who (according to the Times report) wrote: "Poor people can't expect to drive a Rolls Royce or to eat in a fine French restaurant, so why should they expect to receive the Cadillac of analgesics for free?" As if to head off a public relations disaster, John B. Neeld, Jr., president of the American Society of Anesthesiologists, deftly situated the talk in a direction away from fancy cars and restaurants and aimed directly toward principles. "It's unethical," he asserted, invoking one of the hallowed pillars of principlism, "to withhold services because of reimbursement." End of story?

A narrative bioethics—attentive to situations and emotions—would not regard the case closed when one character invokes a hallowed principle. Why was it invoked? Whose interest did the invocation serve? Narrative thrives on conflict, and narrative bioethics can helpfully illuminate the conflicts that stories thrive on. Moreover, all stories include gaps—no narrative tells *everything*—and so a narrative bioethics might stress the gaps in our knowledge of Mrs. Chavez, John Neeld, Jr., and the unnamed anesthesiologist. Not-knowing, that is, matters as much in ethics as in law, where it is important to recognize not only to what is said but also what may be unsaid. Or unsayable. Marxist narratologist Pierre Macherey insists that ideologies always make some statements unsayable, if not unthinkable, much as Victorian ideologies of gender produced *the love that dare not speak its name* (1978, pp. 77–78). John Neeld doesn't say (is it almost *unsayable*?) that, according to the American Pain Society (1995), pain relief is withheld daily in America—and not just for inability to pay. Fifty percent of dying hospitalized patients spend at least half their time in moderate to severe pain (SUPPORT Principal Investigators 1995). Such medical undertreatment for pain has been well-known for many years, despite prinicplism and do-no-harm, but its ethical implications have gone largely ignored even among bioethicists (Rich 1997). A narrative bioethics is concerned not to assign blame but to elucidate the stories in such a way that, when all the voices are heard, it is possible to do the right thing.

Narrative bioethics in effectgives*medicaleros* a significant role in protecting the sick and in redressing injustices that work special hardships on the ill. A focus on feeling and on situatedness helps expose a mostly untold story in which the pain of certain people—such as the "dramatically undertreated" pain of AIDS patients—is held of lesser account (Stephenson 1996). Stigmatized groups are at special risk for pain. Of course, stigma is a social fact for which medicine is hardly responsible, but stigma can infiltrate medical settings in ways that narrative bioethics can help to oppose. Some narratives, that is, are clearly harmful, as philosopher Richard Kearney explains in describing ubiquitous *Us/Them* narrative*s* that divide people— Irish and English, Catholics and Protestants, Cowboys and Indians—into hardened opposing camps (2001, pp. 91–117). Stories help perpetuate racial and ethnic divisions. They help create stock characters—like the infamous GOMER, who carries the acronymic stigma "get out of my emergency room." Mrs. Chavez, for example, is poor, Hispanic, and female. Race and ethnicity, which often overlap with socioeconomic status, in fact have a direct relation to the undertreatment of pain (Green et al. 2003). Even in emergency departments, the evidenceis clear that race and ethnicity have an effect on pain treatment (Todd 2001). Sickle-cell disease in the US, for example, affects mainly African Americans, whose requests for pain medication intersect with powerful social narratives about drug-seeking behavior. In New York City, pharmacies in white neighborhoods are three times more likely to carry adequate supplies of opioid analgesics (Morrison et al. 2000). The wildly uneven figures for worldwide use of morphine serve as a reminder that many patients are denied adequate pain medication in part because of the well-storied American "war" on drugs (DePalma 1996).

Finally, however, narrative bioethics focuses our attention on what is *said*. Speech, like action, is layered with ethical significance. *Medicaleros*, in concert with narrative bioethics, would point out that Mrs. Chavez (while insisting that she's no wimp and that it was a painful delivery) didn't complain about feeling pain. She said she felt *like an animal*.

Narrative bioethics does not necessarily tell us who is right. In fact, it at times it may actively undermine the confidence—born of rationalist, objectivist, principle-driven theories of morality—that a "right answer" is what will best resolve ethical dilemmas. The action called, at times, may be inaction—or, when principles collide, waiting it out—much as the pleasures of narrative may, at times, lead to a rejection of pleasure or the abandonment of narrative. What matters most is how narrative enlists and honors the varied emotions, from joy to grief, that *medical eros* takes into account. What matters most is how narrative competence—in Rita Charon's term—lets us hear and respond to Mrs. Chavez's muted protest against dehumanized treatment. Principles are often not enough—in fact, they can be a smokescreen—when sound reasons, as we will see, can serve as hidden tools for inflicting pain or for silently condoning its infliction.

7.5 *The Great Moment*: The Infinity of the Face

Intense pain is often regardedas a force powerful enough to disintegrate human consciousness and to dissolve the boundaries of the self. Bataille makes a similar claim for eros, however, and even chronic pain embeds a potential threat to identity (Eccleston et al. 1997). *Medical eros* is concernedless with tracking the consciousness of the person who feels pain than with asking—as narrative implicitly asks—what *call* does pain make (what *obligation* does pain incur) on the person who observes it. This is the question that Susan Sontag posed concerning the specific role of photography (2003). It is a question of particular concern for medicine, where the pain of others is a daily presence, and it is addressed with surprising skill in the 1944 biographical film *The Great Moment*: the story of William Morton and the mid nineteenth century invention of surgical anesthesia.[3]

The Great Moment—written and directed by playwright Preston Sturges and loosely based on René Fülöp-Miller's historical novel *Triumph over Pain* (1938)—tells how Morton supplies the expertise and the technology that allow chief surgeon John Collins Warren on October 16, 1846 at Massachusetts General Hospital to perform the first public demonstration of pain-free surgery. The date ranks among the few genuine worldwide turning points. Effective anesthesia delivered patients from the monstrous pain and often lethal consequences of previous surgery. It let surgeons develop slower, more intricate procedures impossible with unanesthetized

---

[3]*The Great Moment* is available on DVD. Paramount edited Sturges's screenplay (Sturges 1995) before it released the film.

patients. Morton's achievement thus warranted scientific honor and financial reward, but, as with Darwin and Wallace, controversy and counterclaims soon embroiled his justified quest for recognition. The film in fact begins with a flash-forward that shows Morton as an old man, worn out with poverty, frustration, and continual setbacks, unrewarded and even vilified. The emotional impact of the film intensifies as we understand that Morton dies a ruined man as the result of a fateful ethical action that he undertakes—as Sturges makes very clear—in order to prevent one patient's pain.

Medical eros brings more than emotional pathos to the narrative of Morton's discovery. In contrast to rationalist claims that another person's pain is always private and unknowable, which of course subverts the claim (to know) that it unravels consciousness, *medical eros* represents pain as more than strictly private, more than locked away in an unknowable single consciousness. Pain, as *medical eros* sees it, belongs to social codes as intelligible as SOS. We may not be able to answer every SOS, but it is self-deception to pretend that we have no idea what response it calls for. Stories too reveal much about the shared social meanings, public beliefs, and collective codes often inseparable from the individual experience of pain (Morris 1991). Once familiar religious narrativesinterpreted pain as divine punishment, much as patients today understand pain within a reductivenarrative of tissue damage and mis-firing neurons. What goes unnoticed is how such narratives dovetail with specific emotions, much as (fictive) stories of divine punishment once evoked (real) fears of Hell. With some clear exceptions, narratives work on us by engaging emotion as well as intellect, which is why Plato banished poets from his ideal republic, where fictions and feelings no longer trouble the all-rational state.

Emotion, as Plato knew, is double-edged and dangerous, no guarantee of right action. Nazi Germany showed how narratives of racial purity could mobilize mass emotion for vicious ends. Emotion is not, however, synonymous with error and irrationality. The biblical narrative of the Good Samaritan memorably enlists emotion on the side of goodness as the pain of an enemy nonetheless calls forth in the Samaritan an ethical act of compassion.

The Great Moment, as it recounts the story of Morton's discovery, turns pain into the arena for an ethical contest between *medical eros* and *medical logos*: which power will do the right thing? While excited crowds and newspaper reporters throng outside Mass General where Warren, the patriarchal chief surgeon, is scheduled to perform the first public pain-free operation, in private *medical logos* is at work to stop the proceedings. Delegates from the Massachusetts Medical Society are meeting with Warren behind closed doors, in protest, citing the ethical principle that holds physicians may not use medicines with unknown ingredients. The delegates have a valid point: the principle of non-maleficence specifically protects patients from quack potions, while Morton has disguised his pain-killing discovery under the classical name Letheon. Morton's personal dilemma is simple: he cannot patent ether, which is a natural substance, so his only financial reward will come from his still-unpatented ether inhaler. His fortune depends on not revealing the ingredients of Letheon prematurely. If his motives are financial, however, the upper-crust delegates of the Medical Society are hardly spotless. Their invocation of principle is less about patient safety than about the disdain that society physicians feel for a lowly dentist who is grabbing the medical spotlight. Power (disguised as principle) clearly resides with the delegates, who remain adamant: no operation. Morton faces a stark choice. His fortune will be made—his insecure family secure —if he refuses to disclose the secret of Letheon, but his refusal means that an anonymous patient will undergo a harrowing leg amputation performed (as Warren puts it dryly) "in the old way."

The conflict between *medical logos* and *medical eros* now movesto a new level. As Morton hesitates, Warren yields to the ethical protest of his colleagues and proceeds directly to the surgical theater. The camera, in a lingering portrait of his isolation, follows Morton as he walks down a long hallway. The *Ave Maria* plays softly on the soundtrack while a priest ministers to the young girl on a stretcher who awaits the operation. Morton ends his long walk at the stretcher and mumbles a few words of concern to the girl (Fig. 7.3).

She responds (one big Hollywood tear glistening on her cheek) that a gentleman has made a new discovery and the operation doesn't hurt any more. No one has told her that the Massachusetts Medical Society, on purely ethical grounds, has just blocked the use of Letheon and doomed her to the fully conscious amputation of her leg.

"Not to relieve pain optimally," asserts Edmund D. Pellegrino, a giant of modern bioethics, "is tantamount to moral and legal malpractice" (1998, p. 1521). The Massachusetts Medical Society has opted for the principle of non-malificence over pain relief. What Morton will *do*? An equally compelling question, however, is *how*

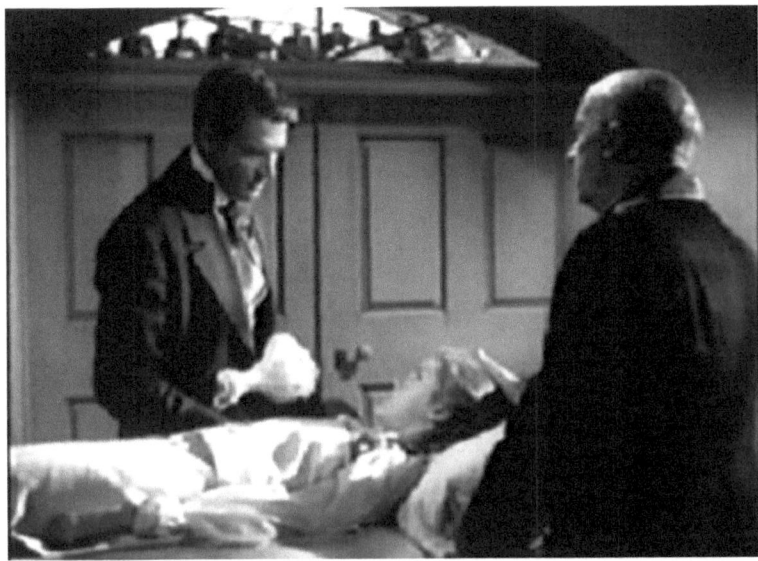

Fig. 7.3 Screen capture from *The Great Moment* (1944), directed by Preston Sturges. William Morton played by actor Joel McCrea

will he decide. Looking into the girl's eyes, as if in possession of a sudden epiphany, Morton makes his choice. The stirring musical crescendo tells us that girl will be spared. The doors of the operating theater fling open, as if by magic, and a near celestial light floods the space. The great moment promised in the title is at least a shared moment: the triumph over pain but also—for Hollywood, moreso—Morton's solitary ethical decision. It is a decision in which *medical eros* in effect affirms the spirit of the law, while medical logos persists in blind, self-interested adherence to the letter. It is not entirely a happy ending. We already know that Morton's brave and lonely act of moral heroism will also entail the defeat of all his worldly hopes.

The film in its bittersweet conclusion raises two final issues fundamental to our thinking about *medical eros* and an ethics of pain: the claims of emotion and the power of the face. It is emotion, not reason, that proves to be the driving force behind Morton's ethical decision. The film, that is, represents moral action not as a product of rational argument—sifting evidenceand weighing principles—but instead moral action proceeds almost on impulse. Unlike the chair of anesthesiology, Morton knows what the right thing to do is—and he does it, almost spontaneously. It is not only a triumph over pain but also a classic Hollywood triumph of heart over head: emotion tells us instinctively what the right action is, while reason gets lost in the thickets of rationalization. As narrative works on us in part through its alliance with emotion, Morton's emotion-driven decision certainly invites a shared emotional response in the audience. It is a legitimate question, however, whether pain here is a special case and whether the spontaneous decision to relieve pain can stand as a paradigm for every other great moment in the history of bioethical decision-making.

Pain may be less a special case than a touchstone instance of a general need to reappraise the role of emotion in ethical decision-making. Films are in the business of selling narratives, and narratives that affirm emotion help to sell more films, but cognitive neuroscience offers a less circular revaluation of emotion. Neuroscientist Damasio (1994) describes a patient with a localized brain injury that impaired the ability to experience emotion, while leaving intact the ability to reason. Significantly, this emotionless reasoner performed well on tests of moral judgment but lost the power to make decisions. Emotion, in short, is necessary for moral action. Even if reason had persuaded him what was the right thing to do, in the absence of feeling Morton could not have done it. Emotion, in short, is indispensable to an ethics that allows us not only to know goodness but also to choose the good and to act upon our choice. Pain, then, offers a useful instance to reject, for good, the long tradition that depicts reason as manly and decisive, while emotion is feminine and hysterical. *Medical logos*, it suggests, cannot act without the assistance of *medical eros*. *Medical eros* has an especially valuable contribution to make because it calls into question an informal ethical imperative that tends to govern medicine. "The ethic under which I toiled," as Rafael Campo recalls his days in medical school, "was that anyone who had time to write about his feelings certainly was not spending enough time searching the medical literature for relevant articles and memorizing the data" (1997, p. 132). If doctors are legendary for subordinating emotion to reason in medical decision-making, they also have earned a reputation for ignoring the place of feeling in their professional self-formation. Martha Nussbaum, classicist and philosopher, points to an ancient argument that emotion is vital to the cognitive activity implicit in ethical knowledge: "We discover what we think about ... events," she writes, "partly by noticing how we feel; our investigation of our emotional geography is a major part of our search for self-knowledge" (1986, p. 15). Self-knowledge, a central concern of ethics, is important to the respectful care of patients, who might otherwise be left in the protection of robots or bookworms, as Campo implies, but even self-knowledge and emotion may prove insufficient to the ethical challenge of pain. Here too *The Great Moment* provides a touchstone occasion for thinking not so much *about* stories as *with* stories. Recall the moment when Morton gazes into the face of the young girl on the stretcher: an episode that a bare-bones structuralist approach to narrative might reduce to the x-ray of a primal face-to-face encounter.

The power of the face—which both calls forth and depends on emotion—is a concept fundamental to philosopher Emmanuel Levinas. Ethics for Levinas is not, as traditionally practiced, a rationalist enterprise either deduced logically from higher principles or erected on foundation of theory. Instead, ethics for Levinas is where philosophy starts. Ethics, in his formula, is "first philosophy." If philosophy cannot get ethics right, it is useless in the world, so why not start with ethics. Ethics for Levinas starts, first and foremost, with the *otherness* of the other person. In particular, his view of otherness emphasizes the inherent, ineradicable, inexhaustible *differences* that make each human being not just unique (as the cliché has it) but irreducible to any knowledge or intellectual content that might summarize or "contain" them. The face as a philosophical concept, for Levinas, is not a unique ensemble of physical features: eyes, lips, nose. It is not an object of vision or an object of thought. The face for Levinas necessarily involves an experience of not-knowing. It evokes the always uncontainable, untotalizable, unknowable *infinitude* of the other person.

Doctors look into the faces of their patients every day. How often do they recognize in that face-to-face meeting an encounter with the *infinitude* of the other person? The face of the person before us, whether we like it or not, makes for Levinas an instantaneous ethical claim. Our relation to the face is—as he puts it in a repeated phrase—"straightaway [*d'emblée*] ethical" (1985, p. 87). The face simply exerts a kind of "call." In what Levinas regards as its nakedness and destitution, it connects us to *the other* in an ethics that precedes reason or principle, an ethics of immediate contact, akin to what happens between William Morton and his young patient: an ethical bond created in the impact that occurs, so to speak, face-to-face. In carefully chosen words, Levinas describes the impact of the other person as a "shuddering" (*frémissement*), and in a note he explains that "shuddering" translates the term *phrike* from *Phaedrus*: the Platonic dialogue where Socrates calls love a "divine madness" that lifts the soul toward truth. Even minus its Platonic echoes, the "shudder" indicates how far this face-to-face encounter taps into emotional strata more primal than logic or reason. "The neighbor assigns me before I designate him," Levinas writes. "This is a modality not of a knowing, but of an obsession, a shuddering of the human quite different from cognition" (1981, p. 87). This pre-rational and impassioned relation—the call of *the other*—ultimately for Levinas initiates a move into language. "The face speaks," he explains. "It speaks, it is in this that it renders possible and begins all discourse" (1985, p. 87). The response of the face, even in silence, creates an implicit relationship of ethical *responsibility*. "The face," as Levinas describes an ethics prior to reason and deeper than principle, "opens the primordial discourse whose first word is obligation...." (1969, p. 201).

Medical eros participates in this unspoken ethics of the face and follows the moral responsibility as it breaks into language. "Are you the girl, the girl for the operation?" Morton asks hesitantly, as he gazes into her face? Her future pain hangs in the balance between them. The shudder of emotion implicit in their face-to-face contact—which Sturges signals with a full orchestral score—is not the opposite of reason, not some trite, frenzied juice squeezed out of the limbic system. *The Great Moment* shows how face, emotion, speech, and responsibility coalesce in a direct concern for *the other*—consistent with the principle of do-no-harm—that Levinas calls "straightaway ethical."

Pain and its cognate states of destitution are never far from Levinas's concept of the face. Hostage, stranger, exile: these repeated Levinasian metaphors for *the other* embody a primordial vulnerability—a helplessness running back to the dawn of time. For Levinas as an east European Jew, the destitution of the face is never remote from memories of the Holocaust. Morton's eyes as he looks into the girl's face have nothing to do with a molecular gaze. In a face-to-face encounter, Morton's doubts and conflict suddenly melt away in an immediate acceptance of his personal responsibility for the pain of the other. The face, of course, will not resolve all the difficult ethical questions surrounding pain. Levinas distinguishes, for example, between our obligations to another person and our responsibility to social justice. (Does the morphine that a wealthy patient gets in San Diego reduce the morphine available to a poor patient in Zaire?) Skeptics may prefer to read Morton's heroism against the grain, alert to the dialectic by which cinematic displays of male virtue so regularly depend on displays of female helplessness, or reflecting that *The Great Moment* speaks to a World War II audience that values male sacrifice in the name of an attractive girl with no name and no history: a figure of national innocence. No matter. Skepticism has slipped us back into thinking *about* stories. What clarifies Morton's action remains as primal today as in 1944: pain and the face of the other.

Medical eros, with its respect for emotion and for the value of narrative, is well suited to recognize pain as, like the face for Levinas, constituting an ethical call: an obligation based on relations prior to reason. *Medical eros*, thus, offers an incentive to regard pain as more than a chartable fifth vital sign. Reason alone and principle alone cannot reproduce the shudder that comes through an encounter with the unknowable infinitude of the other person. *Medical eros*, finally, provides a context for understanding the ethical consequence implicit in the increasing lack of direct face-to-face contact between physician and patient. In fact, modern institutional and government-regulated health caregives added impact to a Levinasian emphasis on straightaway face-to-face ethics. Institutions aren't just impersonal as a byproduct of size and complexity. They often cultivate a bureaucratic facelessness: silos and phone trees engineered to eliminate personal contact and to obscure responsibility. They encourage, as to their advantage, the moral twilight in which personal stories and emotional response lose all standing. Neglect of the face even takes on a literal meaning when physicians spend almost an entire visit peering into their computer screens. *The Great Moment* deploys the pleasures of cinema and the resources of narrative in a manner particularly useful in a medical era of absent faces, when decisions are made by committee and communicated by memo, when individual physicians melt into rotating teams, when the pain of others, in their infinitude, is reduced to entries in the patient's chart as a changing number from one to ten.

Medical eros serves as a salutary reminder that most ethical decisions do not choose good over evil—principle over violation of principle—but rather honor one value or story over other values and stories deemed less urgent. The ultimate goal of an attention to narrative is not to skew ethical decisions in any particular direction but rather to get the stories into the open, to examine their values, to discuss their conflicts, and to explore their various powers to work on us. With all due respect to the conflict of interpretations, no focus group that I can imagine would endorse a conclusion to *The Great Moment* in which Morton glances briefly at the girl, shrugs his shoulders helplessly, and strolls away. *Medical eros* would find it intolerable and worse than unprincipled. Sturges, as a credit to his storytelling skills, crafts a narrative about the discovery of surgical anesthesia in which the emotion of a face-to-face encounter—including an encounter with the infinite otherness of the patient and with the prospect of harrowing pain—prompts a straightaway ethics that makes it impossible, short of self betrayal or a perverse fall into evil, for Morton *not* to do the right thing.

References

American Pain Society Quality of Care Committee. (1995). Quality improvement guidelines for the treatment of acute pain and cancer pain. *The Journal of the American Medical Association, 274*(23), 1874–1880.

Barthes, R. (1975). *The pleasure of the text* (1973, French). (R. Miller, Trans.). New York: Hill and Wang.

Basso, K. H. (1996). *Wisdom sits in places: Landscape and language among the western Apache.* Albuquerque: University of New Mexico Press.

Bataille, G. (1986). *Erotism: Death and sensuality* (1957, French). (M. Dalwood, Trans.). San Francisco: City Lights Books.

Bayer, T. L., Baer, P. E., & Early, C. (1991). Situational and psychophysiological factors in psychologically induced pain. *Pain, 44*(1), 45–50.

Beauchamp, T. L., & Childress, J. F. (1994). *Principles of biomedical ethics* (4th ed.). New York: Oxford University Press.

Breitbart, W., Rosenfeld, B. D., Passik, S. D., McDonald, M. V., Thaler, H., & Portenoy, R. K. (1996). The undertreatment of pain in ambulatory AIDS patients. *Pain, 65*(2–3), 243–249.

Brena, S. F., Sanders, S. H., & Motoyama, H. (1990). American and Japanese chronic low back pain patients: Cross-cultural similarities and differences. *The Clinical Journal of Pain, 6*(2), 118–124.

Brody, H., & Clark, M. (2014). Narrative ethics: A narrative. *Hastings Center Report, 44*(1), S7–S11.

Campo, R. (1997). *The desire to heal: A doctor's education in empathy, identity, and poetry.* New York: Norton.

Carr, D. B., & Bradshaw, Y. S. (2014). Time to flip the pain curriculum? *Anesthesiology, 120*(1), 1–3.

Chambers, T. (1996). From the ethicist's point of view: The literary nature of ethical inquiry. *Hastings Center Report, 26*(1), 25–32.

Chambers, T. (1999). *The fiction of bioethics: Cases as literary texts.* New York: Routledge.

Charon, R. (2001). Narrative medicine: A model for empathy, reflection, profession, and trust. *The Journal of the American Medical Association, 286*(15), 1897–1902.

Charon, R., & Montello, M. (Eds.). (2002). *Stories matter: The role of narrative in medical ethics.* New York: Routledge.

Coles, R. (1990). *The call of stories: Teaching and the moral imagination.* Boston: Houghton Mifflin.

Damasio, A. R. (1994). *Descartes' error: Emotion, reason, and the human brain.* New York: G. P. Putnam's Sons.

DePalma, A. (1996, June 19). In Mexico, pain relief is a medical and political issue. *New York Times.* www.nytimes.com/1996/06/19/world/in-mexico-pain-relief-is-a-medical-and-political-issue.html.

Eccleston, C., A., C. De C. Williams, & W. S. Rogers. (1997). Patients' and professionals' understandings of the causes of chronic pain: Blame, responsibility and identity protection. *Social Science and Medicine, 45*(5), 699–709.

Ellos, W. J. (1994). *Narrative ethics.* Avebury, UK: Ashgate Publishing.

Fillingim, R. B., King, C. D., Ribeiro-Dasilva, M. C., Rahim-Williams, B., & Riley, J. L, 3rd. (2009). Sex, gender, and pain: A review of recent clinical and experimental findings. *Journal of Pain, 10*(5), 447–485.

Fordyce, W. E. (Ed.). (1995). *Back pain in the workplace: Management of disability in nonspecific conditions.* Seattle: IASP Press.

Foster, N. E., Bishop, A., Thomas, E., Main, C., Horne, R., Weinman, J., & Hay, E. (2008). Illness perceptions of low back pain patients in primary care: What are they, do they change and are they associated with outcome? *Pain, 136*(1–2), 177–187.

Frank, A. W. (2013). *The wounded storyteller: Body, illness, and ethics* (2nd ed.). Chicago, IL: University of Chicago Press.

Fülöp-Miller, R. (1938). *Triumph over pain: The story of anesthesia.* (E. Paul & C. Paul., Trans.). New York: Bobbs-Merrill.

Green, C. R., Anderson, K. O., Baker, T. A., Campbell, L. C., Decker, S., Fillingim, R. B., et al. (2003). The unequal burden of pain: Confronting racial and ethnic disparities in pain. *Pain Medicine, 4*(3), 277–294.

Herman, D. (2013). *Storytelling and the sciences of mind.* Cambridge: MIT Press.

Hirstein, W. (2005). *Brain fiction: Self-deception and the riddle of confabulation.* Cambridge, MA: MIT Press.

Hunter, K. M. (1991). *Doctors' stories: The narrative structure of medical knowledge.* Princeton: Princeton University Press.

Institute of Medicine. (2011). *Relieving pain in America: A blueprint for transforming prevention, care, education, and research.* Washington, DC: National Academies Press.

Johnson, M. (1993). *Moral imagination: Implications of cognitive science for ethics.* Chicago, IL: University of Chicago Press.

Kearney, R. (2001). *On stories.* New York: Routledge.

Kramer, P. D. (2013, October 18). Why doctors need stories. *New York Times.* http://opinionator.blogs.nytimes.com/2014/10/18/why-doctors-need-stories/.

Levinas, E. (1985). *Ethics and infinity: Conversations with Philippe Nemo* (1982, French). (R. A. Cohen, Trans.). Pittsburgh: Duquesne University Press.

Levinas, E. (1981). *Otherwise than being or beyond essence* (1974, French). (A. Lingis, Trans.). Pittsburgh: Duquesne University Press.

Levinas, E. (1969). *Totality and infinity: An essay on exteriority* (1961, French). (A. Lingis, Trans.). Pittsburgh: Duquesne University Press.

Lindemann, H. N. (Ed.). (1997). *Stories and their limits: Narrative approaches to bioethics*. New York: Routledge.

Loeser, J. D. (1991). What is chronic pain? *Theoretical Medicine, 12*(3), 213–225.

Lyotard, J. F., & Thébaud, J.-L. (1985). *Just gaming* (1979, French). (W. Godzich, Trans.). Minneapolis: University of Minnesota Press.

Macherey, P. (1978). *A theory of literary production* (1966, French). (G. Wall, Trans.). London: Routledge and Kegan Paul.

Mendelson, G. (1992). Compensation and chronic pain. *Pain, 48*(2), 121–123.

Merskey, H., & Bogduk, N. (Eds.). (1994). *Classification of chronic pain: Descriptions of chronic pain syndromes and definitions of pain terms* (2nd ed.). Seattle: IASP Press.

Montello, M. (Ed.). (2014). Narrative ethics: The role of stories in bioethics. Special issue. *Hastings Center Report, 44*(s1), S2-S44.

Morris, D. B. (Forthcoming). *Eros and illness*.

Morris, D. B. (2002). Narrative, ethics, and pain: Thinking *with* stories. In R. Charon & M. Montello., (Eds.), *Stories matter: The role of narrative in medical ethics*. (pp. 196–218). New York: Routledge.

Morris, D. B. (2010). Sociocultural dimensions of pain management. In J. C. Ballantyne, J. P. Rathmell, & S. M. Fishman (Eds.), *Bonica's Management of Pain* (4th ed., pp. 133–145). New York: Lippincott Williams and Wilkins.

Morris, D. B. (1991). *The culture of pain*. Berkeley: University of California Press.

Morrison, R. S., Wallenstein, S., Natale, D. K., Senzel, R. S., & Huang, L. L. (2000). "We don't carry that"—Failure of pharmacies in predominantly nonwhite neighborhoods to stock opioid analgesics. *New England Journal of Medicine, 342*(14), 1023–1026.

Newton, A. Z. (1995). *Narrative ethics*. Cambridge: Harvard University Press.

Nussbaum, M. C. (1986). *The fragility of goodness: Luck and ethics in Greek tragedy and philosophy*. Cambridge: Cambridge University Press.

Pear, R. (1999, March 8). Mothers on Medicaid overcharged for pain relief. *New York Times*. www.nytimes.com/1999/03/08/us/mothers-on-medicaid-overcharged-for-pain-relief.html.

Pellegrino, E. D. (1998). Emerging ethical issues in palliative care. *The Journal of American Medical Association, 279*(19), 1521–1522.

Rich, B. A. (1997). A legacy of silence: Bioethics and the culture of pain. *Journal of Medical Humanities, 18*(4), 233–259.

Rose, N. (2007). *The politics of life itself: Biomedicine, power, and subjectivity in the twenty-first century*. Princeton: Princeton University Press.

Sharon, T. (2014). *Human nature in an age of biotechnology: The case for mediated posthumanism*. New York: Springer.

Schrader, H., & Obelieniene, D. (1996). Natural evolution of late whiplash syndrome outside the medicolegal context. *The Lancet, 347*(9010), 1207–1211.

Sontag, S. (2003). *Regarding the pain of others*. New York: Farrar, Straus, and Giroux.

Stephenson, J. (1996). Experts say AIDS pain dramatically undertreated. *The Journal of American Medical Association, 276*(17), 1369–1370.

Sturges, P. (1995). *Four more screenplays by Preston Sturges*. Berkeley: University of California Press.

Sullivan, M. D. (1996). Pain as emotion. *Pain Forum, 5*(3), 208–209.

SUPPORT Principal Investigators. (1995). A controlled trial to improve care for seriously ill hospitalized patients. *The Journal of American Medical Association, 274*(20), 1591–1598.

Taylor, J. B. (2006). *My stroke of insight: A brain scientist's personal journey*. New York: Viking.

Teasell, R. W. (2001). Compensation and chronic pain. *The Clinical Journal of Pain, 17*(4), S46–S51.

The great moment. (1944). In *Preston Sturges: 7 films*. DVD. ASIN B000HT3Q2S.

Todd, K. H. (2001). Influence of ethnicity on emergency department pan management. *Emergency Medicine,* 13(3), 274–278.

van Middendorp, H., Lumley, M. A., Jacobs, J. W., Bijlsma, J. W., & Geenen, R. (2010). The effects of anger and sadness on clinical pain reports and experimentally-induced pain thresholds in women with and without fibromyalgia. *Arthritis Care & Research, 62*(10), 1370–1376.

World Bank, The. Health Expenditure, Total (% of GDP). Data. Retrieved from www.worldbank.org.

Chapter 8
Shame, Placebo and World-Taking Cognitivism

Phil Hutchinson

Abstract In this chapter, I begin by exploring the status of the claim that shame is pain. What would we be doing in making that claim? Would we be invoking identity or category membership, such that shame is a particular type of pain? Or are we speaking figuratively, invoking 'pain' metaphorically? If we are tempted to the latter characterization of "shame is pain", then what is the status of the metaphor? Is it a conceptual or cognitive metaphor, and thereby deeply embedded in our modes of thought? Or is it a literary metaphor, intentionally employed so as to illustrate and draw attention to certain aspects of shame experiences? These questions then serve to frame the discussion that follows. In that discussion, I want to put into question what I see as prejudice in favour of propositionality. I pursue this task with reference to a widely discussed 'dilemma of adequate explanation' in the philosophy and psychology of emotions and recent attempts to explain the placebo response, in the work of Daniel Moerman, and that of Fabrizio Benedetti. I offer an alternative to propositionality, which respects the data on the placebo response and helps us avoid otherwise seemingly intractable problems—chiefly the dilemma of adequate explanation—in the philosophy and psychology of emotions. Having done so, I return to my question before concluding with some reflections on the questions these considerations raise regarding debates in medical epistemology.

Keywords Cognitivism · World-taking · Biomedicine · Shame · Placebo · Propositionality

In this chapter, I want to explore some parallels between my own work in the philosophy of the emotions and recent work on the placebo effect. Initially, I will pursue this by addressing myself to a question about the status of the claim that shame is pain. However, in offering an answer to that question, I then want to go further and make some broader claims about the implications of the parallels I here

P. Hutchinson (✉)
Department of Interdisciplinary Studies, Manchester Metropolitan University,
Manchester, UK
e-mail: Phil_Hutchinson@fastmail.fm

© Springer India 2016
S.K. George and P.G. Jung (eds.), *Cultural Ontology
of the Self in Pain*, DOI 10.1007/978-81-322-2601-7_8

explore. What I will propose is that this discussion has profound ramifications, not only in the area of moral epistemology and psychology, but for medical episte- mology also, and specifically, what we take to be the boundaries of biomedicine. But this will come some way in.

So, I want to begin by exploring the status of the claim that shame is pain. What would we be doing in making that claim? Would we be invoking identity or category membership, such that shame is a particular type of pain? Or are we speaking figuratively, invoking 'pain' metaphorically? If we are tempted to the latter characterisation of "shame is pain", then what is the status of the metaphor? Is it a conceptual or cognitive metaphor, and thereby deeply embedded in our modes of thought? Or is it a literary metaphor, employed so as to illustrate and draw attention to certain aspects of shame experiences?

To begin, I quote at length a passage from Lawrence Langer's book, *Holocaust Testimonies: The Ruins of Memory.*

> George S. … is unable to separate his own ordeal from the reality surrounding him, and this in turn prevents him from even thinking in terms of a personal recovery. Work and hunger, work and hunger, is how he describes the rhythm of his days in the Lodz ghetto. He was unable to share his bread ration with anyone, he recalls with troubled demeanour: "If I would, then I would die." He tells of mothers concealing their children to avoid a selection. One mother's child was found and taken; she went berserk, and began revealing the hiding places of the other children. The disintegration of basic life supports undermined the very integrity that Améry sought to cling to, especially when the security of one's entire family was at stake. The consequences, as George S. recalls, were devastating, for him and the community as well:
>
> > I was ashamed of the whole thing, it was so shameful. It was so degrading. You were completely turned. Hunger was devastating to the human spirit; it was devastating to the human body, and you didn't know how to function. Families were beginning to, some were even fighting among themselves over a piece of bread. Some were stealing from each other. It was horrible. Some became informers to the Germans for a piece of bread. They thought they would be saved, and [would save] their families. Everybody did what they could, just to save their family.
>
> Lament rather than censure, George S.'s testimony reveals a far more extensive collapse of what we would call dignity than do some of the previous examples, but only to remind us what a privileged word dignity is in the vocabulary of atrocity. Some behaviour cannot be "undone", its finality being its only legacy. The "shame" that George S. feels as he remembers what he cannot approve of now and could not condemn then leaves a permanent scar on his life.
>
> My imagery is probably inexact here: a scar is a reminder of a curable condition, a past injury healed in the present. What we are really speaking of, as the testimony of Leon H. makes clear, is a festering wound, a blighted convalescence. His story of survival is everywhere afflicted by the scourge of his loss and his own remembered inability to hinder it. The infection begins when two SS searching for valuables come to his family's apart- ment in the Lodz ghetto and force his partially paralyzed mother to tear up some floor- boards. Because she moves too slowly, they kick her mercilessly with their boots; she dies a few days later. "That was my anger," he declares, in conjunction with this description. "I am angry at the world. The world stood still, when we were burning." It is not difficult to

discern from this scenario, however, a more specific rage, directed first at the gratuitous cruelty of his mother's murderers, and then at himself, for being forced to remain mute witness to that deed. He speaks at length of the anger that remains on his face today; it frightened his children, he insists, as they were growing up (Langer 1994, 91–92).

This is a powerful passage, and Langer's suggestion that we see the persistence of shame not as scar but as a festering wound also strikes me as powerful. In what follows I want to work towards (a) answering the questions with which I began: what is the status of the claim that shame is pain? And (b) from there make some comments about Langer's suggestion based on my answer. To reach this point, I first (Sect. 8.1) want to say a little about shame and emotion, from the perspective of philosophy of emotion. I then (Sect. 8.2) want to talk a little about the 'placebo' effect. By this point, I hope to have motivated the readers to let go of any resistance they might have to seeing shame as a member of the category of pain, in a non-metaphorical sense. I will argue that it is entirely plausible to argue that shame is a particular variety of pain, with a very specific set of existential properties.

8.1 Shame and World-Taking Cognitivism

In my book *Shame and Philosophy* (2008), I suggested a framework for understanding emotion, which I there called world-taking cognitivism. I had sought to argue against the widely held idea that we needed a theory of shame, or of the emotions in general. Instead, I suggested, what was required was a framework through which we could make sense of shame, as a particular type of embodied response to the meaningful world (the conceptually-available social world: the life-world).

Philosophical reflection on emotion is often framed by what might be depicted as a dilemma of adequate explanation (see, for example, Deigh 2004 and Prinz 2004). For emotions seem to be both meaningful and characteristically intentional while also, in many cases, being common to both humans (linguistic beings) and non-human animals (non-linguistic creatures). Philosophers and psychologists of emotion who have taken meaning and intentionality as central to their accounts of human emotion—often called cognitivists—have tended to produce explanations which identify an emotion with thoughts of a particular variety, invoking construals, judgements, evaluative beliefs, etc. While philosophers and psychologists who have taken the trans-speciesality of emotion—that some emotions seem to be common to creatures of different species, traversing species divides—as primary and central have tended to produce more biologically oriented explanations, focussing on patterned changes in the autonomic nervous system, neurological changes, etc., which are *caused* by sense impressions. In the case of the complex emotions, such as shame, these explanations might be further embedded in an evolutionary narrative that provides an adaptive rationale.

As has been noted (see Griffiths 1989, 1997; Deigh 1994, 2004; Prinz 2004; Hutchinson 2009), these two approaches are marked by their combining of explanatory strength and explanatory weakness. Those who emphasise thoughts—cognitivists—are strong on meaning and intentionality, but are weak in their ability to account for the trans-speciesality of many emotions. Where those theorists who situate biological mechanisms as their central explanatory factor are strong on trans-speciesality, they have little to contribute to an explanation of an emotion's intentionality and meaningful content in humans (at least without bolting-on a bit of speculative metaphysics in the shape of computational psychology (e.g. Prinz 2004).

I'm here interested in cognitivism. The critique of cognitivism as being fatefully weak in explaining trans-speciesality, as advanced by authors such as Deigh (2004), Griffiths (1997) and Prinz (2004), takes its place alongside other alleged short-comings of the approach, such as the "problem of emotional recalcitrance" (Griffiths 1997; D'Arms and Jacobson 2003). This second criticism is based in the observation that some emotions persist not only in the absence of a constitutive judgement or belief, but in the presence of a belief which might be (if cognitivism were true) expected to absent or mitigate the emotion. The oft-cited example of such a recalcitrant emotion is the fear of flying, where that fear is characteristically experienced while the person holds the recalcitrant belief that flying is the safest mode of transportation. The clash between true beliefs about hazards and true beliefs about risks is another way of putting this. Our emotion-perception privileges, is directed toward, hazard rather than risk on this understanding.

What is common to both these criticisms—the criticism from the trans-speciesality of emotion and the criticism from recalcitrance—is the assumption that the cognitive constituents of emotion, which are invoked in cognitivist explanations, must have propositional structure. Unfortunately, the critics of cognitivism are not unique in holding this assumption. Many prominent defenders and advocates of cognitivism in the philosophy of emotions share the same assumption (I am thinking here of authors such as Martha Nussbaum and Gabriele Taylor, but there are many others who might reasonably face this charge). What if we forgo this assumption? Can we preserve the skeleton of the cognitivist account, its strengths, and thereby the ability to account for the meaningfulness and intentionality of emotion, while not being exposed to criticisms that are based on that theory being committed to propositionality? I have argued (2008 and 2009) that we can do so. What is required is an account of emotion which can preserve meaningful takings of the world operative sub-propositionally. If we can provide this, we avoid the dilemma of adequate explanation by showing there to be no dilemma, and, moreover, we provide the resources for making sense of apparent cases of recalcitrance. Such an account would make sense of what appear to be recalcitrant emotions because we would no longer be committed to the propositionally structured thoughts necessarily playing a constitutive role in the emotion. If meaningful takings of the world are operative sub-propositionally, then these can elicit the emotion in the presence of propositionally structured thoughts that might pull in another direction, so to speak.

Let us look briefly at three ways such a view might be motivated.

8.1.1 The Radical Contextualist Challenge
to Propositionality

One could build-up from certain insights one deems pertinent in post-Wittgensteinian philosophy of language. I am thinking here of the sort of radical contextualism advanced, albeit with slightly different emphases, by Baz (2012), Hertzberg (2001) and Travis (2008). Here one might, persuaded by the treatment of examples one finds in the work of a philosophers like Baz, Hertzberg and Travis, hold that a proposition has no semantic content when treated separate from an occasion of use and the point, or purpose, of its use.

The key here—and on this occasion I am invoking Baz (2012), primarily—is that we are misguided if we take the proposition, or its component words, to be what is pertinent to meaning. Rather, what is pertinent is the point of the utterance: the particular human interest of which the (linguistic) act is expressive. The emphasis on propositions, therefore, comes under a dual attack:

1. Taken alone, extracted from context and devoid of purpose, the proposition simply has no sense. The sense of a proposition is the sense of a proposition expressive of some particular human interest on an occasion.
2. The proposition is, therefore, part of a schema: (i) particular person, (ii) proposition, (iii) occasion of use, (iv) point of use and (v) life-world. Now, the question is this: for meaning to be attributable here, is the proposition element of the schema necessary? Why might particular human interests demand expression uniquely in and through propositions?

If one is persuaded by such arguments, as am I, then it makes little sense to explain the content of emotions by reference to the propositions that, it is claimed, constitute them, for propositions have no content separate from the occasions on which, and the purposes for which, they are put to use. What we need is some kind of characterisation of the emotion, which emphasises the embeddedness of that emotion in a context, and further, that this embeddedness is what confers content along with interests. An emotion is not to be thought of as a mental state, but as a state of a person with particular interests, given their *Bildung*, on occasions. Furthermore, that emotional state is responsive to aspects of the life-world, which are 'live' for that person, given their interests and their enculturation.

I want to suggest that one takes this as *challenge one* to propositionality, and that we call it the radical contextualist challenge.

8.1.2 The Framing Challenge to Propositionality

Here is another way to bring into question the insistence on propositionality. This we might call the "framing argument". Conceptual metaphors are pervasive in our talk about abstract domains (see Lakoff and Johnson 2003). So, for example, concepts taken from the source domain of travel or journeying are employed metaphorically, as conceptual or cognitive metaphors, in the target domain of discussions of a human life. Much of our discussion of life is framed by these metaphors. It is reasonable to assume that in doing so these metaphors both serve to import the structure and carry the traces of their use in the original, source domain. So, we talk of being in a rut, coming to a dead end, having taken a wrong turn, our life being an uphill struggle and so on. A therapist might well point out a person's employment of these metaphors, and seek to facilitate awareness of their metaphorical nature, as a way of showing the way out of the 'rut', and so on.

Now, to illustrate further, consider the metaphors employed in the context of testing for an infection, particularly one subject to stigmatisation, such as HIV. Here one often finds the words 'free' and 'clean' employed to indicate a negative test result. In being so employed, such metaphors can 'smuggle-in' moral judgement, or an evaluation, which might otherwise not be present. Here meaning is conveyed by the metaphorical frames and preoccupation with propositions is apt to lead one away from that which is pertinent to the characterization of the emotional state. A patient might well feel shame on being given a positive test result for a sexually transmitted infection, but in a typical example of what some have called recalcitrant emotions, she might well believe herself to have nothing about which to feel ashamed. Here it is reasonable to assume that one possible source of the shame is the moral judgement smuggled in by metaphors such as 'clean', which serve as moral, or at the least evaluative, frames to a medical procedure.

8.1.3   Misbegotten Ontologizing and Propositionality

The final argument is the one I introduced in my 2009 paper. This we might call the misbegotten ontologizing argument. This argument goes as follows: the preoccupation with propositions is an artefact of analysis, chiefly Fregean, where thoughts are represented as propositions for the purposes of analysis. What some cognitivists in the philosophy of emotions can *seem* to be committed to, and what some of their critics seem to assume they are committed to, is that thoughts *have* propositional structure. Where the methodological claim was that propositions be employed to represent thought, for the purposes of analysis, that claim's status becomes transformed through the "for the purposes of analysis" clause dropping out of the picture. What begins as a methodological recommendation, is ontologized. Thoughts are no longer merely represented as propositions for the purposes of analysis but thoughts are now taken to have propositional structure. This becomes an identity-requirement for thoughts.

Such philosophically-inspired reflections on propositionality led me to propose my concept of world-taking cognitivism. "World-taking" because I want to emphasise that when we seek to make sense of a particular emotional expression, that with which we need concern ourselves is the way the person expressing the emotion has taken-in the life-world: how they have read the world, or the situation. How they have conceived it. "Cognitivism" because I want to emphasise the way our emotions track the (life-)world. The word 'cognitivism' is, therefore, employed in the way that term is used in analytic meta-ethics and not in cognitive psychology or cognitive science. The term invokes no appeal to cognitive processes. The work the term is doing here is that of indicating a commitment to the idea that thoughts track the world, or are answerable to the way the world is.

My proposal is, therefore, that one makes sense of emotional expressions as being based in a person's takings (often but not exclusively perceptions) of loci of significance in a meaningful world (life-world), to which those emotions are answerable. To understand an emotional expression we might reconstruct the (internal) relationship that holds between a person's conceptualization of a situation (including her conceptualisation of self) and the concept of the emotion. So, for example, shame stems from a person's perception of a situation involving her *as* characteristically shameful, and her being, who she takes herself to be, is tainted in and through this perception. To stick with shame, we might say that it emerges from meanings encoded in our language and world often residing at a more basic level than is captured by a focus on propositionally structured beliefs.

So, how might this look? Well, when one sees an event as (for example) shameful, one has perceived an *internal relation* between one's way of taking or seeing that event and one's conception of shame. What is meant by this is that one's perception of the life-world cannot be reduced to representation of facts, even social facts, but must be evaluative perception of the life-world under a particular aspect. We might depict this as one's conceptual characterization of the life-world. One contributing factor to the particular aspect of the world through which you perceive that world on this occasion, is your enculturation and particular human interest on this occasion. The internal relations holding between (a) our evaluative perception of the world under this aspect, and (b) our conception of shame, can emerge as live for us through the forming of both our human and second nature (*Bildung*) and the interplay between those and our interests on this occasion. In those situations, where we might not be alive to such aspects at a particular time, we might come to be so at a later time by means of the dawning of an aspect, through further development of our second nature or through the coming to prominence of certain interests.

Emotions are meaningful and they are about the (life-)world, but that is not to argue that they are constituted by propositionally structured thought. Rather, it is merely to make the claim that they are conceptually mediated takings of the life-world, under an aspect, by an embodied, enculturated being with interests.

Having proposed this way of understanding emotion I want now to turn attention in a different direction. Why I do so will, I hope, become clear. I now turn to recent arguments about placebo responses and meaning responses.

8.2 'Placebo' Effects and Meaning

In testing biomedical interventions, one wants clear evidence that the intervention is effective. Trial design seeks to control factors so we might arrive at clear evidence for or against the intervention's efficacy. We could do this with a surgical, a biochemical, or a therapeutic intervention. Let us here consider a biochemical medical intervention. There are a number of things we need to do to ensure that any results of trials we undertake do, in fact, demonstrate the biochemical efficacy of the intervention being tested.

Trials typically have the following structure: A group of individuals with a medical condition are selected for a trial and they are randomized. This does not mean that they are randomly allocated groups, but rather that they are deliberately allocated groups in a manner that ensures each group is non-biased. A random allocation, like drawing lots, might lead to a biased group. The goal is for the groups to be *randomized*, so that they are not biased in terms of such factors as age-group, sex, ethnicity, socio-economic background, exposure to specific environmental factors, underlying overall health and so on.

We might, therefore, randomize our cohort into four groups, where group one will be administered the drug being tested, group two are administered the current market leading drug for the medical condition, group three are left untreated and group four will be the placebo control group. (One can fruitfully add more groups and one can switch the groups over time, but we will not complicate our example here.)

Groups one, two and four will be 'blind' as regards the medicinal properties of the intervention they receive, as will be those administering the 'drug'. This is why the term 'double blind' is used. So, for example, all subjects might be administered two blue pills each day, in identical packaging. The idea being that the placebo control group has just the same grounds for believing that they are receiving a pill with biochemical properties as do members of groups 1 and 2. However, here is where things become more interesting. We might also design our trials so that we have control groups where placebos are administered differently packaged and coloured (perhaps plain packaging and plain white chalk-like pills). We might also do the same with the drug: have one group administered it in one colour and package while another receives a plain colourless pill in plain packaging. We might, further, have a group that receives pills which have deliberately added foul taste, or that produce a noticeable side-effect.

The reasons for randomisation, inventive control design and blinding are two-fold:

1. The "placebo effect/response", and
2. The role of selection bias, confirmation bias and the like

Blinding and randomisation are there to overcome the second reason. Control design and blinding are there to help those conducting the trial differentiate the results of 'placebo' effects from the effects caused by the biochemical intervention. For the purposes of this chapter, I want to discuss that which has traditionally been labelled the placebo effect/response. I will not here spend time detailing the significant studies, but will seek only to say enough to progress the discussion: put simply then, the 'placebo' effect (a term we will ultimately wish to forgo) is the measurable, observable or felt improvement in health or behaviour not attributable to a medication or invasive treatment that has been administered. Put another way: (quoting Daniel Moerman from his excellent: *Meaning, Medicine and the Placebo Effect* 2002) "the pills were inert; but taking a pill wasn't inert, and the brand name wasn't inert" (Moerman 2002, 19).

I will now discuss the range of proposed explanations for what has traditionally been referred to as the placebo effect. In doing so I will be building up to the reasons cited by Moerman (2002, 2013) in concluding and proposing that we drop the term 'placebo' and instead turn our attentions to the "meaning response". I agree with Moerman, and moreover, I think what Moerman brings out can be rendered further intelligible through invoking the term I introduced: world-taking cognitivism. My discussion will therefore draw primarily on Moerman's (2002) book and a later paper (2013), but his conclusions find support in the work of Benedetti (2014), who complements Moerman's arguments with neuroimaging data.

So, that which has traditionally been referred to as the placebo effect/response tends to be explained in one of two ways:

1. As a conditioned response, which therefore has the character of a mechanism, a little like a reflex response, only one that emerges from conditioning.
2. As an expectancy response, which is therefore characterized on the model of belief and expectation: belief that 'x' leads to expectation that 'x'.

A number of readers will be ahead of the text here, and no doubt will already have noticed how these two candidate explanations for placebo effect/response map onto two prominent accounts of emotion: affect and traditional cognitivist approaches. Authors writing on placebo, such as Moerman and Benedetti, do not invoke this parallel, chiefly (I assume) because it falls outside their purview. This is what I want to draw attention to. So, let us look at each of these candidate explanations for the placebo effect/response and the problems it faces.

8.2.1 Psychological Conditioning

For those whose background is medical science, psychological conditioning can seem like the most natural explanation. I want to suggest that its prominence as a way of understanding placebo responses is based in it being a spontaneous explanation, as opposed to one based on careful consideration of the phenomena. What I mean to do by talking of 'spontaneous explanation' is to invoke the notion of spontaneous philosophy, which is philosophy that emerges from those who do not seek to engage in, and/or who deny that they are advancing, a philosophical explanation. Perhaps they are uninterested in the discipline of philosophy and mistakenly equate that lack of interest with avoiding philosophy. Of course, lack of interest falls short of rejection and avoidance. What lack of interest often leads to is spontaneous philosophizing: philosophical theses and claims, which are spontaneously advanced without knowledge or understanding of their philosophical status, and thereby often serving to reproduce (philosophical) prejudice. I make these remarks regarding spontaneous philosophizing by way of proposing an explanation for the prominence of the conditioning explanation as an explanation for the placebo response. The conditioning explanation fits with a generally empiricist worldview that is natural to—emerges spontaneously from—much medical practice.

Most people have heard of the placebo effect, and they often seem to default to conditioning in order to provide a rational explanation (as opposed to magical thinking of some description: e.g. homeopathy). The *locus classicus* here is Pavlov's dogs, which is the most widely-known example. This conditioning comprises patterned causal sensory stimuli (a) that are reliably associated with another distinct set of sensory stimuli (b) over time, which results in the development of a psychological trigger mechanism that, once developed, becomes operative in the presence of sensory impacts (a) but the absence of (b). In the case of the dogs of the classic example, the auditory sensory impact caused by the ringing of the bell (a) was associated with the sight, scent and then the taste of food (b). These distinct sensory impacts became fused into something akin to a mechanism, what is sometimes referred to as a stimulus-response mechanism, through reliable repeated association over time: conditioning. When the dogs subsequently heard the bell they salivated in anticipation of food, despite the absence of food.

Does this explain the placebo effect/response?

Moerman argues no, and I agree. His reasons for arguing so primarily draw upon studies which do not allow for conditioning as an explanation, while a 'placebo' response is clearly present. What these studies show is that the conditioning response explanation faces two problems:

a. The problem of the absence of the conditioning stage, and
b. The problem of cultural variance: studies where the same experiments with the same conditioning produced significantly different outcomes when conducted on different groups from different cultures, or invoking the language I employed in *Shame and Philosophy*: significantly different *enculturation*.

Perhaps surprisingly, that cultural variance even includes those groups one might take to be, culturally, quite similar, such as German and Danish, as was the case in the duodenal ulcer endoscopy experiments (see Moerman 2002, 81). Even where one finds grounds for claiming conditioning has taken place, it cannot alone be the explanation, because that which is the same in both groups, the conditioning, cannot be what accounts for the difference in the response of each group.

Those who have wrestled with this problem faced by the stimulus-response conditioning explanation, or those whose predilections make them lean towards cognitivist, as opposed to mechanistic, explanation of psychological phenomena have therefore proposed the response expectancy explanation.

8.2.2   Belief and Expectation (Kirsch's Response Expectancies)

Consider the following (perhaps familiar) scenario: you *expect* to find it hard to sleep after a strong cup of coffee taken too late in the day and you *do* find it hard to sleep. Unknown to you, that coffee you were given on this occasion was actually decaffeinated coffee. The expectation was based on—we might say internally related to—your *belief that* the coffee was caffeinated and, perhaps, that the strength of the coffee indicated a high dose of caffeine. Your poor night's sleep was a response to this (these) belief(s) (see Kirsch and Weixel 1988). One can see that while this explanation introduces cognitive constituents (belief) into the explanation, it still invokes a mechanistic relationship between those constituents—belief that the coffee contained a large dose of caffeine, along with the (true) belief that caffeine is a stimulant—and the response: disrupted sleep.

Response expectancy faces the problem that it logically implies propositionally structured belief, or to put it another way, it presupposes *belief that*. There are strong philosophical arguments against such a presupposition (I proposed three in the previous section) but here, in the context of placebo effects, we have further reason to be sceptical about assuming expectation and thus propositionally structured thought (belief that).

The point is that 'placebo' effects have been demonstrated time and time again to operate where there is no articulable belief regarding the relevant factor in the effectiveness of the intervention on behalf of the patient. This is not a point based simply on a patient being unable to state her belief that intervention x is effective, it is rather that studies show that those eliciting a 'placebo' response do not have the resources required to form the belief as to the benefit of the relevant factor. If packaging, pill colour, pill taste or side-effects contribute to the non-biochemical therapeutic effects of a pill then is it really plausible to hold that the patients in question believe, for example, that blue pills are better than white pills for certain ailments? Studies have shown that tablet (or tablet packaging) colour has an impact, that surgical intervention often rates higher than drug administering and so on. What these studies show is that sub-propositional meanings, which are often indexed at high degrees of cultural specificity, provide that which makes sense of the specific placebo effects. Put another way, ways we take our life-world determine effectiveness.

Think, for example, about the extent to which touch, as an effective therapeutic factor, is culturally indexed. The question is not what people believe about the health benefits of having a tactile doctor. If that was the relevant factor we could just have doctors' receptionists give patients questionnaires, asking them whether they want a hug, or a hand on the shoulder as reassurance, and so on.

No, it is, rather, that we want to know the extent to which the meanings encoded in us and our life-world by our enculturation, encoded in our *Bildung* or our second nature, lead us to react positively in a medically significant way to certain sorts of touches. For example, I do not have to believe that certain sorts of touching are acts of compassion and that compassion has therapeutic efficacy, I merely have to feel comforted by the warmth of the hand of another resting on the back of my own hand, I merely need to take it this way. As a secondary question, we then want to know at what level of cultural specificity this is indexed: do we think it simply part of human nature, or is it something specific to certain cultures and not others.

8.2.3 Meaning

So, what we seem to be left with is placebo effects being understandable or explainable as effects emerging from takings of the meaningful (life-)world, that cannot be reduced to either expectations and thus propositional knowledge (judgements, beliefs and the like) or conditioned stimulus-response mechanisms.

That is not to deny that there might be some effects, which can be explained in terms of conditioning or expectation. However, even if one were to concede this, there are still many documented cases of strong or medically significant 'placebo' effects, which cannot be so explained and for these we need a way of talking about the way we meet the meaningful world in all its normative richness.

This is the point where I think World-Taking Cognitivism as a framework for understanding might help us out. It provides for us a way of making sense of our taking of the world. It takes the meaning view of placebo, advanced by Moerman, and provides a little more detail, which might help us gain a deeper understanding. The reason this might help is that we do not stop at the observation that the placebo effect is more than conditioning and expectation, by simply saying it is a 'meaning response'. We go on to say a little about the way in which that meaning response is structured, through our embodied worldliness, and our enculturation, and through thoughts about perception of the life-world (as opposed to say being subject to causal impacts from a Brute Given, disenchanted, world).

8.3   Shame as Pain and the Boundaries of Biomedicine

Taking full account of the role of meaning responses, as documented by Moerman and Benedetti, provides us with a much richer conception of health, illness and therapeutic intervention than we might have if we stick with mechanistic explanation. Biomedicine does not benefit as a science by allowing itself to be constrained by mechanistic explanation of physical systems. Similarly, taking full account of how our emotional responses are meaning responses to the life-world, makes sense of our emotional lives in ways simply unavailable to Jamesian-empiricist theories of emotion and cognitive accounts which invoke propositionally structured thoughts. Psychology does not benefit as a rigorous discipline by allowing itself to be constrained by an empiricist conception of the relationship between mind and world. What is apparent is that there is something of a convergence here, between what we have observed about emotion and what we have observed about placebo. Both are varieties of meaning responses. Where the difference between pain and shame might initially have struck one as a difference in type, between a family of largely physiological phenomena on the one hand and a largely psychological phenomenon, on the other, it now seems difficult to motivate such a view. I want, therefore, to make a modest proposal such that shame is a variety of pain experience, and is so non-metaphorically.

Where would such a view take us in our reflection on the quote in the opening section of this chapter? There Langer corrected his own earlier suggestion that shame was the scar left by an earlier wound, by instead suggesting that shame is better conceived as an open festering wound. If, as I am proposing, we see shame as a variety of pain, then the metaphor of a festering wound works better than that of a scar.

However, as I have already gestured, the implications of this conclusion go beyond the question I set out with and which has hitherto framed the discussion. I want to suggest it goes to the heart of questions and debates in medical epistemology.

From the perspective we are now afforded, we can see that many critics of biomedicine, such as those critics who take themselves to draw upon Michel Foucault's writings on biopower,[1] and many defenders of biomedicine, particularly those who are advocates and promoters of evidence-based medicine (EBM), have a tendency to draw the disciplinary boundaries of biomedicine too narrowly. Both EBM 'friends' and post-structuralist foes can seem united in their depiction of biomedicine as little more than applied biochemistry (complemented by some applied physiology). This, I propose, is what leads many medical practitioners to have misgivings about EBM's impact on their own practice of medicine and what motivates many of the critiques, advanced by those who invoke thinkers such as Foucault and Deleuze.

To explain further, the pages of journals such as *The Journal of Evaluation in Clinical Practice*, *The European Journal of Person-Centred Healthcare* and others are replete with papers which are often authored or co-authored by practicing biomedics. In these papers, the authors seek to argue that EBM's preoccupation with biostatistical methods and its claim that evidence in medicine should be understood almost exclusively as the results of biostatistical analyses of randomized controlled trials, at best only partially captures the actual practice of biomedicine. Such papers often draw upon philosophical arguments, such as arguments about tacit knowledge, arguments about the plurality of knowledge types, about how knowledge claims relate to specific contexts and about the appropriateness of different forms of evidence and evidence gathering methods in different domains of inquiry. What I want to put forward as a preliminary suggestion is this: what many

---

[1]For example, see Michael and Rosengarten (2012). Such critiques sometimes invoke Foucault implicitly via the work of Judith Butler; this is often supplemented with insights drawn from the writing of Gilles Deleuze and occasionally buttressed by a nod to Whiteheadian process philosophy.

of these papers implicitly share is a strong sense that what medical doctors do cannot be captured by what EBM seems to suggest they do and should be doing.

And what of the critics of biomedicine, I mentioned above? Here biomedicine might be depicted as a location where power is produced and exercised, serving to reduce persons to their purely biological existence (bare life): denying or destroying their status as persons. Alternatively, biomedicine might be depicted as forming a discursive field, actively constituting entities (bodies, diseases and so on). It seems to me that depicting biomedicine as operative according to one logic, as forming a discrete discursive field, based on little more than an application of a theory and the identification of some terminology, is to do violence to the complexity, the multifarious contexts, sub-cultures, motivations and so on, which are in play in biomedical practice. The critics see biomedicine as a discrete monoculture.

My proposal is that when we gain better understanding of that which has historically been called the placebo response, we do not merely gain a more satisfactory explanation of those responses, but we gain a better understanding of the practice of medicine and its possibilities. One of the responses to the EBM movement's preoccupation with biostatistical analysis via randomised controlled trials, is that it can seem to relegate the role of the doctor to that of collator and communicator of relevant data sets. But the doctor is, and needs to be, much more than this. A doctor needs to understand patient psychology, understand that the importance of the relationship between doctor and patient, and understand that the relationship between patient and world as not purely one of cause and effect, but that of meaningful takings of a conceptually available world that can have a demonstrable impact on that person's health. When we understand biomedical practice in its true breadth and richness, then the presentations of it by EBM friends and post-structuralist foes seem overly restrictive, and therefore unrepresentative.

References

Baz, A. (2012). *When words are called for: A defence of ordinary language philosophy*. Oxford: Oxford University Press.

Benedetti, F. (2014). *Placebo effects: Understanding the mechanisms in health and disease* (2nd ed.). Oxford: Oxford University Press.

D'Arms, J., & Jacobson, D. (2003). The significance of recalcitrant emotion (or, anti-quasijudgementalism). In A. Hatzimoysis (Ed.), *Philosophy and the emotions, Royal Institute of Philosophy Supplement: 52* (pp. 127–146). Cambridge: Cambridge University Press.

Deigh, J. (1994). Cognitivism in the theory of emotions. *Ethics, 104*(4), 824–854.

Deigh, J. (2004). Primitive emotions. In In R. C. Solomon (Ed.), *Thinking about feeling: Contemporary philosophers on emotions* (pp. 9–27). Oxford: Oxford University Press.

Griffiths, P. E. (1989). The degeneration of the cognitive theory of emotion. *Philosophical Psychology, 2*(3), 297–313.

Griffiths, P. E. (1997). *What emotions really are*. Chicago: Chicago University Press.

Hertzberg, L. (2001). The sense is where you find it. In T. McCarthy & S. C. Stidd (Eds.), *Wittgenstein in America* (pp. 90–102). Oxford: Oxford University Press.

Hutchinson, P. (2008). *Shame and philosophy: An investigation in the philosophy of emotions and Ethics*. Basingstoke, Hampshire: Palgrave Macmillan.

Hutchinson, P. (2009). Emotion-Philosophy-Science. In Y. Gustafsson, C. Kronqvist, & M. McEachrane (Eds.), *Emotions and understanding: Wittgensteinian perspectives*. Basingstoke, Hampshire: Palgrave Macmillan.

Hutchinson, P. (2011). Facing atrocity: Shame and its absence. *Passions in context: Journal of the History and Theory of Emotions I, I*(1), 93–117.

Kirsch, I., & Weixel, L. J. (1988). Double-blind versus deceptive administration of a placebo. *Behavioural Neuroscience, 102*(2), 319–323.

Lakoff, G., & Johnson, M. (2003). *Metaphors we live by* (2nd ed.). Chicago, IL: University of Chicago Press.

Langer, L. (1994). *Holocaust testimonies: The ruins of memory*. New Haven, CT: Yale University Press.

Michael, M., & Rosengarten, M. (2012). Introduction: Medicine: Experimentation, politics, emergent bodies. *Body & Society, Special Issue: Medicine, Bodies, Politics: Experimentation and Emergence, 18*(3–4), 1–17.

Moerman, D. E. (2002). *Meaning, medicine and the placebo effect*. Cambridge: Cambridge University Press.

Moerman, D. E. (2013). Against the 'placebo effect': A personal point of view. *Complementary Therapies in Medicine, 21*(2), 125–130.

Prinz, J. (2004). Embodied emotions. In R. C. Solomon (Ed.), *Thinking about feeling: Contemporary philosophers on emotions*. Oxford: Oxford University Press.

Travis, C. (2008). *Occasion sensitivity: Selected essays*. Oxford: Oxford University Press.

Chapter 9
Self and Suffering in Buddhism and Phenomenology: Existential Pain, Compassion and the Problems of Institutional Healthcare

John Russon

Abstract By bringing together the Buddhist notion that suffering is intrinsic to all forms of our self-experience with Merleau-Ponty's phenomenological interpretation of selfhood in terms of the "habit-body," I show that vulnerability and meaningfulness go hand-in-hand. I then use this developed understanding of the nature of selfhood and suffering as the basis for a critique of various foundational aspects of contemporary, institutionalized healthcare. In particular, I consider ways in which oppressive social and political practices are instituted when the existential dimensions of pain are ignored and a medical model, based on the vision of pain as an alien threat to be eliminated, is adopted instead.

Keywords Merleau-Ponty · Buddhism · Pain · Healthcare ethics · Phenomenology · Selfhood

We are very accustomed as individuals to thinking of ourselves in terms of "I" and imagining "the self" to be something independently real, and the political and cultural endorsement of this idea has been central to much of the modern world.[1] The tradition of European philosophy from Kant through Merleau-Ponty, however, has demonstrated, through phenomenological description of the forms in which our experience is "lived", that this is not a true picture of human reality. Instead, the "self" should be understood as a variable phenomenon rooted in dynamic processes of embodied interaction with an environment.[2] In demonstrating this, phenomenology has

---

[1]For the classic modern statement of the "substantial" notion of the "I", see Descartes (1979, Second Meditation). On the relevance of this notion to Early Modern political theory, see Macpherson (1962). I have discussed political problems integral to this interpretation of persons in Russon (2015).
[2]For a rich and full account of the phenomenological account of the "self," see Marratto (2012) and Costello (2012). I have studied the formation of self-experience in Russon (2013b) and Russon (2014).

J. Russon (✉)
University of Guelph, Guelph, Canada
e-mail: jrusson@uoguelph.ca

© Springer India 2016
S.K. George and P.G. Jung (eds.), *Cultural Ontology of the Self in Pain*, DOI 10.1007/978-81-322-2601-7_9

confirmed the oldest affirmations of the Buddhist tradition.[3] The phenomenon of the "self," the Buddha argues, should properly be understood not as a permanent, independent reality, but as a set of habituated ways of *upādāna*, "grasping" what is happening in experience.[4] These ways of grasping "the self" are simultaneously ways of grasping the world: the determinate forms of self and world are a *paṭicca-samuppāda*, "dependent co-arising" (*Saṃyutta Nikāya* II.1–133).[5] Unlike the phenomenological approach, however, which initially takes its motivation largely from questions of knowledge and method, the Buddhist account has its roots in an attempt to address the *dukkha*, "suffering," that the Buddha argues is attendant upon all the varying forms of "grasping" and "co-arising." Though I will not specifically take up a study of the Buddha's prescriptions for alleviating suffering, I will pursue the idea that suffering is intrinsic to all the forms of our self-experience. By bringing together this Buddhist theme with the phenomenological interpretation of selfhood and experience, I will show that vulnerability and meaningfulness go hand-in-hand, and I will use this developed understanding of the nature of pain and suffering as the basis for a critique of various foundational aspects of contemporary, institutionalized healthcare.

9.1 Phenomenological and Buddhist Perspectives on Selfhood and Action

Merleau-Ponty's phenomenology centrally revolves around the notion that our experience is inherently embodied. The familiar meanings of our world, that is to say, are *essentially* such as to pertain to our condition of having hands, joints, eyes, etc. This is immediately clear with such notions as "chair", for example, for that word precisely names something upon which we sit. Merleau-Ponty argues, though, as does Husserl before him, that that is similarly true of our notions of, for example,

---

[3]For a range of contemporary perspectives on the relationship between Merleau-Ponty's phenomenology and Buddhism, see Park and Kopf (2009).

[4]Compare *Saṃyutta Nikāya* III.114–15. (Conze 1995, p. 75): "The instructed discipline of the Ariyans does not regard material shape as self, or self as having material shape, or material shape as being in the self, or the self as being in material shape. Nor does he regard feeling, perception, the impulses or consciousness in any of these ways. He comprehends each of the *khandas* as it really is that it is impermanent, suffering, not-self, compounded, murderous. He does not approach them, grasp after them or determine 'Self for me [attā me]' —and this for a long time conduces to welfare and happiness."

[5]See especially II.28 (Davids and Woodward 1917): "That being, this comes to be; from the arising of that, this arises; that being absent, this is not; from the cessation of this, this ceases"; and II.65: "That which we will, and that which we intend to do, and that for which we have a latent tendency, this is an object for the persistence of consciousness. If there is an object, there is a support for consciousness." See also I.62 and IV.95. See Berman (2004), on the relationship between this notion (which Berman translates as "relational origination") and Merleau-Ponty's notion of "reversibility."

thing and space. Within perception, we encounter things, but the thing in perception only ever shows us specific profiles (*Abschattungen*) of itself. When we see such a profile, however, we precisely see it *as* the profile *of* a thing. Our perception presents us, as it were, with more than what it simply present: indeed, with more than could possibly be present, for the thing "as such" could never fully present itself in any act of perspectival perception.[6] This difference between the profile actually present and the thing as such presented through the profile is the space of expectation and, indeed, the space of embodiment: when we see the profile of the thing we see it *as* something that promises a "back side" that *would* be there, were we to investigate further, and this further investigation would precisely be a bodily matter of using one's hand to feel the backside, or of walking around to see it from behind. The experience of the thing is possible for us because our perception is situated for us in a space of bodily possibility: the ability to perceive a thing as a thing varies directly with one's experience of oneself as able to go behind bodily and investigate. Like the chair, then, the thing is a meaning that is essentially available to bodily experience. And, as our analysis has already suggested, the same is true of space inasmuch as the very significance we just recognized presupposed our existing with a spatial world given *as* the domain within which one can move.[7] Through these examples, then, we can see the fundamental sense in which the meaningfulness of our experience is an inherently embodied meaningfulness.

Just as the sense(s) of the things of our world emerge(s) from the possibilities for bodily engagement, so, according to Merleau-Ponty, is our sense of self rooted in our embodiment. Prior to being experienced as one object in the world alongside others, our body is, for each of us, our fundamental experience of our possibility for engagement with the world and, consequently, the foundation of our sense of self is the experience of "I can" that is the original meaning of our embodiment. Our sense of self emerges from our developing experiences of competency (and incompetency) in the engagement with the world. Within our developing, worldly negotiations, it is our negotiations with other people that offer the sense of competency and incompetency that is ultimately most important for defining our sense of self.[8] Our growing sense of self is fundamentally premised upon our success (or lack thereof) in finding a "fit" with the world, and most especially with the other people in that world. The "fabric" of our sense of self, then, far from being a "given" bit of ontological furniture, is rather the habituated sense of confidence we have in

---

[6]One of the best statements of this is Husserl (2001, pp. 39–62). Compare Merleau-Ponty (2012, pp. 378–9): "When I say that I see an ashtray and that it is over there, I presuppose a complete unfolding of the experience that would have to go on indefinitely and I open up an entire perceptual future." These themes from Husserl and Merleau-Ponty are richly developed in Howell (2015).

[7]For the theme of space, see Husserl (1997), and Merleau-Ponty (2012), Part I, Chap. 3, "The Spatiality of One's Own Body and Motricity.".

[8]For the "I can," see Merleau-Ponty (2012, p. 139). I have studied the development of personality in these terms in Russon (2003). On the significance of this notion of "I can" in healthcare, see Schenck (1986).

historically established ways of cultivating a confirming sense of equilibrium with our natural and interpersonal surroundings. There are many ways in which the embodied character of this self-world equilibrium offers important insights about our human condition,but I will particularly emphasize one: to the extent that the meaningfulness of our world depends on the *determinateness* of our (mortal) bodies, that meaningfulness is inherently *vulnerable*. More precisely, "to be meaningful" and "to be vulnerable" cannot be separated, with the result that suffering is inherent to the developed forms of our meaningful human lives. This is a point powerfully made by the Buddha.[9]

In his first sermon, the Buddha offers a systematic list of the forms of *dukkha*, "suffering":

> Birth is *dukkha*; ageing is *dukkha*;
> sickness is *dukkha*; death is *dukkha*;
> sorrow, lamentation, pain, grief, and despair are *dukkha*;
> association with what one dislikes is *dukkha*;
> separation from what one likes is *dukkha*;
> not to get what one wants is *dukkha*;
> in short the five groups of grasping are *dukkha* (*Saṃyutta Nikāya* V: 420).

The Buddha does not treat suffering as something reducible to one domain of our experience, but as something that permeates every aspect of life: whereas the first set of "sufferings" pertains to organic conditions—birth and death, ageing and illness—the second group pertains to what we might call relatively passive psychological states (emotions) and the third to more active attitudes rooted in our beliefs and desires. Indeed, the concluding line of the quotation makes explicit that *dukkha*, suffering, pertains intrinsically to all of those "graspings" that constitute our very experience of being someone.[10] And, whereas the first group (birth, ageing, sickness and death) pertains to circumstances that basically "befall" us, the last group—matters of what one dislikes, likes or wants—pertains to matters that we have a large role in shaping.

The Buddha himself specially emphasized the idea that our action is decisive for shaping our lives. This is evident at one level in the whole doctrine of *karma*, "action," according to which we are responsible for shaping our own destiny.[11] More immediately, we have the capacity to change the ways in which we feel likes, dislikes and so on through our *kusala*, "skilful" (or, alternatively, through our

---

[9]In this paper, I write for convenience as if the words and ideas of the sermon are those of Siddhattha Gotama; in fact, of course, these are teachings handed down by tradition, and they may very well be the concentrated insight of generations of Buddhist thought, rather than ideas coming directly from any single individual. See Harvey (1990, pp. 3–4, 15–17).

[10]For the five "graspings," see Harvey (1990, pp. 49–50).

[11]See *Majjhima Nikāya*, III. 203 (Horner 1954–1959). Within the Buddhist tradition, there is a strong emphasis on the theme of our active role in shaping matters even of birth and death; I do not extend my paralleling of Merleau-Ponty and Buddhism to this level. On this divergence with respect to Buddhist soteriology, see Berman (2004, pp. 134–135). I discuss below my understanding of the philosophical importance of the notion of *karma*.

akusala, "unskilful") action.[12] Skilful action is rooted in non-greed, non-hatred and non-delusion, and is conducive to the development of wholesome states of mind, rather than causing spiritual or material harm to oneself or others. Buddhist practice generally is oriented to encouraging "the purification, development and harmonious integration of the factors of personality, through the cultivation of virtue and meditation" through skilful action.[13] Precisely *because* there is no given, substantial "self" as an ontological ingredient in our makeup, we necessarily face the responsibility of shaping "who" we will be: "the self" is a matter of *how* the forces constitutive of our experience are navigated, resulting either in a greater or a lesser sense of truly "free" agency.

More specifically, the path of development outlined in the Buddhist tradition is one of separating oneself from a kind of servitude to that which one "craves." Typically, we understand our "self" (behaviourally, but often also conceptually) in terms of dimensions of the world to which we have strong attachments. In a typical day, for example, "I" appear when "I am hungry" or when "I want that," or even when "I must get that done." Generally, the things of the world in which we have invested our desire set the terms for our experience. Kant referred to this as the "heteronomy" of the will (Kant 2005: Part II): when we live in this way, it is the things of the world that are essentially the "agents" in our experience, and we are pushed to and fro by the vicissitudes of those things to which we are intimately attached. We notice this especially pointedly in our "addictions" to drugs: if I am a smoker, the cigarette effectively "calls" me to smoke it, and my day is significantly ruled by the presence or absence of cigarettes, (and hence, politically and economically, by the makers of the cigarettes). The Buddha's point is that an analogous "addiction" to the world generally is characteristic of the normal formation of our personalities, and Buddhist practice is largely devoted to recognizing and removing the "craving" or "thirst" [*taṇhā*] that defines our normal situation, thus liberating us from the domination of these forces, a domination that is ultimately *dukkha*.[14]

This notion that, through our actions, we can transform our navigation of the forces constitutive of our personality, and that "the self" is essentially the established "how" of this navigation corresponds closely to Merleau-Ponty's understanding of the self as fundamentally a phenomenon of habit. As we noted above, the core sense of self is found in the experience of "I can." The "I can" is our embodied sense of possibility—our sense of how the world allows us to engage with it—and, as we

---

[12]See *Majjhima Nikāya*, 1.115, 415–16, II.114 (Horner 1954–1959).

[13]Harvey (1990, p. 50). On ethics and "spontaneous right action" in Merleau-Ponty and Buddhism, see Mazis (2009), especially 196–203.

[14]The core principles of Buddhist practice are found in "the Holy Eightfold Path," which is "the Middle Way"; see *Saṃyutta Nikāya* II.43 and *Majjhima Nikāya* III.71–8. Compare also Krishna's advice to Arjuna: "Be intent on action, not the the fruits of action; avoid attraction to the fruits and attachment to inaction! Perform actions, firm in discipline, relinquishing attachment; be impartial to failure and success—this equanimity is called discipline" (*Bhagavad Gita* 1988: Book 2, Verses 47–8). On the resources of Buddhism for dealing with pain in a medical context, see Kabat-Zinn et al. (1985).

develop, this sense of possibility develops accordingly. As children, we are largely powerless in our engagement with the world, and we are heavily dependent upon the support of adults to ensure our very existence, let alone our well-being. In appropriately supportive environments, however, we quickly develop enhanced capacities for engaging with the world. With the passage of time and through considerable effort, children learn to engage more powerfully with their bodies and the spatial world through walking, they learn to engage more powerfully with other people through talking, they learn to focus their attention and thereby learn theoretical and other truths, and so on. Crucial to these experiences of learning are processes of habituation. In the case of walking, for example, the child must repeatedly attempt to balance until at some point she succeeds in holding herself upright as she traverses the floor; she must subsequently enact this practice repeatedly until her limbs and the floor no longer confront her as challenges, but she instead can easily and automatically walk. She acquires a new ability—a new "level" in her relation to the world, in Merleau-Ponty's language (Talero 2005)—by becoming so habituated to a pattern of relating to the world that the worldly challenge is transcended and she approaches the world with a new ease. In this new situation, the very terms of her relation to the world have changed: the habituation now allows her to disregard the experiences of limbs and floor that were formerly salient, and instead focus her attention on the new sorts of tasks and projects—such as running, skipping, going to the back of the yard, etc.—that are available to one who can walk. Whereas formerly she had to struggle with a more or less alien body and alien space, she has now become a "walker," one who travels quickly with the cooperation of her limbs and her space. Through this process of habituation, she has developed—she has become—a new "I can," a new self, as the "how" of the navigation and coordination of the forces constitutive of her experience has changed.

When we reflect on this notion of habituation, we can recognize that action has the peculiar character of building upon itself: as the Buddhist notion of *karma*, "action," affirms, our actions do not just happen in a moment, but continue their formative impact long after the moment of their initial enactment.[15] A first attempt at whistling does not produce the perfect whistle, but something of it "sticks," with the result that a second attempt, and a third and a fourth gradually accumulate— somewhat like a snow-ball grows when rolling down a snow-covered hill—until one can whistle. The first attempt did not completely accomplish whistling, but it nonetheless had a continuing efficacy that, coupled with the continuing efficacy of the second and the third attempt, enabled the fourth attempt not just to be another futile attempt identical to the first, but one that could complete a movement towards whistling begun, but not finished, with the first. Indeed, in every subsequent experience of whistling, that first, awkward attempt at blowing air through pursed

---

[15]The notion of *karma* is in fact inherited by Buddhism from earlier forms of Indian religion, and it is a notion shared with, for example, Hinduism. On this ancient notion, see Doniger (2009, pp. 168–170).

lips continues to live on, or, we might say, we continue to inhabit that time.[16] And what is true at this very local level of pursuing one's lips and blowing is equally true at the global level of how one acts in general: through the repeated enactment of a way of living, we precisely develop a character, a personality. Our earlier actions—actions often undertaken blindly or one-sidedly—continue to act through us in and as our developed personalities. Further, the world into which we integrate ourselves through our childhood and subsequent development is also not a neutral world, but is a world intrinsically shaped by the actions of those who preceded us: at the level of the family, we "inherit" through our upbringing the healthy or unhealthy forms of interpersonal interaction that have shaped the parenting practices of our parents and, they, of course, similarly already carried within themselves an analogous legacy from their parents[17]; again at a cultural level, when we learn, for example, to drive according to the rules of our traffic laws, we are effectively taking into ourselves—our "selves"—the principles of action and interpretation that led our forebears to establish our particular legal system.[18] Ignoring the "metaphysical" theories about re-birth that provide the ancient context for the notion of *karma*, we can nonetheless see that the basic notion of *karma*—that action has a continuing formative effect—is profoundly true of our experience, precisely because "the self" is not given, but is rather a matter of our habituation to ways of navigating the forces constitutive of our experience.[19]

At the level of our developed, adult personalities, this primacy of habituation shows itself in the distinction, in Merleau-Ponty's terms, between the "habit body" and the "body at this moment." To make this distinction clear, Merleau-Ponty draws on a peculiar experience of pain—the pain of a "phantom limb."[20] It is a well-documented phenomenon that various individuals continue to "feel" a limb after it has been amputated. This cannot simply be a "psychological" phenomenon of denial or something similar, for the experience can sometimes be eliminated through physiological intervention; on the other had, it cannot simply be a physiological matter, because the experience can typically be initiated by perceptions or memories, i.e., "psychological" stimuli. Merleau-Ponty argues that this failure of

---

[16]For these themes of temporality, see Merleau-Ponty (2012, p. 85).

[17]I have given a phenomenological analysis of this "family" inheritence in Russon (2003), especially Chaps. 4 and 5. The stories of "blood-guilt" and its legacy in the classical Greek tragedies offer a particularly powerful reflection on these "karmic" effects. On the psychologically formative effects of families and other institutions, see Leder (2005, pp. 110–112).

[18]Compare Pierre Bourdieu's notion of the social *habitus*: "The *habitus*, a product of history, produces individual and collective practices—more history—in accordance with the schemes generated by history. It ensures *the active presence of past experiences*, which, deposited in each organism in the form of schemes of perception, thought and action tend to guarantee the 'correctness' of practices and their constancy over time, more reliably than all formal rules and explicit norms" (1980, p. 54; emphasis added).

[19]On the relevance of traditional Hindu notions of *karma* for the treatment of pain in medical contexts, see Whitman (2007).

[20]I have discussed Merleau-Ponty's analysis of the phantom limb and the implications of this analysis in Russon (2013a). See also McMahon (2014).

the isolated terms of mind-body dualism to account for the experience reveals, in fact, that there is something inherently embodied about "the mind," and something inherently psychological about "the body."[21] Specifically, "the body" is not a machine that reacts mechanically to stimuli, but is a matter of behaviour, of intelligent responsiveness to situations: our embodiment—our embodied "I can"— is an habituated way of holding onto the *meanings* of situations. Correspondingly (as we saw above), our "consciousness" is not a free-floating, self-possessed mind; instead, we perceive and understand *as* a (typically non-self-reflective) bodily, behavioural engagement with the world. "Beneath" my immediate, reflective self-experience, then, (and as the Buddha's notion of *paṭicca-samuppāda*, "dependent co-arising" maintains), is an anonymous, accomplished, habitual enmeshment with a meaningful situation, a habitual self that effectively carries out most of the work of my meaningful engagement with the world "behind my back" such that, as we saw above in our discussion of habituation, most of the terms of my engagement with the world can be ignored by my explicitly self-reflecting "I." This, according to Merleau-Ponty's analysis, is what is revealed by the experience of "phantom limb" pain: though my "body at this moment" [*le corps actuel*] has lost a limb, at a more basic level I continue to live from my "habit body," [*le corps habituel*], that is, I live from an experience of the world in which "I can" grab with my arm or step with my leg (Merleau-Ponty 2012, p. 84). My "I," most fundamentally, is defined by the habituated forms of commitment to engagement with the world upon which the meaningfulness of my immediate experience is built.

Because our "selves" are not given in advance as ontologically independent components of our reality but are, instead, the cultivated ways we have of navigating the forces constitutive of our experience, the meaningfulness of our lives will always be embodied, will always rest upon the developed forms of our bodily engagement with the world.[22] Our bodily organism and the physical world with which we interact bodily are inherently vulnerable to damage, however.[23] For that reason, the meaningfulness of our lives will itself always be vulnerable. As we saw in our reflection on the child, I become the "I" that I am through developing such habits as navigating the bodily-spatial world through walking and navigating the interhuman world through talking. I depend upon being a walker, and I can lose this ability. Whether or not I experience this as an organic, or phantom-organic, malady, I suffer through the fundamental impairment of my developed form of being in the world. Again, I depend upon my interactions with others, and the loss of my parents or of my friends through their death, or the loss of my ability to interact with them through my own loss of speech induces in me a particular kind of suffering:

---

[21]For Merleau-Ponty's analysis of the phantom limb, see (2012, pp. 78–85). On this theme of the insufficiency of mind-body dualism, see Leder (2005).

[22]On the strong parallels between Merleau-Ponty's notion of embodiment and the Buddhist rejection of a substantial notion of self, see especially Mazis (2009; especially, 186–189).

[23]Compare *Saṃyutta Nikāya*, I.135, and II. 66–68 on the inherently "non-self" character of all things.

a suffering, not in the sense of the alien imposition of an uncomfortable sensation, but in the sense of a crippling of my very being, an existential blow to my very sense of being able to be myself.[24] Because I am who I am through my habituated engagement with those worldly or interpersonal others, my very sense of "I" is inherently vulnerable to their loss. There is necessarily a unique form of suffering that attaches to every "level" of our experience; hence the ubiquity of suffering, *dukkha*, of which the Buddha spoke.

9.2 Existential Pain and the Politics of Healthcare

From our analysis above, we can see that suffering takes as many forms as meaning takes. Indeed, suffering itself is essentially a meaning: it is an actualization within the realm of possible significance to which we are open.[25] As the drink on a hot day beckons to me, attracting my attention and inciting me to drink, so does the sudden reminder of my father's death repel me, inciting me to turn my attention away from it even as it holds me in its spell, or the soreness in my legs urges me to stop running even though I know that I must carry on to the top of the hill.[26] These pains occur at a site where another, different meaning could have occurred, and they "say," essentially, "turn away," even though turning away is not in fact possible. In whatever domain a range of possible meanings opens up, possibilities for pain open up and the character of the pain will vary with the character of the domain of meaning ranging from unpleasant sensations felt in my body, through the emotional agony of existential longings and torments, to the depths of an unmasterable anxiety that challenges my very ability to maintain a coherent relationship to meaning in general. This understanding of the nature of human suffering is crucial for allowing us to be appropriately compassionate and caring in our dealings with ourselves and others. Starting from this understanding, I want to identify three problems in principle that are constitutive of much contemporary, institutionalized healthcare.

The first problem is that the theoretical core of contemporary Western healthcare, which itself is becoming more and more the "global" reality of institutional healthcare, is the so-called "medical model" of pain according to which pain is the uncomfortable feeling associated with strictly physiological processes which are

---

[24]On the theme of intersubjectivity in Merleau-Ponty and Nagarjuna, and on the relation of this to language, see Berman (2004, especially 137–141).

[25]On the idea that pain is a meaning, see Honkasalo (2000).

[26]I have given a phenomenological analysis of the internal dynamics of "attention" in Russon (forthcoming). See also Casey, "Attending and Glancing," Chap. 9 (2007; especially 311–335); Vermersch (2004, pp. 52–54); and Bredlau (2006).

understood to be the true, causal reality.[27] This "medical model," which opposes the reality of physiological causality to "merely subjective" experiences, precisely relies, of course, upon the dualism of mind and body that phenomenology and Buddhism challenge. The practical impact of this approach is, effectively, to differentiate between "legitimate" and "illegitimate" claims to be experiencing pain: whereas, from the perspective of the suffering individual, the reality of pain is the first-person experience of discomfort, from the perspective of the institution, (which means, immediately, the healthcare institution but also, more ultimately, the insurance companies who will determine which care-practices will and will not be funded), it is demonstrable physiological causality that is the reality of pain. In fact, "pain-claims" are notoriously not easy to correlate with specific physiological "causes," and this "subjective" nature has often made it difficult for individuals to get adequate treatment and support.[28] The reliance on the "medical model" thus introduces a barrier in principle between those in need of care and the institutions of care. And, in addition, the requirement that patients be able to prove the legitimacy of their claims results in those suffering from pain being subjected to the practical burden and discomfort of undergoing tests and the psychological burden of living under the suspicion of making fraudulent claims and of being "illegitimate."[29]

A second problem is the operative, institutional presumption that experience is an attribute of individuals, a theoretical reliance upon precisely the notion of a permanent, substantial "self" that is challenged by phenomenology and Buddhism. What phenomenology and Buddhism have shown is that the self is established through relations with the world and with other persons. This constitutive relationship to other persons in particular entails that our self-experience is inherently intersubjective and, indeed, "communal," in the sense that we are able to be the "selves" that we are only through the ongoing, practical endorsement of this self-experience by others.[30] The theoretical commitment to the individualist

---

[27]The International Association for the Study of Pain, for example, defines pain as "an unpleasant sensory and emotional experience associated with actual or potential tissue damage, or described in terms of such damage." On the problems with the "medical model" in dealing with pain and suffering, see Cassel (1982). For a related argument that pain is an "extra-medical" and "biocultural" phenomenon, see Morris (1991). See also Coulehan (2012), and Rawlinson (1986). On problems with the "medical model" in general, compare Goldenberg (2010).

[28]On the limitations of this "somatogenic" model of pain, see Okifuji and Turk (1998). As they report: "The psychophysiological bases for many chronic pain syndromes are elusive. For example, no pathology is identified in over 80 % of patients with chronic back pain" (Okifuji and Turk 1998, p. 142). See also Wilde (2003), for the idea that chronic pain does not just "occur in their physical body but also in their embodiments. For such patients, dualistic (mind-body) notions of the body as object and mind as subject can devalue experiences that are necessary for healing and for managing everyday problems related to their illness or injury" (Wilde 2003, p. 170).

[29]See Okifuji and Turk (1998, p. 143): "Many patients report that stigmatization associated with the psychogenic ["hysterical"] and motivational ["money-seeking"] models substantially adds to their suffering.".

[30]On the intersubjective and communal dimensions of self-experience, see Stolorow (2013); see also Russon (2003), Chap. 4.

interpretation of our experience—a principle integral to Western culture and politics broadly, and thus integral to the legal and cultural "background" of healthcare as well as to the specific policies of healthcare institutions—results in a number of related problems. (a) As family therapists such as Salvador Minuchin and systems theorists such as Gregory Bateson have shown, many so-called "psychological" problems, such as anorexia nervosa and alcoholism, are properly consequences of interpersonal—and, typically, familial—systems. In other words, the problematic form the behaviour of a particular individual takes is actually simply one part of a dynamic system unfolded throughout a larger network of persons, with different individuals taking on different functional roles in the system.[31] The "individualist" interpretation of persons that is operative in institutional situations of healthcare wrongly identifies the malady as belonging to the individual, rather than recognizing the family- or social-group as dysfunctional, resulting in the individual's suffering being misdiagnosed and mistreated and leaving the dysfunctionality and suffering of the group untreated. (b) Inasmuch as our ability to "be ourselves" is premised upon our participation in the appropriate interpersonal and social networks, separation from those relevant other persons can produce a pain as real and significant as that caused by any physiological tissue damage. There is suffering experienced by immigrants or, more severely, refugees who have been separated from their familial, social, cultural and religious contexts that is caused by damage to the intersubjective bases of their identities, but an individualist approach to healthcare can neither recognize nor appropriately treat this damage to the very "tissue" of self, but can at best treat this, again, as a "subjective," psychological discomfort.[32] (c) The presumption that persons are unambiguously individual also translates into the demand that persons behave as individuals. While it can, of course, be important to defend the ability of women, for example, to function as self-responsible individuals in legal or other contexts where this "right" might not be recognized by other members of her family or social or religious communities, it can also be an unwelcome imposition to require a woman to assume this status if her very sense of self is premised on her participation in a social world that does not recognize her as having this status.[33] In these ways, then, the premises of modern, institutionalized healthcarework against the adequate recognition of human suffering.

A third and final problem is a related presumption of "individualism", this time registered at the level of body rather than the "mind". This is the approach to the person that imagines the individual to be detachable from all other things and

---

[31]See Minuchin et al. (1978), and Bateson (1972, pp. 225–243), "The Cybernetics of 'Self': A Theory of Alcoholism." See also Laing and Esterson (1990). On the need for care itself to take the form of an intersubjective network, see Fritsch (2010).

[32]On the suffering faced by immigrants due to separation from family, town and homeland, and the problems intrinsic to living in a new land from which one is always "absent," see Sayad (2004).

[33]See Fadiman (2012), for the related issues of the clash of cultures in the experience of a Hmong family's struggle with the American hospital system following the diagnosis of epilepsy in one of their daughters. On the ambivalent value of the notion of "individual rights" in the context of different religious cultures, see Hoff (forthcoming).

spaces that are not "one's own body". In fact, the attachments we considered immediately above that bind our sense of self to other people are themselves paralleled by bonds of attachment to a worldly, material "home".[34] As we saw in the context of Merleau-Ponty's analysis of the "habit body", it is essential to our sense of self that we have "behind" us a developed way of being in the world to which we are habituated. This "habit body" is essentially the way we have made for ourselves a home in the world, on the basis of which we are able to engage in the moment-by-moment activities of daily life. This lived sense of "home" draws centrally upon the interpersonal and social relationships mentioned in the preceding point but also upon spatial and material realities, such as a house, a yard, furniture, a street, photographs, etc. As with the failure to recognize the intersubjective tissue of selfhood, so does the failure to recognize the spatial tissue of selfhood lead to a number of problems. (a) Kirsten Jacobson, for example, has done substantial work to demonstrate that existential maladies such as agoraphobia, hypochondria and anorexia should be understood as "disorders of dwelling," but the presumption of the ontological isolation of the person to the individual body entails that these forms of suffering that are rooted distinctly and definitively in problematic relationships to "home" are not recognized as such and resulting in mistaken diagnoses and inadequate treatments.[35] (b) Suffering that is rooted in "tissue damage" to our lived spatiality is not recognized as such, but, if acknowledged at all, is seen only as a "subjective discomfort". These are problems, again, characteristic of immigrants or refugees who suffer from their separation from their homes, and again of the elderly, for whom the spatial (and, to be sure, the interpersonal) world in which they made their home—"the old neighbourhood," for example—disappears with time.[36] (c) Virtually by definition, to be "institutionalized" is itself a painful separation from one's home, and thus is itself a kind of suffering.[37] This is a significant reality in any case, but it is especially significant for those persons, such as the chronically ill and the very old, for whom life in the hospital becomes a permanent reality and the failure of healthcare workers to recognize and understand this compounds the sufferings of these individuals.[38] Here again, then, we can recognize from a variety of angles ways in which the premises of contemporary healthcare preclude it in

---

[34]For the theme of "home" in the phenomenological interpretation of the person, see Jacobson (2009).

[35]See Jacobson (2004, 2006). For a reflection on the political implications of this interpretation of agoraphobia, see Jacobson (2011).

[36]On the pain of "homesickness," pertinent as much to interpersonal as to spatial relations, see Russon (2013a).

[37]On the experiential implications of hospital architecture, see Adams et al. (2010).

[38]On the significance of hospital architecture in general, see especially Ulrich (2000, pp. 49–59). On the stress faced by children and youth in hospital environments, see Pillitter (1987, pp. 567–578), and Korpela (2001). On the theme of permanent institutionalization of the elderly as an undermining of the experience of home and the forms of suffering related to this and to the failure of healthcare practitioners to recognize this, see Young (2005). On the distinctive experience of coming to find oneself at home in the sickbed, see Van den Berg (1966), especially Chap. 1, "The Meaning of Being Ill".

principle from adequately recognizing and addressing the real forms of human suffering that are revealed by a phenomenological or Buddhist analysis of our experience.

9.3 Conclusion

It is the definitive mandate of the healthcare profession to show compassion and to care for persons in their suffering. The most prominent forms of contemporary healthcare, however, are premised on an interpretive model of the human person that fundamentally distorts the phenomenon of suffering and, consequently, care. The long-standing insights of Buddhism and the contemporary analyses of phenomenology offer a compelling, alternative vision of the nature of human experience that offers rich resources for criticizing contemporary healthcare practices and for developing alternative approaches to healthcare that are simultaneously more appropriately compassionate and more effective.

References

Adams, A., Theodore, D., McLaren, C., & McKeever, P. (2010). Kids in the atrium: Comparing architectural intentions and children's experiences in a pediatric hospital lobby. *Social Sciences and Medicine, 70*(5), 658–667.

Bateson, G. (1972). *Steps to an ecology of mind*. Chicago, IL: University of Chicago Press.

Berman, M. (2004). Merleau-Ponty and Nagarjuna: Relational social ontology and the ground of ethics. *Asian Philosophy, 14*(2), 131–145.

Bourdieu, P. (1980). *The logic of practice*. (R. Nice, Trans.). Stanford, CA: Stanford University Press.

Bredlau, S. (2006). Learning to see: Merleau-Ponty and the navigation of 'terrains'. *Chiasmi International, 8*, 191–198.

Casey, E. S. (2007). *The world at a glance*. Bloomington: Indiana University Press.

Cassel, E. J. (1982). The nature of suffering and the goals of medicine. *New England Journal of Medicine, 306*(11), 639–45.

Costello, P. (2012). *Layers in Husserl's phenomenology: On meaning and intersubjectivity*. Toronto: University of Toronto Press.

Coulehan, J. (2012). Suffering, hope and healing. In R. J. Moore (Ed.), *Handbook of pain and palliative care: Biobehavioral approaches to the life course* (pp. 717–732). New York: Springer.

Davids, C. A. F. R., & Woodward, F. L. (Trans.). (1917). *Saṃyutta Nikāya (The book of kindred sayings)*, 5 Vols. London: Pāli Text Society.

Descartes, R. (1979). *Meditations on first philosophy*. (D. A. Cress, Trans.) Indianapolis: Hackett.

Doniger, W. (2009). *The Hindus: An alternative history*. New York: Penguin.

Conze, E. Horner, I. B., Snellgrove, D., & Waley, A. (Eds. & Trans.). (1995). *Buddhist texts through the ages*. Oxford: One World.

Fadiman, A. (2012). *The spirit catches you and you fall down: A Hmong child, her American doctors, and the collision of two cultures*. New York: Farrar, Straus and Giroux.

Fritsch, K. (2010). Intimate assemblages: Disability, intercorporeality, and the labour of attendant care. *Critical Disability Studies, 2*, 1–14.

Goldenberg, M. (2010). Clinical evidence and the absent body in medical phenomenology: On the need for a new phenomenology of medicine. *The International Journal of Feminist Approaches to Bioethics, 3*(1), 43–71.

Harvey, P. (1990). *An introduction to Buddhism: Teachings, history and practices*. Cambridge: Cambridge University Press.

Hoff, S. (Forthcoming). Hegel and the possibility of intercultural criticism. In N. Robertson & S. Dodd (Eds.), *Unity of opposites?. Hegel and Canadian political thought*. Toronto: University of Toronto Press.

Honkasalo, M. L. (2000). Chronic pain as a posture towards the world. *Scandinavian Journal of Psychology, 41*(3), 197–208.

Horner, I. B. (Trans.). (1954–1959). *Middle Length Sayings (Majjhima Nikāya)*, 3 Vols. London: Pali Text Society.

Howell, W. (2015). Learning and the development of meaning: Husserl and Merleau-Ponty and the temporality of perception and habit. *Southern Journal of Philosophy 53*, 1–27.

Husserl, E. (1997). *Thing and space: Lectures of 1907*. (R. Rojcewicz, Trans.). Dordrecht: Kluwer.

Husserl, E. (2001). *Analyses concerning passive and active synthesis: Lectures on transcendental logic*. (A. J. Steinbock, Trans.). Dordrecht: Kluwer.

Jacobson, K. (2004). Agoraphobia and hypochondria as disorders of dwelling. *International Studies in Philosophy, 36*(2), 31–44.

Jacobson, K. (2006). The interpersonal expression of human spatiality: A phenomenological interpretation of anorexia nervosa. *Chiasmi International, 8*: 157–73.

Jacobson, K. (2009). A developed nature: A phenomenological account of the experience of home. *Continental Philosophy Review, 42*(3), 355–73.

Jacobson, K. (2011). Embodied domestics, embodied politics: Women, home, and agoraphobia. *Human Studies, 34*(1), 1–21.

Kabat-Zinn, J., Lipworth, L., & Burney, R. (1985). The clinical use of mindfulness meditation for the self-regulation of chronic pain. *Journal of Behavioural Medicine, 8*(2), 163–190.

Kant, I. (2005). *Groundwork for the metaphysics of morals*. (T. K. Abbott, Trans.; revised; L. Denis, Ed.). Peterborough: Broadview Press.

Korpela, K. (2001). Children's environment. In R. B. Bechtel & A. Churchman (Eds.), *Handbook of environmental psychology* (pp. 363–373). New York: John Wiley and Sons.

Laing, R. D., & Esterson, A. (1990). *Sanity, madness and the family: Families of schizophrenics*. Harmondsworth: Penguin.

Leder, D. (2005). Moving beyond 'mind' and 'body'. *Philosophy, Psychiatry, and Psychology, 12*(2), 109–113.

Macpherson, C. B. (1962). *The political theory of possessive individualism: Hobbes to Locke*. Oxford: Clarendon Press.

Marratto, S. (2012). *The intercorporeal self: Merleau-Ponty on subjectivity*. Albany, NY: State University of New York Press.

Mazis, G. (2009). The flesh of the world is emptiness and emptiness is the flesh of the world, and their ethical implications. In J. Y. Park & G. Kopf (Eds.), *Merleau-Ponty and Buddhism* (pp. 183–208). Lanham MD: Lexington Books.

McMahon, L. (2014). *The Phantom Organic: Merleau-Ponty and the Psychoanalysis of Nature. Chiasmi International 16*, 275–90.

Merleau-Ponty, M. (2012). *Phenomenology of perception* (D. A. Landes, Trans.). New York: Routledge.

Miller, B. S. (Trans.). (1988). *Bhagavad Gita*. New York: Bantam Books.

Minuchin, S., Rosman, B. L., & Baker, L. (1978). *Psychosomatic families: Anorexia Nervosa in context*. Cambridge, MA: Harvard University Press.

Morris, D. B. (1991). *The culture of pain*. Berkeley, CA: University of California Press.

Okifuji, A., & Turk, D. C. (1998). Philosophy and efficacy of multidisciplinary approach to chronic pain management. *Journal of Anesthesia, 12*(3), 142–52.

Park, J. Y., & Kopf, G. (Eds.). (2009). *Merleau-Ponty and Buddhism*. Lanham MD: Lexington Books.

Pillitter, A. (1987). *Child health nursing*. Boston: Little Brown and Company.

Rawlinson, M. C. (1986). The sense of suffering. *Journal of Medicine and Philosophy, 11*(1), 39–62.

Russon, J. (2003). *Human experience: Philosophy, neurosis, and the elements of everyday life*. Albany, NY: State University of New York Press.

Russon, J. (2013a). Haunted by history: Merleau-Ponty, Hegel, and the phenomenology of pain. *Journal of Contemporary Thought, 37*, 81–94.

Russon, J. (2013b). The virtues of agency: A phenomenology of confidence, courage, and creativity. In K. Hermberg & P. Gyllenhammer (Eds.), *Phenomenology and virtue ethics* (pp. 165–179). New York: Bloomsbury.

Russon, J. (2014). Between two intimacies: The formative contexts of individual experience. *Emotion, Space and Society, 13*, 65–70.

Russon, J. (2015) On secrets and sharing: Hegel, Heidegger and Derrida on the economics of the public sphere. In V. Sanil & D. Dwivedi (Eds.), *Public sphere from outside the west* (pp. 41–57). New Delhi: Bloomsbury.

Russon, J. (Forthcoming). Freedom and passivity: Attention, work and language. In K. Jacobson & J. Russon (Eds.), *Perception and its development in Merleau-Ponty's phenomenology*. Toronto: University of Toronto Press.

Sayad, A. (2004). *The suffering of the immigrant* (D. Macey, Trans.). Cambridge: Polity Press.

Schenck, D. (1986). The texture of embodiment: Foundation for medical ethics. *Human Studies, 9*(1), 43–54.

Stolorow, R. (2013). Intersubjective systems-theory: A phenomenological-contextualist psycho-analytic perspective. *Psychoanalytic Dialogues, 23*(4), 383–389.

Talero, M. (2005). Perception, normativity, and selfhood in Merleau-Ponty: The spatial 'level' and existential space. *Southern Journal of Philosophy, 43*(3), 443–461.

Ulrich, R. S. (2000). Effects of healthcare environmental design on medical outcomes. In *Design and health—The therapeutic benefits of design, Proceedings of the 2nd Annual International Congress on Design and Health*. Stockholm: Karolinska Institute.

Van den Berg, J. H. (1966). *The psychology of the sickbed*. Pittsburgh, PA: Duquesne University Press.

Vermersch, P. (2004). Attention between phenomenology and experimental psychology. *Continental Philosophy Review, 37*(1), 45–81.

Whitman, S. M. (2007). Pain and suffering as viewed by the Hindu religion. *The Journal of Pain, 8*(8), 607–613.

Wilde, M. H. (2003). Embodied knowledge in chronic illness and injury. *Nursing Inquiry, 10*(3), 170–176.

Young, I. M.. (2005). A room of one's own: Old age, extended care, and privacy. In I. M. Young, *On female body experience: "Throwing like a girl" and other essays* (pp. 155–70). Oxford: Oxford University Press.

Chapter 10
Many Faces of Woman's Pain

Shefali Moitra

Abstract The present essay begins with a mapping of the types of pain endured by women in a patriarchal structure, and the efforts made to transform the situation and reduce negative forms of pain as well as covert and overt suffering. Justice is commonly invoked as a remedial measure for woman's pain. Two approaches to justice have been discussed: 'Justice as sameness', which is a pro-status quo theory, and 'justice as difference' which is a revisionary theory. Each system of justice gives rise to its own pain. One such problem is woman's lack of means for communicating her needs. The inability to make oneself understood is a major source of pain. Having discussed the taxonomy of pain as located in the context of patriarchy and as located in some of the remedial measures, an account of a few classical explanations of woman's oppression such as those given by Engels, de Beauvoir, Tagore and Freud have been stated in the hope that identification of the problem may lead towards solutions.

Keywords Justice · Power · Suffering · Difference · Sameness · Patriarchy

10.1 Structures of Patriarchy

Pain is a necessary corollary of being positioned in a patriarchal culture. A patriarchal culture is identified, among other things, by its power structure. It is also characterized by its masculine and feminine role definitions. Both the power structure and the role definitions of patriarchy are guided by a clear-cut either/or disjunction. So one either enjoys a position of power in the overarching patriarchal

Shefali Moitra is a Former Professor of the Jadavpur University

S. Moitra (✉)
Jadavpur University, Kolkata, India
e-mail: smoitra22@rediffmail.com

© Springer India 2016   197
S.K. George and P.G. Jung (eds.), *Cultural Ontology*
of the Self in Pain, DOI 10.1007/978-81-322-2601-7_10

structure, or one does not—one is either empowered, or one is disempowered. In like manner, either a particular gender role is expected of someone or it is not. The roles are also divided on the basis of an either/or binary.

When a role is not attributed to someone, then its negation is attributed. For instance, if the role of a powerful protector is not attributed to 'x' then the role of being protected is attributed to 'x'. This does not mean that individuals cannot, or do not, change roles; it means that the changes are treated as aberrations, or as exceptions to the rule. Thus, if the roles attributed to a woman are appropriated by a man then we come across expressions such as the 'effeminate' man, and if a woman follows the male-role model she is perceived to be a 'manly' woman. In this way, the change in role performance is seen as an acquired mannerism; whereas the original role ascription is perceived as natural, or as 'behaviour in conformity with nature'.

One of the things that keeps patriarchy firmly entrenched as an overarching structure is the overt and covert system of role ascriptions and associated positions of power. The regimentation takes place both through abstract and concrete forms. Abstract tools for keeping an individual on the prescribed dotted line often do not meet the naked eye. Language, literature and various art forms are the commonly used mediums to ensure conformity to role expectations. The entire value system in patriarchy is geared towards the preservation of the role-status-quo. Whatever freedom is exercised by the individual must remain circumscribed by the limits laid down by patriarchy's role expectations. Freedom has to be enjoyed within the scope of the metaphorical 'elbow room'. A structure regulated by rigid norms is meant to guarantee efficiency.

The power structure in patriarchy is a top-down power structure. The path from the position at the bottom to the position at the top is linear. The only way to gain power in patriarchy is by imbibing the virtues of the powerful at the top. For instance, if 'knowledge' is power then the only way to gain power is through the means of 'knowledge'-acquisition. Similarly, if power is gained by 'physical strength' then those at the bottom are at the bottom because they lack physical strength and those at the top are there by virtue of their physical strength. In cases where physical strength is considered to be the key to power there knowledge will not have the same empowering capacity and vice versa. These are just two examples to illustrate how the top-down power configuration operates. There may be many other virtues that replace physical strength and knowledge as instruments of power. For instance, being born a biological male may provide the passport to power. The position at the top is not necessarily characterized by a single instrument of power.

Patriarchy often speaks of a cluster of characteristics that equip one for the position of power. Some of the commonly acknowledged power-yielding charac-teristics are physical strength, control over emotions and capacity for abstract thinking and rationality. Patriarchy may take many forms depending on the char-acteristics that are attributed to the powerful individual. Patriarchy is defined in terms of the top-down power structure and not in terms of the choice of coveted characteristics. The choice of characteristics may vary from one patriarchal culture to another. Whatever be the prized characteristics they must belong to the male-gendered individual. Further, patriarchy is not a monolithic structure of power. It intersects with other structures of power based on class, caste, religion, economic status and so forth.

The top-down power structure coupled with a gender division forms the basis of patriarchy. The purpose of this structure is to control woman's productive and reproductive labour so as to bring forth an efficient system of production and inheritance. Patriarchy is grounded in a kind of dualistic rational practice. As a result the 'bottom' or the 'other' is defined in terms of a negation of the characteristics possessed by the 'top'. Thus the 'bottom' or the 'other' is neither characterized nor assessed independently on the basis of its unique attributes. The 'other' is always characterized as the negation of a primary position. So if man occupies the primary position at the top then woman is treated as the 'other' and positioned at the bottom. This means that she is not identified independently. She is identified by the negation of the master's traits. Her traits are seen as a 'lack'. The only way she can be empowered is by gaining the master's virtues and being included in the master's house. She has no stand-alone-virtues. If man gains power through possessing the virtues of physical strength, abstraction, control over emotions and rationality then woman will be characterized as the 'other' or as lacking these virtues. In order to reach the pinnacle of power she must acquire the master's virtues.

Before examining the possibility of woman's acquiring power we need to outline her given position in patriarchy. Perceived as a 'lack' or the 'other' or as complementary to man woman is initially bereft of the male-gender virtues by definition. This means she lacks physical strength, capacity for abstract thinking, control over emotion and a proclivity towards rational thinking—or she lacks whatever attributes are considered to be manly by a particular patriarchal culture. Thus the virtues she possesses will be the opposite, e.g. she will have the capacity for concrete thinking, she will be emotional and she will use emotion as a guiding principle. Once the respective role expectations are laid down in terms of clear-cut binaries the social relationships and institutions are then accordingly organized.

10.2   Heads I Win, Tails You Lose

Woman's position as the 'other' in patriarchy is precarious. On the one hand she is expected to nurture certain traits which will qualify her to be a 'good woman'; on the other hand the very same traits disqualify her from occupying a position at the 'top'. To gain power she has to acquire a contrary set of characteristics. This gives rise to a tension. She is never at ease. If she remains at the bottom and conforms to her feminine-role-ascription she is bereft of power, and if she is positioned at the top then her feminine-role-ascriptions are incompatible with the expectations attached to her status. Women often try to cope with this tension through a fine balancing act. The balance is never perfect and this causes the woman to suffer from uneasiness and a sense of guilt. Guilt arises because the woman feels she is not able to do justice to either the prescribed feminine role or the acquired masculine role. A constant sense of pain is associated with such guilt. The conflict of roles not only gives rise to guilt-related pain, the existential conflict leads to a paralysis of judgment which is painful.

In the public eye women appear to be indecisive, weak, vacillating, inefficient and decorative pieces. None of these evaluations is complimentary. They all lead to low self-esteem and a painful state of dejection. It is expected that woman will transcend her allotted position at the bottom and rise to a position at the top. Since the transcendence is never total the 'inclusion' leads to an incongruity which is painful. While going through the process of being included or absorbed into the top, the tension of being pulled between two value-paradigms—the masculine and the feminine—causes pain. The 'top' is a constructed space. One can only enter that space and become a member by acquiring male gender virtues. Male members of society dominate this space as there is an absolute 'fit' between their role ascriptions and the specifications of this space. Men are comfortable in this location as the fish in water. But, for the woman she has to gain another kind of accomplishment and at the same time not lose her femininity (Beauvoir 2010, p. 296).

The way out of this conflict is not by shifting from patriarchy to matriarchy. Matriarchy is based on the same top-down power structure.[1] There is only a shift in the position of man and woman. Woman with her gender virtues will be placed on the top in matriarchy and man will subsequently be treated as the 'other', the 'lack'. As long as the top-down power configuration persists and the 'other' is treated as a lack, the other will be in pain. This is so, irrespective of whether the 'other' is situated at the bottom of the power structure as in the case of the 'feminine' woman or is included in the top as in the case of the 'masculinized' woman.

The patriarchal status quo is often enforced by denying the right of inclusion. Members situated at the bottom are denied entry at the top. Similar mechanisms are also adopted by the caste-hierarchy. In patriarchy the non-inclusion may be on account of an exclusion imposed by those at the top or it may be a refusal opted for by those who are at the bottom. The members at the bottom may feel that the top is not a coveted position. They may feel the bottom is a location that holds a greater promise for improvement, freedom and empowerment. Thus, working for an improvement of the situation at the bottom may be more desirous than an exodus from the bottom. Such a stance is characterized as an essentialist position since it is pro-status quo. The pain felt by the citizens at the bottom in the essentialist account is not the same as that of the 'inclusionist' account.

Patriarchy is an oppressive system. It tries to coerce people into predetermined slots. Those situated at the margins or at the bottom of the structure are the worst

---

[1]Whether matriarchy was ever present in history is a debatable issue. Engels held, there was a transition from matriarchy to patriarchy leading to the 'great historical defeat of the feminine sex'. Simone de Beauvoir contests this point. According to her, "in reality this golden age of Woman is only a myth" (Beauvoir 2010, p. 80). We may also note that historical experience of matrilineal and matriarchal societies like the Khasi-Jaintia and Garo communities of Meghalaya and the Nayars of Kerala are once again heavily weighed against women. They have been societies that entitle women but relieve men of their responsibilities, ending up like in the modern cases of double burden for the working women.

affected because they are the victims of all forms of deprivation. Being confined to the bottom means being subjugated to pain and suffering. Ironically being at the top also entails suffering, of course, of a different form.

Those who are in positions of power have to constantly 'perform' in order to hold on to their position. They always suffer from the anxiety of not being able to project the image of an all-knowing, fully rational and strong individual. No doubt much of their power is derived from supporting institutions, like being the head of an institution or receiving the protection of powerful institutions, like, political parties and religious institutions. Powerful institutional support is frequently employed to alleviate one's anxiety of losing control. Since institutions and their associated power are transient they fail to give a dependable prophylaxis for anxiety. Being in the driver's seat may be a coveted position but remaining there is problematic. An apt account of this situation can be found in the proverb 'uneasy lies the head that wears the crown'. The only permanent way out of this crisis is to change the ball game, in this case, change the configuration of power. Only a shift from a top-down configuration to a power-sharing configuration can solve the problem. Unless such a structural change can be brought about pain and suffering will remain an integral part of the top position in patriarchy. Patriarchy not only brings about suffering to the margins it also impacts the core.

So far we have identified two categories of sufferers: (1) those who are deprived and are at the bottom and (2) those who are anxious as well as afraid and are at the top. There could be a third group who are happy with their assigned role but object to its devaluation. They are historically positioned at the margins. Their pain and suffering is caused by non-recognition of their autonomous existence. They deny being the 'other'. They claim to be 'different', not in terms of being a negation of the original, or in terms of being a lack. In a disjunctive framework that accommodates only one position and its negation there is no room for 'radical difference'. Difference is always reduced to a derivative of the 'same'.[2] This model of interpretation poses a stumbling block for the upholders of radical difference it leads to a communication failure between the respective supporters of the two models. The failure of communication is painful and it causes suffering. The communication failure is a result of a conflict of world views. The proponents of radical difference accuse the former group of imposing discrimination by interpreting 'difference' in terms of a 'lack'.

10.3   Difference and 'Justice as Sameness'

When one group defines the masculine–feminine difference in terms of a derivative of the original and expresses the difference in the following symbolic form 'p versus ∼p' and the second group speaks of radical difference and expresses it in the

---

[2]"The proposition "p" and "∼p" have opposite sense, but there corresponds to them one and the same reality" (Wittgenstein 1961, p. 4.0621).

symbolic form 'p versus q' and they both claim that their understanding of the masculine–feminine difference is correct, then we are left with a choice between the two, that is, either (p versus ∼p) or (p versus q). The former interpretation may be referred to as the derivative theory of difference and the latter as the radical theory of difference. The logic of bivalence will demand that one has to be a true account of difference and the other has to be false. Historically there have been feminist proponents of both interpretations of difference. Each interpretation has far-reaching consequences for the understanding of gender injustice and pain.

When these two interpretations of difference are translated into their related forms of practice the stark disparity between the implications of these two views comes to light. It may be added that a way of evaluating the differentiated members is associated with each of these interpretations. In the former one side of the disjunction is given more value than the other, because, one is taken to be the original and the other is its lack. So it is not only that 'p' is different from ' ∼p', it is also the case that 'p' is more worthy or more complete than ' ∼p'. By contrast the interpretation of difference in terms of 'p v q' also attaches a value tag to the two members of the disjunction but unlike the former interpretation the value tags may have the same valence.

The practical implications of the two interpretations of difference can now be compared and contrasted in the domain of gender justice. Gender justice is a major issue in feminist theory and practice. All feminists agree that gender injustice is one of the primary sources of pain and suffering. Therefore, the achievement of gender justice is the central aim of feminist theory and activism. Commonly gender justice is equated with gender equality. Those who interpret the difference between masculine and feminine in terms of 'p versus ∼p' will forward a theory of gender equality which will be very different from the theory of gender equality propounded by the advocates of radical difference, that is, in terms of 'p versus q'.

The difference between the two positions could be highlighted by their respective responses to Aristotle's famous dictum: 'like cases to be treated alike and different cases differently'. The derivative theory of difference may use Aristotle's dictum to undermine the theory that woman's subordination is unjust (Kiss 1998, p. 487). Since 'p' is different from ' ∼p' their respective treatments should also be different according to Aristotle's dictum. Equal treatment is legitimate in cases where the members are equal. Two members are equal when the same predicates can be attributed to them. The way patriarchy has defined gender-roles the same predicates cannot be attributed to men and women. They can be equal only if they are the same.

To be the same, ' ∼p' will have to overcome her lack and 'become' the same as 'p'. Often 'differential' treatment is encouraged to bring the deprived-party up to the benchmark so that justice can be equally meted out to them. Many concessions could be sanctioned with a view to creating a level playing-field. Once this is attained, justice can be 'properly' implemented. After all the Greek Goddess of justice is portrayed as blindfolded and holding a pair of scales in her hand that is not tilted to any side. This reminds us of the Hindi expression '*andha kanoon*' or 'the law is blind'. This does not mean the law is unseeing it means the law is unbiased.

An unbiased law is projected as an impartial law. Feminists who are not in favour of 'justice as sameness' acknowledge that the aim of such theories is to do away with difference and pluralism in the eyes of law so that justice can prevail. They point out that doing away with difference would create a monolithic culture where the voice of the powerful will form the normative standard. All other voices will then be subsumed under that one voice. The fear is, a subsumption of the different to the same cannot be gained through the normal course of action. Without coercion and violence all the different voices cannot be brought under one umbrella-voice. If this feminist understanding of justice as sameness is correct then this model of justice must accept violence to be an integral part of justice. This gives rise to a paradox. The concept of justice as sameness was initially invoked to do away with injustice since that was the primary source of pain. Now if violence is a part and parcel of justice as sameness then gaining justice will mean opting for justice-inflicted pain. This would be a situation of moving to the fire out of the fry pan.

Those who speak in favour of 'justice as sameness' may argue that what is being termed 'violence' is actually a form of disciplining meant for the improvement of humankind. Disciplining may not be appealing to all. It may even seem unpleasant and in that sense painful. One may want to persist with the argument and say, 'this kind of pain is beneficial to all'. Pain may be of two types: positive pain and negative pain. The former yields positive results, like, growing pain. Many painful feelings are delightful, for instance the hardships of difficult and complex thoughts (Rorty 2009, p. 83). One may be reminded of John Stuart Mill's famous pronouncement, 'better to be Socrates dissatisfied than a fool satisfied'. This kind of pain should not be equated with suffering.

Suffering is a form of negative pain. We began by discussing the syndrome of pain in woman's lived experience and now we have used the expression 'suffering'. This is a significant shift. One of the definitions of pain given by *The Concise Oxford Dictionary* is 'mental suffering or distress'. So pain may also be understood as suffering. However, all cases of pain are not instances of suffering whereas all sufferings are painful. Thus all pains do not call for remedy, but, all sufferings do. In other words, negative pains are synonymous with suffering and need remedy; whereas, positive pains are not cases of suffering and they do not call for remedy or cure.

10.4 Justice as Difference

The supporters of 'justice as difference' would argue that their objection to 'justice as sameness' has been grossly misunderstood. They admit the fact that there are pains that are not synonymous with suffering. They object to the indiscriminate elimination of difference. Not because difference is a value in itself but because the freedom of choice is greatly cherished and cannot be bartered for justice-as-sameness without reservation. The indiscriminate curbing of freedom is a negative pain and a cause of suffering. 'Justice as sameness' propagates the agenda of regimentation which is not a pro-choice agenda.

The feminist opponents of the theory of 'justice as sameness' are divided into two groups: one group wants to redefine justice and the other group seeks to opt out of the justice framework altogether and look for other alternatives for addressing gender discrimination. The ethics of care is forwarded as one such alternative to justice as sameness. The ethics of care will not be discussed in the present essay. The focus will be on the attempt to avoid pain through an alternative model of justice. The alternative to 'justice as sameness' is 'justice as difference'. The latter attempts to continue with the feminist commitment to justice and acknowledges the recalcitrant nature of difference. The proponents of 'justice as difference' accuse the supporters of 'justice as sameness' of throwing the baby with the bath water. In the name of delivering gender justice they do away with the category of gender itself. In an economy of sameness there is no room for gender-difference. This is achieved by shifting their focus from the categories of man and woman to the category of human which according to them is a neutered category. The very possibility of acquiring a neutered identity is questioned by the upholders of 'justice as difference'.

Feminists who are engaged with a theory of 'justice as difference' do not give up their allegiance to justice as equality. Obviously, the proponents of 'justice as sameness' consider this to be a contradiction in terms. They ask, 'how can a commitment to equality be fulfilled without a commitment to sameness'. In other words, how can equality and difference be coherently accommodated in a single system of justice? In response to this question, theorists championing 'justice-as-difference' argue, this is the only way in which pain related to regi-mentation and the denial of freedom can be redressed.

Theorists who champion 'justice-as-difference' begin by redefining equality. As Elizabeth Kiss reports, "indeed recent feminist arguments about gender and equal treatment deepen our understanding of equality under the law as 'lack of hierarchy not sameness'" (Kiss 1998, p. 489). The lack of hierarchy in the case of a comparison between man and woman would mean that their being different does not legitimize a discriminatory value-judgment. There is no scope for introducing a hierarchy between two different relata. Justice as sameness diligently holds on to the Aristotelian law of identity where 'a = a', whereas the justice as difference theory is willing to uphold the possibility of 'a = b'. Without going into the question of whether 'justice as difference' is a proper explanation of justice or not let us accept it as a coherent alternative to 'justice as sameness'.

Having a plausible alternative theory of justice does not ensure the implemen-tation of that theory. The first step towards implementation is to be able to convey the theory to possible implementers. A problem arises when the concepts contained in the new theory are so novel and different from the existing views that they are not comprehended by the dispensers of justice. This is an instance of speaking from two different conceptual frameworks. In one framework equality means sameness and in the other equality means non-hierarchy.

10.5   Overt and Covert Suffering, Positive and Negative Pain

To borrow an expression from Quine, the speakers representing two different conceptual frameworks are not merely 'words apart', they are 'worlds apart'. When two individuals desire each other's companionship and there is total communication failure the situation is frustrating to say the least. If an individual feels that the communication breakdown can never be repaired then there is either a resignation to the situation or a persistent dissatisfaction with the situation. Resignation leads to covert suffering and dissatisfaction leads to overt suffering. The issue may be further elucidated by the help of an example.

According to the mainstream modernist account there exists a mind/body dualism—mind is qualified by consciousness and body lacks consciousness. Further, philosophy is associated with a purely mental activity by the modernist. This has led to 'philosophy's bodiless commitment to thought' (Zita 1998, p. 309). Radical feminists who want to bring in the discussion on body and sexuality into mainstream philosophy find this to be an obstacle. As a result most feminist reconceptualizations of sexuality have by and large occurred outside of mainstream philosophy (Zita 1998, p. 307). There remains that dissatisfaction of not being allowed to raise philosophical questions about issues that are central to woman's lived experience. Feminists feel, by disallowing a philosophical discussion on sexuality a kind of silencing is being imposed. Silencing leads to a communication breakdown of a different kind. The communication crisis discussed above in the context of two theories of justice was related to a semantic problem, namely, 'what is the meaning of equality?'. The communication problem related to the non-recognition of sexuality as a philosophical problem is not a semantic problem. The question is one of accommodating or not accommodating a lived experience in philosophy. Philosophy is commonly defined as 'the love for wisdom'. Feminists who push for the inclusion of sexuality into philosophy feel pained at mainstream philosophy's refusal to do so. The struggle for the recognition of sexuality as a legitimate concern of philosophy continues. This is a case of communication failure due to stonewalling. Here the resulting suffering is overt. The suffering increases manifold because sexuality and related abuses lie at the root of discrimination against women. The continued avoidance of critical engagement with this problem and its consignment to silence is part of the problem.

Stonewalling is one side of the problem. The other side is woman's lack of conceptual apparatus. In the absence of an existing platform for discussing such issues threadbare an adequate vocabulary and means of expression need to be developed. The little that is being formulated is not receiving a patient hearing. What emerges is not a case of communication failure; it is a case of non-communication or a communication non-starter. A second group of feminists prefer to remain resigned to the situation. Instead of pushing for the reconceptualization of philosophy and the inclusion of sexuality into philosophy, these feminists have called for a reprivatization of the personal (Zita 1998, p. 307). This means the problems associated with sexuality will never be critically discussed. Individuals will be left to fend for themselves. Since truth-telling is part of the solution redemption of this problem will never be forthcoming. Each will have to depend on one's individual resources to find a way out of sexual oppression. The resulting pain will have to be suffered in silence. An invisible silent pain may become an unrecognized covert pain.

Patriarchy places women in a place where sexual abuse is a regular feature. Women are subjected to progroms of rape, witch hunt and female feticide. Privatizing the personal is compatible with the patriarchal design. Patriarchy requires the adaptation to the pain accruing from these and similar practices. An accompanying insensitivity is a highly prized response as that could further entrench the power status quo. We had made a distinction between 'positive pain' and 'negative pain' and concluded that positive pain is facilitating and negative pain is debilitating and is a form of suffering. Progroms against women are an instance of negative pain and suffering. Adaptation and cultivated insensitivity to negative pain could be ways of alleviating such pain. A common prescription for women is to try and forget and open a new chapter in life. Some women may feel that finding an escape route from negative pain is the only option and forgetting provides such a way out.

Moira Gatens does not support an escapist stance. She admits that remembering deeds of violence can be extremely painful. She also admits that forgetting helps overcome pain. Yet she thinks there are certain things that cannot be forgotten and more importantly should not be forgotten. She says, "But *how* they are remembered is important for the present and the future. We need to understand and remember how we became what we are, not in order to live what we have become as our 'truth' but rather as our conditions of possibility for that which we may become" (Gatens 1996, p. 77).

Thus a distinction needs to be made between the pain suffered due to a program, which is a negative pain and the memory of that progrom which is a positive pain. Remembering helps us to be self-consciously political and work for a change (Gaten 1996, p. 77).

10.6 How Did This Happen?

In a male-dominated, male-produced culture woman's autonomous identity is lost. The recurrent question is 'how did this happen?' or 'why did this happen?' Why did woman not assert her identity and claim a role in formulating culture? De Beauvoir tells us whenever they intervened in history it was from a masculine point of view (Beauvoir 2010, p. 149). The question continues to haunt us, 'how did man succeed in moulding woman according to his design?'

When feminists try to 'understand and remember how we became what we are' they come up against disparate accounts of history forwarded by male protagonists. Human culture has been constructed by men and has been dominated by men. Of the various explanations forwarded by men some explanations of woman's subjugation have been appropriated in principle by feminists. Some of the more commonly accepted explanations are the Freudian, the Marxist and the existentialist explanations of the subjection of women.

The Marxist thesis has been clearly explained in Engel's *The Origin of the Family, Private Property and the State* (1972). He explains how male power grew out of economic dominance and sexual authority over women. Engels speaks of the 'world-historical defeat of the female sex'. He believes there was a time when 'each was master in his or her own field of activity'. But when production became more valued than household work then 'the wife became the first domestic servant'. All feminist thinkers do not agree with Engel's account of the beginning of woman's subjugation and suffering. We shall not enter into this debate here.

Simone de Beauvoir's position on the history of gender discrimination is similar to the Marxian position. She too thinks that history was written by man in his own interest and women's interests were never taken into consideration. De Beauvoir believes that it is man's interests, concerns, fears and needs that counted (Beauvoir 2010, p. 148). In the picture she draws, woman's subordination is somewhat a matter of convenience for her. So there is a kind of unholy alliance between the dominating male and the subordinated female.

This point is often missed by the readers of *The Second Sex*. Readers tend to believe that according to de Beauvoir women were pushed to the margins by men who ganged up to 'make' woman what she is today, even though she was not born that way. This is a misinterpretation of the opening sentence of Part Two of *The Second Sex*, 'one is not born, but rather becomes, a woman'. Simone's careful choice of words needs to be noted, she says 'becomes' she does not say 'is made'. Women's choices made on the basis of bad faith are largely responsible for her marginalized position. De Beauvoir says: "Hence woman makes no claim for herself as subject because she lacks the concrete means, because she senses the necessary link connecting her to man without positing its reciprocity, and because she often derives satisfaction from her role as *other*" (Beauvoir 2010, p. 10).

De Beauvoir points out that this top-down relation between man and woman has been present throughout history. There was never a time when woman was not subordinate to man. She also says that the subordination did not take place at any fixed point of time. Had that been so a change in the power equation could also be undone at a fixed point of time. This does not imply that history is an immutable given according to Simone. She squarely holds woman responsible for not transforming the situation (Beauvoir 2010, p. 8).

Tagore has a similar but more charitable view about the male dominance of culture. According to him in the initial stages of civilization women were preoccupied with the chores of child rearing and the responsibility of reproduction. This kept women fully preoccupied whereas men had more leisure on their hands. Therefore, men could invest their energies in abstract activities like propagating culture, law, literature, art and philosophy (Tagore 1968, p. 380). As a result woman had no role in the making of history.

Tagore addresses the question 'how did man succeed in moulding woman according to his design?' He says when man loves a woman he wants to see her, in her entirety, in the form of his creation. Woman's entire form is created in man's mind and in his imagination. This is what Tagore calls, *chitter drishti* and *bhaver drishtti*. Having created a mental image of his beloved he solicits her response to his prayer or *prarthana*. He desires the fulfillment of his prayer in its entirety. But, what does he achieve by merely soliciting a certain disposition or behaviour? Does such solicitation or prayer ensure a desired response?

Tagore holds that solicitations and entreaties have a great productive force especially if their focus is unambiguous and clearly expressed. He feels if what is asked for is clear and unambiguous then one can pretty well predict what one will receive. For him solicitations do have a creative force. When confronted with such entreaties women try their level best to live up to the expectations. He says by repeatedly wanting woman to behave in a certain manner man has in a way constructed woman. Tagore says that is why women hang so many metaphorical curtains of secrecy in so many places so as to hide their 'selves'. In this way, they only project the kind of self that is solicited by men.

Bashfulness is that mode of behaviour by which women can conceal so much from the public gaze and create an impression of available empty space ready for inscription. Tagore holds that an individual who conceals one's self appears to the outer world to have no self. The self then appears to be a vacant tablet on which anything and everything may be inscribed. But why would woman subject her self to such abnegation? Tagore feels basically woman desires companionship. For the sake of companionship she is willing to decorate herself with all kinds of attributes even at the cost of concealing herself (Tagore 1968, p. 386). A similar explanation of woman's plight is found in Carol Gilligan's writings. "Women often sensed that it was dangerous to say or even to know what they wanted or thought—upsetting to others and therefore carrying with it the threat of abandonment or retaliation" (Gilligan 1993, p. ix).

Both Tagore and Gilligan speak of woman's predicament of wanting to remain related and having to pay a heavy price in order to remain related. The price has to be paid in terms of tears and unilateral adaptation. A rough prose rendition of one of Tagore's songs is as follows, "I am bound in a relationship, from which I want to come out, but coming out is painful" (Tagore 1986, p. 82; translation mine).[3]

The way de Beauvoir interprets woman's acceptance of subordination in patriarchy is very different from that of Tagore. Tagore's version may seem quite poetic. As if the male partner creates an image through desire and imagination and the female partner strives to fit the imagery by withholding her autonomy and agency. The entire process of projection and reciprocation is presented by Tagore with a romantic overtone, without a trace of pain. There is no reference to the role of power in Tagore's explanation of how man succeeded to mould woman. On the contrary, both in Marx/Engels and in Simone de Beauvoir power is a major determining factor of woman's subordination.

---

[3]*"Jaraaye aachhe baadhaa/chhaaraaye jete chai/chhaaraate gele byathaa baaje."*

Through the above discussion. I have tried to highlight the complexity of woman's position in patriarchy and some of the different ways in which the situation has been understood. Whichever way the problem is seen it is clear that woman is in a disadvantageous position in patriarchy. She may be responsible for this, a position to which de Beauvoir subscribes, or she may not be responsible. Marx and Engels believe the circumstances may be responsible for woman's degradation. Woman's nature is responsible for her degradation in society according to Freud. He explains woman's disadvantageous position in terms of biological determination. He goes on to say, "We must not allow ourselves to be deflected from such conclusions by the denials of the feminists, who are anxious to force us to regard the two sexes as completely equal in position and worth" (Freud 1991, p. 342).

10.7 Conclusion

Depending on the way we see the problem the 'cause' of woman's suffering, the 'nature' of her suffering and the 'location' of her suffering may change. In this essay, an account of the locations and types of pain suffered by women in a patriarchal structure has been outlined. Subsequently, several forms of reprisal have been examined. The pro-status quo supporters try to find some room within patriarchy where they feel secure and comfortable. A high price has to be paid for this. In order to adapt to the situation one has to accept being crippled. An extreme response to the shackles of patriarchy is to walk out of the power setup and champion, the cause of 'care'. The pain associated with this position is associated with loneliness and a form of ghettoization. A third alternative is sought through 'justice as difference'. This position also has its accompanying problems. Non-oppressive tools for dispensing justice need to be manufactured and the plan has to be implemented—both tasks are formidable. Once the problem of charting the overt and covert sources of pain is accomplished it will be easier to weigh the options.

References

Beauvoir, S. (2010). *The second sex*. (C. Borde & S. Malovany-Chevallier, Trans.). New York: Alfred A. Knopf.

Engels, F. (1972). *The origin of the family, private property and the state*. (A. West, Trans.). New York: International Publishers.

Freud, S. (1991). Some psychical consequences of the anatomical distinction between the sexes. (J. Strachey, Trans.). In S. Freud, *On sexuality: Three essays on the theory of sexuality and other works*. A. Richards (Ed.), *The Penguin Freud Library* (Vol. 7, pp. 331–343). London: Penguin.

Gatens, M. (1996). *Imaginary bodies*. New York: Routledge.

Gilligan, C. (1993). Letter to readers. In C. Gilligan, *In a different voice* (pp. ix–xxvii). Cambridge, MA: Harvard University Press.

Kiss, E. (1998). Justice. In A. M. Jagger & I. M Young (Ed.), *A companion to feminist philosophy* (pp. 487–99). Oxford: Blackwell.

Rorty, A. (2009). Spinoza on the pathos of idolatrous love and the hilarity of true Love. In M. Gaten (Ed.), *Feminist interpretations of Benedict Spinoza* (pp. 65–85). University Park, PA: The Pensylvania State University Press.

Tagore, R. (1968). *Paschim Yatrir Diary* (1929; in Bengali). In *Rabindra-rachanabali* (Vol. 19). Kolkata: Viswa-Bharati.

Tagore, R. (1986). *Gitabitan (1930)* (Vol. I). Kolkata: Viswa-Bharati Granthanbibhag.

Wittgenstein, L. (1961). *Tractatus Logico-Philosophicus* (1922). (D. F. Pears & B. F. McGuiness, Trans.). New York: Routledge and Kegan Paul.

Zita, J. (1998). Sexuality. In A. M. Jaggar & I. M. Young. (Eds.) (pp. 307–320). *A companion to feminist philosophy*. Oxford: Blackwell.

Chapter 11
Pain and Agency: On the Essential Importance of Vulnerability and Transgression

Shannon Hoff

Abstract This chapter argues that human action is inherently accompanied by various kinds of pain and that the status of the pain ensuing from action is ambivalent, both positive and negative in its significance. It begins with a description of the essentially active aspect of human experience, that character it has that involves it essentially with the world and the objects, people, and environments encompassed by the world. On the basis of that description, the chapter investigates the different kinds of pain that result from openness to this world, distinguishing between those kinds of pain to be avoided and those that are key aspects of human development, and identifying that pain that results from our separation from the intersubjective and objective conditions of agency. The chapter aims to develop a nuanced approach to the human experience of pain, arguing against the tendency to overlook and oppose certain kinds of pain.

Keywords Pain · Suffering · Action · Vulnerability · Transgression · Exclusion

This chapter argues that human action is inherently accompanied by various kinds of pain, and that the status of the pain ensuing from action is ambivalent—namely, it is not straightforwardly negative, but can also be positive. I will begin by showing the way in which action is central to the execution of a human life, or the fact that human life has an essentially active aspect, and that it thereby essentially involves the objective world, constituted by objects, environments, and others. Second, I will describe the various kinds of pain that result from our vulnerability to other people and to the world, arguing that this pain, while in some cases a danger to be avoided, is in other cases a symptom of human development and thus positive in its significance. Third, I will describe another kind of pain that is due to our intrinsic connection with the agency of others and the support of objective reality: that pain that results from our separation from intersubjective and objective realities.

S. Hoff (✉)
Memorial University of Newfoundland, St. John's, NL, Canada
e-mail: shoff@icscanada.edu

The chapter aims to develop a nuanced approach to the human experience of pain, arguing against the tendency to overlook certain kinds of pain and to too quickly oppose other kinds.[1]

11.1 The External and Intersubjective Conditions of Human Agency

To be and to persist as a human being, one typically operates in light of various goals: the goal of meeting one's immediate needs, of "making a living" or engaging in a fulfilling career, of experiencing various kinds of pleasure, of training oneself for specific activities, of educating oneself, of making and maintaining relationships with other people, of shaping one's life in light of the vision one has for oneself, and so on. Further, the accomplishment of any of these goals requires specific actions in the world: the actions of acquiring the immediate goods necessary for survival, of producing the resources that will give one access to these immediate goods, of putting oneself in specific pleasure-inducing situations, of enrolling in training and educational programs and attending classes, of talking and interacting with other people, and so on. To be human, that is, requires *enacting* oneself as human, which involves acquiring property, making a place for oneself in the world, carrying out projects in the world, and expressing oneself. It involves shaping external reality such that it circles and supports our lives and our agency, in all the manifold ways in which we exist—as animal and needy, as desiring of success, honor, and recognition, as oriented toward the production and revelation of meaningfulness. Human life is essentially externalized in this way; our lives are essentially enacted in external space and in relation to objects.[2]

The fact that there is an essentially active aspect of human life means that to be myself I must interact with that which is not me, that which does not immediately take shape around my desire, and that which may not in fact acquiesce to my will or "cooperate" in my self-enactment: namely, objects, environments, and other people. Both to sustain my physical existence and to enact a life that answers to a basic desire for meaning of some kind, I have to learn how to consume life-sustaining materials; how to move around in space with the help of my body, other vehicles, and traffic systems; how to acquire housing, employment, and money; how to deal with the various systems in which phenomena such as food, housing, employment, and money are embedded, and so on. Further, to perform these actions I emerge into a space that is shared with others; I act on and appropriate objects that are also real for them; I participate in contexts, situations, and procedures that also include them.

---

[1]On the rich variety of the forms of pain, see Wilde (2003) and Schenck (1986).

[2]For a phenomenological discussion of the ways in which action is essentially outside of our control insofar as it brings us into relationship with an external world and the judgements of others, see the section called "The Spiritual Animal Kingdom" in Hegel's *Phenomenology of Spirit*.

Being myself, therefore, always affects and implicates other people, since the objects, environments, and situations that I touch or produce in my self-enactment are also real for them.[3] But my action does more than affect others; rather, it is effectively *constituted* by them. On the one hand, the actions of others have shaped the world that becomes my domain of activity, and I have objects, situations, and realities to engage with on the basis of their activity, and on the other hand I am reliant on other people to help create in me the capacity for activity, to guide me to the point at which I can act and to continue to improve my capacity for specific kinds of action. I learn the skills of activity primarily through the help of other people, which means that I rely on their cooperation even prior to developing the ability to request it, and my own early ideas about the shape that my development should take are largely unreliable. I am fundamentally dependent on them for my capacity to be myself, since I do not emerge in the world as a capable being and I do not have the capacity to choose or reject their intervention or to judge whether or not their guidance is responsible, reasonable, or good.[4]

While enacting ourselves implicates objects, environments, and other people, we do not typically obtain their consent for that self-enactment. In cultivating in another person the capacity to act, for instance, we do not gain consent from her, but forcefully shape her without her consent. In fact, one of the capacities we typically aim to develop through such cultivation, whether we are conscious of it or not, is the capacity *for* consent, the capacity to make choices for oneself and interact with other people in a self-directed way; this capacity itself needs formation. In other ordinary contexts, we extend constantly beyond the boundaries of our own bodies and psyches without asking the consent of others—in flagging down an auto rickshaw, in writing an essay, in selling a house, in commenting on someone's behavior, and so on. It is impossible to live while remaining within individual physical and psychical boundaries; living essentially involves their traversal. We rarely ask people if they will allow this extension of our bodies and purposes into the world, inserting ourselves into domains that are also the domains of their action and interacting with objects that are also for them without their explicit permission.

We do, of course, attempt to deal with this inevitability in various ways. In teaching people to be mature, for instance, and in taking on the aim of maturity ourselves, we aim at forms of action that would fit the general trajectory of other more or less reasonable people, meaning that it is likely that we would be able to obtain consent from them for the things that we want to do. The development of mature understanding is to some extent the development of a capacity to understand the perspectives of others and take them into account in formulating our own purposes and actions; hence, while we may not actually obtain consent for our

---

[3]For a discussion of the idea that in acting in the world we are *ipso facto* implicated in relations with others, see Russon (2009, pp. 98–105).

[4]For treatment of the centrality of recognition by others to the formation of the human person, see Laing (1990), the section called "Independence and Dependence of Self-Consciousness" in Hegel's *Phenomenology of Spirit*, and the Second Theorem (§3) of Fichte's *Foundations of Natural Right*.

actions, we may act in a way that in principle deserves it. Further, our societies are generally shaped in accordance with law, and in living in accordance with law, which we typically do, we are implicitly acting on the basis of the permission and consent of others. Because of the way in which law construes "small business" and "private house," for instance, my access to the business is protected and my access to the house is forbidden, under ordinary circumstances, and this is what its inhabitants or owners effectively desire. In obeying the law, then, I am indirectly acting out of a respect for that desire. In a sense, the law is an embodiment of respect for consent, since the law structures shared reality so as to support collaborative behavior and prevent undesired intrusions and transgressions.[5]

Even with law and the adoption of a basic moral attitude toward other people, however, it is impossible to avoid transgression and conflict completely, and thus also impossible to avoid producing the pain and suffering that come from them. Let us explore some of the forms that that transgression takes, and the various kinds of pain and suffering that attach to each form.

11.2   The Pain of Transgression

We experience a specific kind of pain because of the fact that our action is always embedded in a context shared by others, a pain due to the fact that our actions always have the potential to hinder the effective actions of others, in such a way that they can be anything from a minor irritation to a major obstacle. A person who takes the only available taxi before another person is able to do so may keep that second person from seeing her dying father for the last time or from seeing his child being born. A student who enrolls in a class on a whim may indirectly prevent another from enrolling in that class, hence from completing the requirement of her degree in the intended period of time, and hence putting her family's financial well-being at risk. A woman half-heartedly decides to apply for a job, and she is offered the job and takes it, giving it up after only one year, whereas for the second, rejected and equally qualified candidate on the list, the job was the epitome of all that he wanted. A man decides that the trajectory of his development requires that he move from Lahore to Delhi, even though his partner's life and well-being will be thereby constrained and challenged. Since enacting oneself and one's own purposes requires taking up the world as one's domain, it can involve disrupting the trajectory of others for whom the world is the same and causing them pain associated

---

[5]In his discussion of "tacit consent" in the *Two Treatises*, John Locke implicitly illuminates the way in which the law expresses a certain basic respect for the consenting individual. In principle, reasonable people would seek to avoid rule by the arbitrary self-interest of another and hence consent to the rule of law, which in principle regulates interaction in the name of shared interest. A system of law, further, reflects consent if no law requires the abandonment of self-preservation, for no reasonable person would consent to such a law (Locke 2003, p. 160). On this topic, see Josephson (2002).

with the failure to fulfill their purposes. It can also cause them to feel frustrated, insignificant, and neglected, as though their purposes are of relatively little import.

Second, because we depend on the intervention of others in order to be able to develop as agents at all, we are vulnerable to various kinds of pains associated with that dependence: the pain associated with having learned bad habits of action and interaction from others that prevent us from being able to fulfill our goals, as well as the pain associated with being judged by them and being challenged to change, and so on. We are not automatically and spontaneously fully formed and competent, and to become formed and competent requires dependence on others, who some-how need to alert us to the need to develop. Our purposes, that is, must be sub-ordinated to the purposes that others such as educators, parents, and other caregivers have for us. However, both to discover that one's present capacities need to be transformed, and to undergo activities that would lead to transformation, can be painful experiences—the first because it can suggest to us that there is something "wrong" with us in the present, and the second because it requires deferral of the satisfaction of other kinds of desire. A teacher, for instance—in pursuing the goal of cultivation of her students—may decide that a critical and challenging approach would be most effective, especially when she is dealing with a characteristic in the student that he is stubborn about working through, but this approach can lead her student to feel the pain that comes from confusion about what is happening, from a diminished sense of self-worth, or from a sense of alienation from the teacher.[6] Further, other people are responsible for our cultivation and development, but there is no guarantee that they will do a good job; we can inherit from them bad habits of action and interaction. Some of these habits can prevent effective agency in the world, causing us to be unable to respond effectively to the demands made by personal and interpersonal situations.[7] Our incapacity to function well in certain situations can cause different kinds of pain—pain associated with alienation, rejection, and the sense of not belonging, or with the frustration of fundamental life-goals, and so on.

Thus, because of the way in which agency involves the continuous transgression of boundaries, through the necessarily shared character of its domain and through our unchosen dependence on each other, we inflict and suffer pain of various kinds, the pain involved in having one's own action prevented by another, in experiencing an incompatibility between one's own and another person's development and desires, in being challenged to become different, and in being dependent on people

---

[6]On the emotional challenges intrinsic to the experience of education, see Kirk (2015: Chapter 3).
[7]For example, as Susan D. Calkins explains, if an infant shows a tendency "to be easily frustrated by barriers and restrictions" (1994, p. 63) and this tendency "is met by caregiver attempts to control and coerce the infant," this can lead to the child coming to view "interactions with peers as opportunities to exert control or to achieve the upper hand and... lead to a prevalence of aggressive and antagonistic interactions" (1994, pp. 63–64). For more insight into the ways in which the patterns of interaction that we develop with intimate others in private shape our adult forms of interaction, see Laing's notion of "ontological security" (1990: Chapters 1–3), Winnicott (1986), and Russon (2003: Chapter 5).

who fail to produce in us good habits of action and interaction. Further, this pain is not something to which we consent, ordinarily; it is not something over which we have control, since it is often a symptom of the processes of our development as beings capable of consent, control, and choice and it accrues to us on the basis of relationships—in other words, on the basis of our having made ourselves open to the shaping power of other people.

It is not the case, however, that this pain is straightforwardly negative, something to be avoided and prevented or something against which we should learn to protect ourselves.[8] The transgressive action of other people, the situations in which it is not realistic to expect consent, the experience of pain: all of these can be the conditions of possibility of effective human existence that we should not want or aim to live without. It is only on condition of the independent and transgressive actions of others that we have at our disposal a profound and complex world of significance; because of the creative appropriation and transcendence of existing conditions, we live with the rewards of centuries of human discoveries; because our consent is not required, this world is available to us; because of the guidance, constraint, and criticism of others, *our own agency* is available to us. Our powers and capacities, as well as objects of concern, significance, and meaning, are due not simply to our own actions, and if our consent were a condition of their accruing to us then we would not have them at all. The transgressive actions of others, and our capacity to be transgressed by them, are essential conditions for the development of meaningful human life.

If agency is to some extent and in some ways *due to* the transgressive action of other people, and if the experience of pain is a consequence of that transgressive action, then it is improper, undesirable, and problematic to be absolutely opposed to the experience of pain and to structure personal, social, and political life so as to protect against the possibility of pain by instituting standards for action and interaction that would aim to prevent it. The experience of pain is not straightforwardly positive or negative; it can in fact be either. At times it is rightly avoided, but at other times it is an indication of growth and development or a symptom of the irrevocable and desirable existence of other people, and hence to be embraced.[9] We cannot avoid others and the world in acting; rather, they are the essential contexts of action and its essential ingredients. The development of agency is essentially the development of the capacity to grapple with and appropriate as one's own the domain in which one acts, which essentially involves others, who are doing the same thing, and objective reality, with its own often resistant manner of existing. If it were void of any understanding of the significance of the actions and interventions of others and the nature of objects, an action would be highly ineffective and problematic. Thus the pain associated with becoming involved with others and the

---

[8]Some religious traditions (such as Hinduism, for example) similarly identify pain as an occasion for learning and growth, and thus not as something to be renounced and avoided. See for instance Whitman (2007).

[9]On the positive significance of the experience of vulnerability to other people, see Nortvedt (2003). For related issues in medical contexts, see Gjengedal et al. (2013), Radley (2000), and Toombs (1993).

external world should not be avoided at all costs, and to assume that it should is to deny the necessity of a reality resistant to one's own agency. Let us look more closely, now, at some examples of situations that portray this ambivalence: situations involving pain in which that pain is not necessarily negative, undesirable, or to be avoided.

In educational contexts, what some may perceive as one person's abusive transgression of another person's dignity might be rightly perceived, rather, as a powerful push along a developmental path involving a challenge to that other person's sense of reality and of herself and inspiring in her awareness of the significance of transformation. The actions of various caregivers can be experienced as oppositional and disrespectful, opposed as they are to the *current* state of character and agency of the one who is developing in the name of her possible *future* state, when they are in fact powerful expressions of care and concern. In the domain of education, too much emphasis can be placed on the comfort and affirmation of students and too many restrictions can be placed in the way of certain kinds of educational interventions, such that important kinds of transformative interaction are precluded. Too strict an insistence on the non-transgressible character of human individuals can in fact be an obstacle in the way of their development, and too wary an attitude toward the vulnerability and pain associated with such experiences can result in the failure to develop the capacities to interact effectively with others and the world. Here, what seems to be care and concern for the individual can in fact be neglect of her identity as dynamic and developing, and it shows the importance of the transgressive intervention of other people and the experience of pain to the development of our agency.[10] The Chorus of Aeschylus' *Agamemnon* captures this point when it observes: "Zeus, who guided men to think/ …has laid it down that wisdom/comes alone through suffering" (Aeschylus 1991, lines 176–178).

We identified above the possibility that people can develop bad behavioral habits that prevent effective interaction in certain contexts, due to the negative influence of certain kinds of caregivers in their lives. In these cases, the experience of pain due to not being able to fit in, to feeling alienated and judged as incompetent, and so on, does not have to be the end of the story; it can in fact lead to the identification and treatment of one's bad habits. If other people involved in such contexts were to accept the bad behavior unequivocally, the person exhibiting it would lose the opportunity to change. If the primary motivation of all involved were to avoid the experience of discomfort and pain, the opportunity for development would decrease. Of course, it would be more desirable if the transferral of bad behavioral habits had not taken place, and the pain associated with problematic behavior is in that case unfortunate. This does not mean, however, that it cannot be a trigger

---

[10]Freud observes that because extreme pain can accompany the emergence of unconscious material, the resources of the psyche are mobilized to resist therapy, and that this is a powerful hindrance in the way of its success. See Freud (1949).

leading to the revision of bad habits and the development of better forms of interaction in the future.

In addition to the importance of experiencing a certain kind of pain and vulnerability in relation to other people, it is also important and valuable to be open to experiencing a certain kind of pain and vulnerability in relation to one's environment. We can see a problematic approach to the experience of pain in relation to the increasing surveillance and regulation of the activities of mostly Western children. Over the past couple of decades, the behavior of parents toward children has changed, due partly to fears about possible injury. Children face increasing restrictions in play and decreasing opportunities to move about without surveillance, in the form of increased regulation of in-car seating, more laws concerning the protection of their bodies during play (through mechanisms such as helmets and kneepads and greater restrictions on certain kinds of playground equipments), greater legal and customary restrictions of opportunities to be on their own, and so on. Presuming to protect children through these measures, we effectively do the opposite—that is, we undermine the conditions of possibility of the development of effective agency.[11] Children have fewer opportunities to learn about the dangers and vulnerabilities they are faced with in the world, and thus have fewer occasions to learn, in somewhat protected environments, the skills required in the face of those dangers and vulnerabilities. Regulations reflect the assumption that agency can be produced without reference to and interaction with its domain, without learning how to appropriate as one's own the domain in which one acts; they reflect the assumption that agency is something that happens solely on its own terms, without reference to the outside world. Hence this protection by regulation can actually cripple agency, rather than protect it. The defense of individual boundaries and the fear of their transgression again turn into their opposite—prevention of the development of agency. Because it is not the case that the external world yields to the human will—because it puts obstacles in the way of action against which we collide—to effectively communicate to children that it does so yield is to oppose their learning and development and to endanger them.

We have explored the fact that the development of agency can be accompanied by the experience of pain, both in relation to the external, objective world and in relation to other people, because individual agency is a product of sources that transcend us as individuals. We have also discussed several situations that

---

[11]This issue has recently garnered some attention in media beyond the academy; see, for instance, Tierney (2011). For a discussion of the harmful effects of the overzealous application of safety standards to playgrounds, see Frost (1997). The productive effect of unregulated and unstructured peer-to-peer interactions and disagreement on the playground is discussed in Pellegrini and Bohn (2005). "When peers disagree," they write, "they are confronted by points of view other than their own and, if they want the interaction to continue, they must accommodate their peers' point of view. These sorts of social interaction often occur on playgrounds at recess" (2005, p. 15). Michael Ungar argues that the ways in which we go about keeping children safe are "inadvertently putting them at much greater risk of serious harm" (2007, p. x), and that "children who push to find their limits (and scare us adults in the process) may also be those who are the ones most ready for life" (2007, p. xiii).

illuminate the positive valence that pain can have as a symptom or indication of positive transformation or development. Now let us turn to another kind of pain, that which accompanies the loss or concealment of these objective and intersubjective conditions of our agency, and illuminate the importance of noticing and preventing this kind of pain that accrues to us not by virtue of the transgression of our individuality but by virtue of the transgression of our embeddedness in larger realities.

11.3 The Pain of Exclusion

Because we learn how to be human only in interaction with intersubjective and objective reality, we can experience pain due to being cut off from it. Because our specific communities, cultures, languages, shared practices, and meaningfully articulated worlds of objects provide the platform upon which we develop a meaningful sense of ourselves, or because belonging to specific linguistic, cultural, and social worlds is a condition of agency, we can experience suffering by having our cultural specificity denied, by having our connections with these worlds unacknowledged and unconsidered, by being cut off from interpersonal and "interobjective" interaction. Because we rely on a developed objective reality and on other people for the development of our own agency and for the availability of a world of meaning and significance, we are who we are only in relation to these realities, and can be transgressed in our own identity by being forced to be "abstract individuals" whose import and significance is supposed to be self-contained.

Thus, while we can experience pain by virtue of the transgressive action of others in relation to us, or by virtue of our fundamental intimacy with others, due to our reliance on them for the formation of our very individuality, we can also experience pain by having that fundamental intersubjective reality transgressed or taken away from us.[12] Because the agency of others is linked so substantially to our own, its removal or erasure can be the occasion for suffering; we can experience pain from being cut off from the bonds that have contributed to the development in us of agency and the possibility of a meaningful life, and from the worlds and practices of significance in which we participate—specifically, social, cultural, and religious worlds and practices.[13] Such painful experiences are surely felt by

---

[12]Indeed, various psychosocial, spiritual, and religious variables, including the production of new meaning or a new identity for the one who suffers pain, or the formation of narratives about this identity and experience, can ameliorate the biological and psychological experience of pain in turn. For a discussion of these and related issues, see Moore (2012), especially Wachholtz and Makowski (2012, pp. 697–713), Coulehan (2012, pp. 717–731), Morris (2012, pp. 733–751).

[13]See, for instance, Lear (2006). Lear explores what happens when a culture collapses, or when most or all of the categories through which life had previously been imbued with significance cease to make sense, as occurred to the Crow Tribe in the latter part of the nineteenth century when the buffalo disappeared. He writes that "[h]umans are by nature cultural animals: we necessarily

immigrants and refugees who leave their homes, by people who are forced to live apart from their intimate relations or from those who have established the terms by which their lives are centrally defined, by prisoners placed in solitary confinement, by children without devoted caregivers, and so on.[14] When the explicit intersubjective affiliations constitutive of personal identity—whether social, cultural, or religious— are denied to us, we can experience pain. This pain is often under-acknowledged in societies that operate with a sense that individual identity is discrete and that its claim to its autonomy is ultimate, that to which other kinds of claims should be subordinate, and it also lies behind the suffering involved in the experience of colonialism, in which the "universality" of Western ideals is advanced to the detriment of the specificity of cultural practices.[15] Construing agency as solely individual can cause its own kind of pain, a result, in this case, of the *withdrawal* of the necessary, transgressive agency of others in the lives of individuals.

A similar kind of suffering accrues to the individual by virtue of the withdrawal of objective resources. If we become human on the basis of a certain kind of interaction with objective, external reality, then the absence or removal of that reality can cause us pain—one may require "a room of one's own,"[16] for instance, or a place for play, the means of travel, the conditions of health, and an economic system that allows for the stable production of life-sustaining goods. If we understand the human being to be the product of interaction with an external, objective, and intersubjective world, then its existence and the meaningfulness of its

---

(Footnote 13 continued)

inhabit a way of life that is expressed in a culture. But our way of life—whatever it is—is vulnerable in various ways. And we, as participants in that way of life, thereby inherit a vulnerability. Should that way of life break down, that is *our* problem" (2006, p. 6). On the suffering that comes from being cut off from the material and intersubjective dimensions of one's home, see Young (2005: Chapter 8, "A Room of One's Own: Old Age, Extended Care, and Privacy").

[14]For the suffering faced by immigrants, see Sayad (2004). For a discussion of the necessary role that being with others plays for us and thus the damage that comes from solitary confinement, see Guenther (2013). Guenther writes that "[i]ntensive confinement, whether it is produced through forced solitude or forced contact with others, in the context of the prison industrial complex or the animal industrial complex, commits a form of structural violence against animal ontology. It threatens to break the hinges of an intercorporeality that human animals share with nonhuman animals—not only with the social animals whose forms of relationality most closely resemble our own, but with any other animal that lives and grows by relying on the mutual support of other living, growing beings" (2013, p. 157). For a discussion of the problems associated with "the absence of early coexistential structures" (2013, p. 22), see Simms (2001).

[15]See, for instance, Frantz Fanon's analysis of that experience and his criticism of Western "universality" in *Black Skin, White Masks* and *The Wretched of the Earth*. In *The Wretched of the Earth* Fanon writes that when the colonized "hear a speech on Western culture, they draw their machetes or at least check to see they are close to hand. The supremacy of white values is stated with such violence... is so impregnated with aggressiveness... In the period of decolonization the colonized masses thumb their noses at these very values, shower them with insults and vomit them up" (1963, p. 8).

[16]Here I am using Woolf's phrase (1929).

life rely essentially on ongoing access to and reliance on that world. If becoming human is something accomplished in interaction with an external environment, then we support human beings if we support these external resources and human access to them.[17]

Because human life is essentially lived in relation and in embeddedness with other objects and subjects in a shared reality, its effective enactment requires the continued existence of this relation. The pain that results from removal from these relations, then, operates as a sign that there is something here to be avoided. Again, this pain accrues to human individuals by virtue of the fact that they *enact* their identities and that they do so in relation to other people, environments, and objects, and this pain is to be avoided in the name of the protection of these embedded human identities.

11.4 Conclusion

Being in the world is a matter of enacting oneself with and in others, objects, and environments, who and which make themselves manifest in our agency and in the sense of self that we develop. The individual is not a discrete unit, essentially separable from her environment, and to attempt to protect her completely from intervention by others and the world or to prevent her from certain forms of interaction with them is to misunderstand the nature of human experience and potentially to cause her pain. Her being with others is characterized fundamentally by transgression and by mutually shaping interaction; the intrusion of the other is a basic human reality, the very medium through which we develop as agents. The sources of agency in fact outstrip what seem to be individual boundaries and individual control, and the experience of pain often illuminates this reality. We are not actually in control of our own lives and of the conditions of possibility of our existence, and the vulnerability we have with regard to our environment can be the occasion for pain even as it is the occasion for development. Rather than simply supporting human autonomy, bodily integrity, and self-directed independence, we should support and answer to the precarious and vulnerable conditions under which autonomy, integrity, and independence are fostered, recognizing accurately the kinds of pain that are characteristically experienced in these contexts.

Increased understanding of the kinds of human suffering caused by our essential vulnerability to the world and to other people should also lead to better protection of the determinate conditions that lie at the basis of agency and human development. If the development and sustenance of relations, traditions, and environments are the key constituents of agency in the world, then these relations, traditions, and

---

[17]This is the basis of Marx's position, of course, which explores the way in which the existence or development of capitalism essentially runs contradictory to its principled commitment to the free human being. See, for instance, *The German Ideology* and "The Communist Manifesto" in Engels and Marx (1978), as well as Marx (1992).

environments demand a certain kind of care oriented specifically to them, not simply to the individuals involved in them. Instead of the protection of individual rights, for instance, this would require the protection of the domains of meaning in relation to which we develop as human individuals in the first place, the protection of the integrity of the realities in which we are embedded, which operate as the intelligent limbs and prostheses of human identity and agency. Given that we extend into the world beyond our discrete bodies and individual identities, the trajectory of that extension needs support. The resources and practices by which we sustain ourselves as bodily, creative, transforming, and interacting beings, in relation to which we are intrinsically and necessarily vulnerable but in the absence of which we suffer, require care. And the practices and priorities that threaten our fundamental openness to each other and to the world within these determinate social forms need to be opposed.

References

Aeschylus. (1991). *Agamemnon*. In D. Grene & R. Lattimore (Eds.), *Greek tragedies*, 2nd ed. (Vol. I). Chicago, IL: The University of Chicago Press.

Calkins, S. D. (1994). Origins and outcomes of individual differences in emotion regulation. *Monographs of the Society for Research in Child Development, 59*(2–3), 53–72.

Coulehan, J. (2012). Suffering, hope, and healing. In R. J. Moore (Ed.), *Handbook of pain and palliative care* (pp. 717–731). New York: Springer.

Engels, F., & Marx, K. (1978). R. C. Tucker (Ed.), *The Marx-Engels reader*. London: W. W. Norton & Company.

Fanon, F. (1963). *The wretched of the earth*. (R. Philcox, Trans.). New York: Grove Press.

Fanon, F. (1967). *Black skin, white masks*.(C. L. Markmann, Trans.). New York: Grove Press.

Fichte, J. G. (2000). *Foundations of natural right*. (M. Baur, Trans.). Cambridge: Cambridge University Press.

Freud, S. (1949). *An outline of psycho-analysis* (J. Strachey, Trans.). New York: W. W. Norton.

Frost, J. L. (1997). Child development and playgrounds. *Parks & Recreation, 32*(4), 54–60.

Gjengedal, E., Ekra, E. M., Hol, H., Kjelsvik, M., Lykkeslet, E., Michaelsen, R., et al. (2013). Vulnerability in health care: Reflections on encounters in everyday practice. *Nursing Philosophy, 14*(2), 127–138.

Guenther, L. (2013). *Solitary confinement: Social death and its afterlives*. Minneapolis: University of Minnesota Press.

Hegel, G. W. F. (1977). *Phenomenology of Spirit*. (A. V. Miller, Trans.). Oxford: Oxford University Press.

Josephson, P. (2002). *The great art of government: Locke's use of consent*. Lawrence: University Press of Kansas.

Kirk, G. (2015). *The pedagogy of wisdom: An interpretation of Plato's Theaetetus*. Evanston, IL: Northwestern University Press.

Laing, R. D. (1990). *The divided self: An existential study in sanity and madness*. New York: Penguin.

Lear, J. (2006). *Radical hope: Ethics in the face of cultural devastation*. Cambridge, MA: Harvard University Press.

Locke, J. (2003). I. Shapiro, (Ed.), *Two treatises of government and letter concerning toleration*. New Haven: Yale University Press.

Marx, K. (1992). *Capital,* (Vols. 1–3), (D. Fernbach, Trans.). London: Penguin.

Morris, D. B. (2012). Narrative and pain: Towards an integrative model. In R. J. Moore (Ed.), *Handbook of pain and palliative care* (pp. 733–751). New York: Springer.

Nortvedt, P. (2003). Subjectivity and vulnerability: Reflections on the foundations of ethical sensibility. *Nursing Philosophy, 4*(3), 222–230.

Pellegrini, A. D., & Bohn, C. M. (2005). The role of recess in children's cognitive performance and school adjustment. *Educational Researcher, 34*(1), 13–19.

Radley, A. (2000). Health psychology, embodiment and the question of vulnerability. *Journal of Health Psychology, 5,* 297–304.

Russon, J. (2003). *Human experience: Philosophy, neurosis, and the elements of everyday life.* Albany, NY: State University of New York Press.

Russon, J. (2009). *Bearing witness to epiphany: Persons, things, and the nature of erotic life.* Albany, NY: State University of New York Press.

Sayad, A. (2004). *The suffering of the immigrant.* (D. Macey, Trans.). Cambridge: Polity Press.

Schenck, D. (1986). The texture of embodiment: Foundation for medical ethics. *Human Studies, 9* (1), 43–54.

Simms, E.-M. (2001). Milk and flesh: A phenomenological reflection on infancy and coexistence. *Journal of Phenomenological Psychology, 32*(1), 22–40.

Tierney, J. (2011). Can a playground be too safe? *The New York Times* (18 July).

Toombs, S. K. (1993). *The meaning of illness: A phenomenological approach to the patient-physician relationship.* Dordrecht: Kluwer Academic Publishers.

Ungar, M. (2007). *Too safe for their own good: How risk and responsibility help teens thrive.* Toronto: McClelland & Stewart.

Wachholtz, A., & Makowski, S. (2012). Spiritual dimensions of pain and suffering. In R. J. Moore (Ed.), *Handbook of pain and palliative care* (pp. 697–713). New York: Springer.

Whitman, S. M. (2007). Pain and suffering as viewed by the Hindu religion. *The Journal of Pain, 8* (8), 607–613.

Wilde, M. H. (2003). Embodied knowledge in chronic illness and injury. *Nursing Inquiry, 10*(3), 170–176.

Winnicott, D. W. (1986). *Home is where we start from.* New York: W. W. Norton & Company.

Woolf, V. (1929). *A room of one's own.* New York: Harcourt.

Young, I. M. (2005). A room of one's own: Old age, extended care, and privacy. In I. M. Young (Ed.), *On female body experience: Throwing like a girl and other essays* (pp. 155–170). Oxford: Oxford University Press.

Part III
Social Contexts of Pain

Chapter 12
Dislocations, Marginalizations, Past and Present: Pain-Experiences of Two Marginalized Communities

R. Umamaheshwari

Abstract This essay seeks to locate pain within sites of memory of a *past* that was painful, and sites of destruction of a *present*. It thus seeks to understand pain through two distinct avenues, across historical space, time and cultures. First there is the Tamil Jaina community with a recorded (lived) history in Tamilnadu, a state in India, from the second century BCE onwards, and its steady marginalization over time, which is remembered and reproduced through stories of persecution suffered at the hands of the dominant tradition or communities in different time-periods in history. Then, there are the *adivasis* (tribal communities) by the Godavari River in Andhra Pradesh-Telangana states of India, fighting their own battles against the act of destruction of both their presents and their pasts on account of a dam, the Indira Sagar Polavaram National Project, being constructed over Godavari. However, in exploring pain through these two distinct avenues, the emphasis of the essay is to highlight the need to locate beings in pain through the idea of 'cartographies' that are destroyed and created afresh. This essay, thus locates pain in politics—where histories, communities, cultural spaces are constantly marginalized.

Keywords Adivasi · Tamil jaina · Cartography · Pain-sites · Displacement · Remembering

Could it be said that histories of many nations are built on sites of pain of several communities, and that it takes very little for these sites of pain to be churned up at moments in time? Is it possible to posit the idea of a 'cultural being' of pain or suffering, or the 'being' of pain within culture in terms of the existence of pain or suffering, or in the recognition or acceptance or acknowledging of that pain or suffering? Or to say that there is a layer of pain and suffering hidden within history or histories of communities (especially those marginalized over time) that needs to be extracted and made sense of?

These questions emerge as the outcome of my present essay, and though they are not answered within the space of this particular essay, what is highlighted is the

R. Umamaheshwari (✉)
Indian Institute of Advanced Study, Shimla, India
e-mail: umamaheshwari_1999@yahoo.com

227

importance of understanding pain-experiences within the horizon of such questions. The nature of pain that I seek to address through this essay has usually not found reflection in the academic realm, though the pain of marginalization or becoming targets of xenophobia, of communalism and racism has been addressed in a lot of scholarly writings before, though not constructed in the terminology of 'pain' necessarily, unless the work addressed 'trauma' through the psychoanalytical discourse.

12.1 Two Sites, Past, Present

I look at two kinds of pain, across two very different cultural and historical spaces and each having to do with the nature of political discourse that binds communities within limited historical confines, or confounds them into a present that seems to mock at their pasts with amazing persistence. In both of these cases, I seek to locate the idea of pain or suffering as a constant, a 'refrain', or a constant refrain, to put it simply. The first register in my exploration is constituted by the episodes from the Tamil Jaina history, as understood from within their own experience of marginalization, and as perceived by them—a community that is stuck in moments of their past which was, for them, a violent experience. The second register is the contemporary Indira Sagar Polavaram multi-purpose National Project which is essentially, a mega-dam on Godavari river—and the ensuing story of displacement of the tribal communities of Andhra Pradesh-Telangana (and perhaps extendable to villages of the two other Indian states of Odisha and Chhattisgarh). Specifically, the dam will displace more than 300,000 people, more than 200,000 of them being *adivasis*/Scheduled Tribes. The dam is supposed to generate 960 MW of electricity for a multi-national industrial corridor by the south-east Coast, now in the new state of Andhra Pradesh. This means that, since the project is conceived by the state as a 'public good', the government holds the right to acquire land from the tribal communities, compensating them in terms of cash and land for those who have land, as per the Land Acquisition Act[1] in place. Thus, the sense with which I see or locate or 'feel' pain—through this study—is at two levels: one, within a cultural space where remembering or memory is a 'site of pain' of a painful past, recovered again and again by members of a community marginalized over time in Tamilnadu or Tamil history; the other is a pain of dispossession and displacement or dislocation from sites of belonging (historically, emotionally).

However, in both cases, strangely (since there is nothing that connects the Tamil Jainas with the *adivasis*), there is a 'present' being constructed with the speed of

---

[1]The Right to Fair Compensation and Transparency in Land Acquisition, Rehabilitation and Resettlement Act, 2013. This is today known as The Right to Fair Compensation and Transparency in Land Acquisition, Rehabilitation and Resettlement (Amendment) Ordinance, 2015. The 2013 Act has provisions for compensating loss of land for *adivasis*/Scheduled Tribes with land. The 2015 Ordinance is at present a matter of intense contestation from various quarters in India.

lightning, over several histories of theirs with pain finding its expression through memory and remembrancing. In both cases, there is an experience of pain that emerges through a silent 'watching'. The Tamil Jainas 'watching' over ancient Jaina sites in Tamilnadu being either destroyed, or appropriated at some point by the dominant Hindu tradition and the *adivasis*/tribal communities 'watching' their land and environs destroyed to make way for a new paradigm where they are no longer central. In both these cases, there is the pain of being silent witness to the construction of 'presents' (of whichever time) over destruction of 'pasts', and finding oneself (as a community) on the fringes and vanishing into the oblivion of history.

Incidentally, in the Tamil Jaina case, there is within the tradition, a certain acceptance of a physical aspect of pain, which is self-inflicted, in order to overcome the feeling of it, or the existence of it, in the route towards salvation/liberation. This mode of acceptance of pain is evident in the practices of the naked Digambara Jaina monks who systematically pluck out hair from their heads, eat once a day, walk miles on foot, and accept these extremes to constitute the path towards the ultimate liberation from the body. For them, the body has to be put through these 'tests' in order to bring home the point that the corporeal is ephemeral and just a medium to attain salvation. But the level of acceptance for this pain and its internalization does not seem to help the Tamil Jaina community when it comes to dealing with another realm of pain, which is: a certain dispossession from history through persecution.

In the case of the *adivasi*/tribal people of Godavari, there is a pain that is induced from the outside, or from above through the system to be precise, the invisible and visible state and other hegemonic structures (Kafkaesque, in its many layers of both physical and metaphorical constructions, within and outside of the 'body' of governancing). These are people who become victims of that pain which may be manifest physically in terms of being uprooted from emotional and physical spaces or histories, and sometimes manifest in the bodily wounds inflicted on them, were they to dare to question this uprooting. But emotional scars remain etched and then either make new identities or destroy the identity altogether—of a people, or of a culture, or their history itself.

The nostalgia of a past that was good, but destroyed and now recollected through 'remembrance' of a particular instance or instances of violence with the 'remembering' seeming almost like a performance, is one example of pain-experiences. And then there is the pain-experience of the present being in the process of destruction, talking of these in terms of 'loss' of homes and lives through physical displacement, of what *will be*—of a future uncertain. In both these cases, there is the pain of dislocation, of a certain dismembering; and pain that is expressed in the language of loss, of *what was*, to *what is*. That which *was* is often constructed as a space or site or situation that was built by the community through their agency, and that which *is*—the present—a forced, painful construct. In both cases, the pain is also about having been actors in history to becoming either non-actors or 'beneficiaries' or 'minority' in the state or political structure.

12.2 Locating Pain-Sites in Context

Dispossession is not sufficiently discoursed through the lens of 'pain' in contemporary understanding of 'development' (or even in critiques of it).[2] I have been engaging with contexts where pain or suffering is a constant, at the deeper levels that I speak of here, either in the remembering, almost as a performance, or in real mundane terms of looking out at a blank space, a future that is more an illusion—where the breaking up of a home is imminent, impending and pain that is felt in terms of what was and what will be. In the case of the Tamil Jainas, the pain-experience is in terms of a past that is gone forever, a past that was not pleasant, which led to a present that 'shouldn't have been so'; for the *adivasis* the pain-experience is imminent in the immediate future on account of loss of the present—howsoever challenging the present may be for disadvantaged communities ('disadvantaged' being the ironic appendage given to them in a democracy). There is also the fact of some pains not being either recognizable or acknowledged given that modern institutions are meant to *not* feel pain of communities that have suffered uprooting, dislocation or marginalization for various reasons.

> Pain has no "place" in a regularised landscape, for its uncanny inversions of inside and outside, center and periphery, would upset the linear/lineal structures of social paternalism. That is, in the text of the city as in the textual sublime, pain is an inadmissible disturbance of the clear delineation—of the decisive hierarchisation—of worker and bourgeois, public and private, family and anomie…. (Ramazani 1996, p. 217)

If one were to reformulate the above statement to locate the subject(s) of this essay, one would say that official history has generally ignored or negated the 'pain' inherent in the marginalization of communities and their memories in order that the status quo be maintained. The status quo has generally been one of a 'great Indian tradition', which is accepting of 'diversity' (one should not confuse this for accepting of 'difference') and the power of the great tradition to absorb or be adaptive of various cultural expressions. The persecution of the Tamil Jaina[3] during the early medieval historical time-period and the drastic reduction in their numbers and their settlements across Tamilnadu have generally remained mere aberrations

---

[2]It is thanks to Pravesh and Siby that I have been able to look deeper at the very concept of pain and suffering, or the cultural contexts of it, even though in the course of my longer engagements (with the Tamil Jainas and the *Adivasi* [indigenous tribal population currently referred to in the Indian Constitution as 'Scheduled Tribes'/STs] and Dalit [some of whom were the formerly 'untouchable' castes of the Indian caste hierarchy currently referred to in the Indian Constitution as 'Scheduled Castes'/SCs] communities of Godavari), I have been either 'listening in' to painful pasts or seeing painful presents, all through.

[3]Or, for that matter, Buddhist. Till date, there isn't any history of the Tamil Buddhists and what happened to them. There is no living Tamil Buddhist community tracing their history from the early centuries BCE. We only know of the Tamil literary works such as *Maṇimekalai* and *Kuṇṭalakeci* as being Buddhist. While *Maṇimekalai*, an epic, has been edited and translated into a few Indian languages, and English, the philosophical-poetic treatise, *Kuṇṭalakeci* is not available in its entirety and only some verses are extant.

and mentioned usually in passing in mainstream history writing thus making an entire community invisible. In that, the history of a violent suppression is glossed over and it is not a surprise that very few people are even aware of there being a community called the Tamil Jainas or *naiṉār*, who practiced agriculture in the southern part of India, in contrast to the general Jaina population with stereotypes of being rich businesspeople in the northern parts of India. And then there is the other curious aspect about the relative non-availability (unless there is some dogged pursuit of it) of Buddhist and Jaina literature in Tamil in comparison to the abundance of both, the literature of the *Śaiva* and *Vaiṣṇava* traditions and their critiques, in a culture that has been, by far, the most 'nationalistic' about the Tamil language.

In the case of *adivasis* of Godavari, the 'modernisation project' of post-independence India in the Scheduled Areas has left them with little freedom to choose a lifestyle, that to them, represented a continuity with the past (not the colonial past, but the past of their ancestors before the colonial rulers put a system of governance in place to suppress some of the most consistent revolts in those areas). Their history seems to have been one of interventions and invasions and never 'acceptance' of their ways, and of their refusals to become 'like others' and move to the cities. In general, in mainstream contemporary political and economic discourse, stories of pain or dispossession are disallowed; the tendency is to look at vertical, upward growth where uneasy questions of the past (or present) have no place, for it threatens to upset the system/structure.

Though my essay is not about 'physical' pain, suffered at the level of the human body, it is not to deny such pain-experiences. There are, no doubt, *also* physical pain-experiences, such as when torture is involved. Instances of bodily pain-experiences, was evident in my encounter with some pathetically monetarily poor Konda Kammara tribal people in the villages Chinnabhimpally and Pedabhimpally in the Indukuru Panchayat in East Godavari district. These were Scheduled Tribes who had been granted 'assigned' government land in the early '70s on which they had their small homes along with small cultivating lands where they had been cultivating cashew and other fruit crops. One fine day, the government officials started digging up their lands for the 'R&R'[4] colony of Polavaram dam that would be built there for 'STs' from the submergence villages. When Ekka Rajanna Dora, a 70-year old man asked the officials why his land was being dug up, the policeman beat him up. When others questioned them why the old man was

---

[4]Rehabilitation and Resettlement (R&R) is an important component of projects where the government acquires land; where land is acquired from the Scheduled Tribes, until recently, the Act governing land acquisition required the government to compensate tribal communities not just monetarily but also in terms of land (in case of land-owning tribal people). However, where they were landless, they will be given a housing site and a one-time monetary settlement—150 sq. ft house site and (in case of Polavaram dam) Rs. 150,000/-in cash. All of this is given in installment cheques. For land compensation, the *adivasi* (in official records the 'ST') person would have to show 'proof' of ownership in the form of 'patta' (land documents), failing which she or he will not get any land in compensation for the loss of cultivated fields.

being beaten up, the Revenue official slammed cases (of "Obstructing Government Official on Duty") against a few of them. Pamula Veerasamy, another septuagenarian, told me: "They beat me up. I went to the police station but the S.I (Sub-inspector) did not register an FIR…"[5] Rajanna Dora and Veerasamy were both frail and old Konda Kammaras; illiterate and poor, they had nothing but a 'government assigned land' in their names and tiny homes in the hamlet which they had been struggling to retain and both were physically abused by the arms of the state for having done so. Such pain-experiences that emerge from physical abuse is not the main concern of my essay since their physical wound had healed when I had met them in July, 2007, but they (and the others of their community) were conscious of, and in pain due to, the assault on their dignity and Self. The cashews and mangoes of their years of toil and labour of love, instead of benefitting them, became sites of extreme invasion by the authorities out to complete by all means, fair and foul, the target set for the acquisition of land by the state government of what was then united Andhra Pradesh. The Konda Kammara land was 'taken away' by the Revenue Division Officer for setting up the 'R&R' colony for the 'oustees' of the Polavaram project. However, the compensation for the land thus 'taken away' was given to an upper caste non-tribal and an ex-bureaucrat from an entirely different place since he possessed that fantastically alienating document called 'land deed' in his name, although through foul means. Thus, the government, or its agents, had played a game on the bodies and sites of tribal people. The wounds, more than physical, was thus cultural—for these would be tribal bodies as 'sites' of (cruel) governance and their homes would be sites of constant invasion, physical and structural, by upper caste assertion, or the assertion of machines (literally) and tools of 'modernity' couched in legal, constitutional terms to suit purposes of the dominant or dominating. Both *policying* and policing of the Tribal body or Self has resulted in deep suffering and pain for the *adivasi*/tribal communities of this region. The invasion and intrusion into their homes and lands without their informed consent, in fact, can be equated very well with the method of torture inflicted upon 'criminals', convicted or otherwise, as we well know. There is a 'body' (or bodies) here, and the site of violence; and both the tribal body and the site are the destination of a new modern 'economic development' discourse, which gives the officials in the state, immunity from trials, to set about acquiring land with impunity. The words of abuse, hurled at Rajanna and others of his village at this instance by the Revenue Division Officer (RDO) were later submitted in the form of a petition by the Kammara people, to arrest the RDO under 'Prevention of Atrocities against SCs, STs Act'. The abusive words, in fact, were aimed at the tribal bodies, equating them with wild animals, among other things. A written response was sought from him on the case from the Andhra Pradesh High Court. In his written response he claimed to have "conducted counselling to the innocent ST people who caused the disturbance…" (Umamaheshwari 2014, p. 159). Needless to say, he was never

---

[5]FIR or First Information Report is the first legal procedure filed with the police by the complainant, with which will commence the procedure of a criminal suit in India.

arrested. He was duly promoted in some months and transferred to another place and in a higher position.

Thus, there is a deeper pain ensuing from suffering the pain of the emotion, or the cognition of suffering that is remembered, or something endured or something being lived through. Sometimes emotional scars do translate into the physical if we expand the very idea of the physical from the narrower clinical agenda that restricts the notion of 'pain' from invoking its physical dimension. One can legitimately speak of pain that can be located within studies of marginalization of communities, and questions of race and gender. Such pain lives in, emerges from, and survives, on the canvas of politics and not merely the physical confines of the body. What does it mean to live in the pain of being unimportant to history? To live as permanent marginals in a world order where your knowledge, language, world-view have no place?

In each of the two cases that I have observed, the Self is presented in a permanent and indelible (or inerasable) space of suffering or pain of an event or a series of events that have made their lives what they are. Their being insignificant to the history of a region or nation is a painful realization to them.

When people are displaced from their homes, as in the case of the present ongoing Polavaram dam project on Godavari river (where displacement is underway, if not fully 'realised'), the suffering caused from loss of land which was historically theirs, from other vulnerabilities—poverty and uprooting—can in the course of time also lead to physical ailments and diseases that may well have their roots in an emotional pain. In a village called Mamidigondi in Polavaram mandal of what was West Godavari district, I saw Madakam Kondayya, a Koya[6] woman in a makeshift thatched hut looking out into empty space (even as I captured that moment of those eyes looking out into empty space, in my camera, before getting to know her—the one moment I did not take the permission for clicking a picture) amidst an assortment of utensils, and other household things scattered about her. She was to move out any day from *this*, her home, now a ruin, into an alien space called 'R&R Colony' far away from here. I learnt from her some of the sad politics of 'compensation' money and the fact that women like her had no say in the monetary transactions made on behalf of people like her for that piece of land where will stand (if miracles in history did not happen) the spillway of a mighty dam generating electricity for billion dollar world industries—things Kondayya was not aware of. The only truth that she was conscious of, was that she was stuck between this site, once home—now visible only in bits and pieces of household stuff of a lifetime or perhaps a few generations of Koya history of Mamidigondi—and with no money to complete construction of her new home on another site with which she has no emotional connect. Ironically, the new site on which the 'R&R' home of hers was being built, will not even have the Constitutional protection guaranteed to

---

[6]The Koyas are one of the indigenous communities residing in the region around rivers Godavari and Sabari and their settlements are predominantly located in the Indian states of Telangana (besides in Odisha-Telangana border villages) and Andhra Pradesh.

adivasis like her, since it was not in the Scheduled Area.[7] After a few hours, on my way back from the same lane, I would see Madakam Kondayya squatting on the path, looking skywards. She would tell me, *"maaku anta ayomayam..."* (It is all chaos for us now). At yet another spot in the same village was an abandoned home. It was under construction when I had passed by the previous year (way dreams are constructed) and had an old woman seated outside, feeding the fowls. The following year, the dream had been abandoned, and had given way to a tin board announcing that it was to be the pathway towards the tunnels for the dam. The old woman was no longer part of the scene, which would have been the normal scenario in a normal village in more normal times. The pain here was not limited to the people who never got to construct their dream home with space for all to be. There are hens and goats and a cow, or a buffalo, and birds, and there is a wide-trunked Tamarind tree, or a mango tree, with their own histories, as well, unlike the 'R&R Colony' which is not a village but a 'colony', stated as such in records of the state, with 150 sq. ft four-dimensional space only for the humankind of the category 'Scheduled Tribe' and marked in the records as such, as a mere category with names, but no history to those names. A few kilometers away, a similar story unfolded, of a corn-field belonging to Koya farmer Boragam Rama Rao, crushed and dumped with rubble from the dam construction site. A Koya agricultural land had changed hands with the state and private contractors for a stated 'public good'. Such are the cultural and political sites of pain.

The memory of a painful past, or painful present that surrounds one's life is expressed in many ways by people in zones such as these which are perpetual 'submergence' or 'dislocation' zones. Does it have a recognition or acceptance as something important for theoretical discourse? I locate therein the cultural, social ontology of not pain, per se, but *being in pain*. There are moments, when these pain-experiences transfer onto the onlooker, like it transferred to me through the blank gaze of Madakam Kondayya, making its existence clear. In these cases then, there is something to be said about transference of pain, as well. In my recordings of different sites of pain—where do I belong? Or do I belong? Does that pain touch me too? And do I internalize it?

Not much has been studied on this aspect of displacements from and in history. Pain or suffering is hardly considered a worthwhile angle from which to understand displacement of communities. The term has a level of abstraction inherent which perhaps makes it seem outside the parameters of developmental politics. Similarly, 'loss' is an abstract term. What is compensated for is what is 'taken' (as a commodity), which the government or state can only address through material mitigation of that loss, which is thus in monetary terms, and hardly something that addresses the deeper and in fact more important—even if abstract, or in fact,

---

[7]This essentially means that once Madakam Kondayya's people will be forced out of this village, they will lose out on the identity (Constitutionally fixed) of Scheduled Tribe and thereby education, health-services and other welfare schemes, which are entitlements guaranteed by the Indian Constitution to *adivasis* of the "V Schedule" areas, will also be lost once they start residing in what they call 'Plain area' or non-Scheduled area.

because of its abstraction—human sense of pain and loss and suffering. There is a social pain and cultural location of pain. For instance, sexual offences against women, in the cultural-social realm, cause more than physical pain that many a times leave permanent scars of various natures. These scars are not mere personal scars suffered by the victims but must be seen as societal scars, a collective pain-space that each society has to feel responsible for. There are constant constructions of pain-sites in displacement zones and submergence zones of big dams that show residues and physical remnants of what was, a constant reminder of how new sites of political and economic power can emerge over older ones of shared histories and lives of a village or people.

In his discussion on modernity and the 'topography of the urban space' with its in-built capacity to produce 'forgetting', Connerton remarks:

> For the members of the subaltern group the residential area is where an interlocking network of social relationships is located. This physical area has considerable meaning to the inhabitants as an extension of the home, since various parts of it… convey a sense of belonging. These concrete, locally particular resources provide an experience of familiarity and stability, a sense of continuity through the memory of the locality of place. (Connerton 2009, p. 133)

The dams and the purpose for which dams are constructed are both sites with similar tendencies of erasure of memory, or at least negating of memory of cultural groups, that are at the fringes of this process. Therefore, the pain of uprooting from sites which hold not just certain 'house types' (distinguishable in standard anthropological treatises on the 'tribe') but an entire lived memory, is not felt by people who are the engineers of this process, and who are themselves situated in city spaces that are far removed from (and thence blind and deaf to) homes and lives of the *adivasis*. Connerton remarks:

> Modernity, or at least that component of it represented by the economic expansion of the capitalist process of production, produces cultural amnesia not by accident but intrinsically and necessarily. Forgetting is built into the capitalist process of production itself, incorporated in the bodily experience of its life-spaces. (Ibid,, p. 125)

And, in the process of construction of urban spaces, which has been the experience in the case of India since the last two decades or more, "[t]he scarcity and impoverishment of vast tracts and many groups throughout the world are for the most part forgotten, a mental habit of forgetting generated by the taken-forgrantedness of consumer-availability in the metropolis". (Ibid., pp. 142–143)

Similarly, but at another level of 'forgetting', rests our history, where sites of older Buddhist or Jaina traditions becoming Hindu temples hide pasts of violent repression and persecution and their presence, as a dominant structure, keep reminding these communities of what it means to be marginalized.

Commenting on Martin Luther King Jr.'s assertion that "[o]ur nation was born in genocide…. [and that] we are perhaps the only nation which tried as a matter of national policy to wipe out its indigenous population… elevat[ing] that tragic experience into a noble crusade", Roxanne Dunbar-Ortiz remarks that, "[s]omehow, even 'genocide' seems an inadequate description for what happened, yet rather than viewing it with horror, most Americans have conceived of it as their country's manifest destiny" (Petersen 2014).

The same could be said in the case of most of the marginalized *adivasis*/tribal communities in India. But the genocide here need not be seen in terms of physical extermination of an ethnic group, but as extermination of their language, spaces and ways of life. Recently, the Prime Minister of India, Mr. N. Modi repeated—in Canada—that 'Hinduism is a way of life' (and what was important, at the level of the discourse of modernity, was that he mentioned that the Supreme Court of India says so).[8] His statement was reported with gaiety in the newspapers the next day but for some strange reason, all other religions, including religions of *adivasis*, do not seem to get the credit for being 'ways of life', too. A Gondi king[9] had addressed students in the Hyderabad University (in the February, 2015) and lamented that even after 65 years of Indian independence from British rule, the Gondis (and other *adivasis*) are yet to attain their independence and autonomy, and that in spite of several petitions to include the Gondi language in the "VIII Schedule" of the Constitution of India,[10] and the religion they practice, which is *not* Hinduism, be acknowledged as a separate religion, nothing much has been conceded yet.[11]

---

[8]This was made as part of a speech delivered by the Prime Minister, Mr. Narendra Modi, on April 17th, 2015 at a temple in Vancouver. I heard it over the All India Radio (India's national broadcaster). But his speech and this statement was reproduced on various videos (which can still be found on Youtube) and in newspapers the next day. "The Supreme Court has said that Hindu dharam is not a religion but a way of life… I believe the SC's definition shows the way," the Prime Minister said while visiting the Lakshmi Narayan Temple near Vancouver. (see online report: http://www.thehindu.com/news/international/hinduism-not-a-religion-but-a-way-of-life-modi/article7112383.ece). Also see *The Times of India* report. Online: http://timesofindia.indiatimes.com/india/PM-Narendra-Modi-in-Canada-Hinduism-not-a-religion-but-a-way-of-life/articleshow/46954122.

[9]The Gonds are another indigenous community in India mostly inhabiting the region known as Gondwana which includes parts of the Indian states, Maharashtra and Telangana.

[10]Schedule VIII of the Indian Constitution grants official status to Indian languages. Gondi is not an 'official' language, as per the Constitution. There is no provision of separate religion status for the Gond communities in the Indian Constitution. They are, for all legal purposes, considered 'Hindu'.

[11]*Gondraje*, Dr. Birsha Atram, made this point at a Seminar on "Adivasi Autonomy: Self, Home and Habitat" organized by the Department of History, Hyderabad University, and the Indian Council of Philosophical Research, New Delhi, at the University of Hyderabad—19th–21st February, 2015. Incidentally, many communities, such as the Jainas, had also fought cases for centuries (even in the colonial period) to distinguish their religion, and make it legally a separate religion and not club it with 'Hinduism', which had been the case.

12.3 Sites of Memory, Marginalization and 'Expression' of Pain

I now get to a different pain-canvas: where pain, in many senses, almost defines the 'being' of a community, through memories preserved of events in the past that caused and continue to cause pain.

> Methodologically speaking, memories are at their most collective when they transcend the time and space of the events' original occurrence and take on a powerful life of their own, "unencumbered" by actual individual memory and become the basis of all collective remembering as disembodied, omnipresent, low intensity memory. (Kansteiner 2002, p. 189)

Reverting to the Tamil Jainas, let me give a very brief account of their history in Tamilnadu. The Tamil Jainas are adherents of Digambara Jaina tradition and settled predominantly in northern Tamilnadu—largely north and south Arcot districts, Kanchipuram. Tamil Jaina villages also exist in Tanjavur district, and in recent times a substantial erstwhile agrarian Jaina population has moved into cities such as Chennai seeking other livelihood options. The Tamil Jainas today are categorized as a 'minority' community in Tamilnadu—their population being around 30,000[12] in the year 2000. The community has had a long journey from having flourished as a major religious community in Tamilnadu to a state of relative obscurity (to a microscopic minority) and marginalization. Historians have traced the presence of the Jaina religion in Tamil country from about second and third century BCE, based on the Tamil Brāhmi inscriptional records. The Tamil Jaina community has contributed extensively to the development and enrichment of Tamil language and literature, with compositions such as *Silappadikāram*, *Cīvakacintāmaṇi*, *Nālaṭiyār*, *Nīlakesi*, *Naṉṉūl*, *Tirukkuṟaḷ*, etc. The majority of Tamil Jainas are agriculturists, with very few in government and other work sectors, and the community has been agrarian throughout, as against the general perception of Jainas as being predominantly a mercantile community. The Tamil Jainas that I speak of here are *not* the later migrant settler Jainas of the Marwadi Svetambara Jaina mercantile community found in Chennai or other towns in Tamilnadu and who *may* speak Tamil. The latter are referred to as *'seth'* while the former are locally referred to as *'naiṉār'*.

In its 'identity'—self-perceived notions of being a persecuted community, which is largely corroborated by historical evidence, built over several centuries—the Tamil Jainas locate their present state of being. Conversations with the Tamil Jainas are filled with stories; past and the present seemed at times to merge seamlessly in these stories where the Tamil Jainas placed themselves as both external observers and the ones who experienced these in a past time. The stories and the self-perception may be seen as 'sites' of identity, something preserved almost as a

---

[12]According to the census by the Jaina Youth Forum, Chennai, taken in year 2000. A new Census was recently initiated by the Tamil Jainas in February this year (2015) to enumerate the work-related profile of Tamil Jainas in Tamilnadu.

sacred site of collective memory. In the early stages of history there were substantial Tamil Jaina settlements in the region in and around Madurai, but with the onslaught (or propagation, depending on the way we perceive it) of the 'bhakti' *Śaiva* and *Vaiṣṇava* traditions in the region between the seventh and ninth centuries CE— often associated with proliferation of temples to *Śaiva* and *Vaiṣṇava* gods and goddesses (within the universalized 'Hindu' religious paradigm)—these areas were abandoned and Jaina settlements came up in northern Tamilnadu. The historical vestiges of Jaina religion can still be seen in Madurai, sans Jaina villages. This community has witnessed and lived through change—at times violent. A community that gave to the Tamil language the largest part of its grammar and poetry, besides 'universal' icons such as *Tiruvalluvar* (whose *Tirukkuṟaḷ* verses are still part of school and college syllabus in Tamilnadu) is today waging a quiet battle to be granted minority status on account of its socio-economic and demographic profile. Largely agrarian, the Tamil Jainas are a living example of how a community manages to survive amidst universalised, dominant cultural paradigms, at times negotiating spaces, cultural and social, and at others, resisting these changes, while asserting its identity. They are a living example of how identities are constructed and reinforced and asserted; and also that of non-change, which leads to a community's gradual deterioration though not 'death'. At another level, in the process of negotiating, the community silently accepts the dominant cultural idioms with its own set of explanations for doing so. In modernity's terms, the Tamil Jainas have filed petitions to the government to grant them 'Minority' status on account of their socio-economic profile.

There is a popular story narrated by the Tamil Jainas in the Cenji region, a story popularly referred to as the '*sumantāṉ talai pattu*' ('story of the one who carted ten heads'). I heard the story for the first time at Vilukkam, a Tamil Jaina village. This was the first story that was narrated to me the moment the question of persecution during the bhakti period came up. But instead of the account that many are familiar with, regarding the bhakti bard/'saint-poet' Appar and *Tirugñānasambandar*,[13] I heard a different version of this story belonging to a much later period. Incidentally, *Tirunāvukkarasar*, or Appar, was said to have been a Jaina monk who converted to *Śaivism* after being supposedly cured of a stomach ailment when he prayed to *Śiva*, as advised by his sister. The *Śaivite* bards in fact created an entire sacred geography of *Śaivite* temples wherever they went singing the hymns in praise of *Śiva*. Many local cults—village goddesses and even tribal gods—got

---

[13]These are two bards who have been canonized and deified in the mainstream Tamil culture and their icons can be seen in almost all the temples. The *Śaivite* bards are referred to as 'nāyanmārs' while the *Vaiṣṇavite* bards are referred to as '*āḻvārs*'. 7th–9th centuries CE is considered as the period of the onset and flourishing of the bhakti movement (which focused on the so-called 'personal god-concept'). A large volume of scholarship from the West and within India has emerged on the hymns composed by these bards in praise of a god or goddess. In mainstream scholarship bhakti was apparently anti-caste, but in reality, the bhakti movement (as is historically substantiated), which in fact lent support to the establishment of several temples across Tamilnadu, and land grants to *brāhmiṇs*, was part of the same paradigm. The *Śaivite* *tevāram* hymns are said to contain abusive verses against the Jainas, as noted by scholars of Tamil history.

incorporated into an overarching *Śaivite* temple worship paradigm with the emergence of the bhakti tradition in Tamilnadu. And the Tamil Jainas consider (this emergent, and in later periods—nineteenth/early twentieth century revivalist) *Śaivism* to be their nemesis. Post-bhakti movement, many Buddhist and Jaina sacred centres were converted into either *Vaiṣṇavite* or *Śaivite* religious centres. The Buddhists—institutions and people—of Tamilnadu simply left the cultural-historical space forever while the Jainas survived, perhaps through uneasy negotiations.

Meanwhile, the story of the '…ten heads' goes like this: a ruler of Cenji[14] from a lower caste sought a high caste bride for himself. He went to the *Brāhmiṇs* who told him the Jainas were of a higher caste. He sought a bride from the Jainas. The Jainas, insulted by a low-caste ruler seeking a girl from their community, in turn insulted him by tying a dog to the wedding post on the wedding day, and fled the place. He retaliated by ordering the severing of heads of Jainas in Cenji country. Fearing their lives, many Jainas converted to the *Śaiva* faith by smearing sacred ash on their foreheads and it is these people who are called the *nīr pūci nayinārs* (Jainas who smeared sacred ash). Apparently, the king then got his son married to his sister's daughter. When his daughter-in-law was pregnant, she was blessed by *samaṇa muṇis* (Digambara monks). The king then ordered his men to stop the killing of those with *pūṇūl* (sacred thread) and *candanam* (sandalwood paste) on their foreheads (that is, the Jainas, who wear both these markers). In some versions they say it was the black dog tied to the post, with a note that if that black dog could be made a white one, the Jainas would give their girl to the king in marriage. The enraged ruler ordered beheading of Jainas, whosoever should be seen in the streets. This continued, and many Jainas were killed, until one day the king, who had been married in due course, became father to a son. In that moment of joy, he ordered to stop the killings. In some other versions the king did not stop at ordering beheading of the Jainas. He commanded that the person who beheads ten Jainas should carry the head of every tenth Jaina killed. "They beheaded one, and placed ten heads over one, and thus went on killing Jainas. This is referred to as *sumantāṇ talai pattu* (carried ten heads)" (Sastry 1995, p. 46; my translation).

Thurston has also recorded the story, which is as follows:
In 1478 AD, the ruler of Gingee was one Venkatampittar, Venkatapati (local oral tradition gives his name as Dupala Kistnappa Nayak) who belonged to the comparatively low caste of the Kavarais. He asked the local brahmans (for a girl from their caste to marry, they directed him to the Jainas; they called him to a particular spot; left a dog tied to a post at the marriage place…) Furious… he issued orders to behead all Jains… Meanwhile, another Jain of the Gingee country, Gangayya Udaiyar of Taiyanur, had fled to the protection of the zamindar of Udaiyarpalayam in Trichinopoly, who befriended him and gave him some land… (he fetched back Virasenacarya, made tour of Gingee… got some people to return to their faith). These people had mostly become Saivites, taken off their sacred threads and put holy ash on their foreheads, and the name Nirpuci Vellalas… is still retained. The descendants of

---

[14]In most of these stories recounted to me the community did not mention the king's name. Doing some archival search for the story, I found Thurston referring to the same story and the king's name there is given as one Venkatapathy Nayaka.

Gangayya Udaiyar still live in Tayanur, and in memory of the services of their ancestors to the Jain cause, they are given the 1st betel and leaf on festive occasions, and have a leading voice in the election of the high priest at Sittamur in the Tindivanam taluk. This high priest, who is called Mahadhipati, is elected by representatives from the chief Jain villages. These are, in Tindivanam taluk, Sittamur itself, Viranamur, Vilukkam, Peramandur, Alagramam and the Velur and Tayanur already mentioned. (Thurston 1909, pp. 429–430)

This was one of the two colonial documents (Mackenzie's being another, recorded in the Mackenzie manuscripts, 1837, D 3796) that gave the story a 'written' form, which becomes a permanent archive outside the community memory. I found this material when I went looking for 'more' on the story and to cross-check versions of it after I had heard the story in the Tamil Jaina villages during the course of my doctoral research. Finding it in the colonial record also shows that this story had been in circulation even during that time and the person concerned with documentation had written down the memory of the Tamil Jainas of that time-period. It is amazing that the account has survived in Tamil Jaina minds across generations.

It would help to historically locate this story if I mention some other stories highlighting the age-old Śaiva–Jaina conflict in Tamilnadu, as under:

[1] A story in the *Periyapurāṇam* [composed by *Cēkkiḻār*, a Śaivite bard] talks about *Tiruvoṭṭiyūr*. A *Śaiva* man planted a male toddy tree. Few Jainas questioned him if these male trees could transform into female trees; they questioned *Gñānasambandar*, who sang a *patikam* [verse] and before dawn the trees transformed into female trees. The Jainas fled that village. The *Tiruvoṭṭiyūr Śiva* temple has frescoes showing the impalement of Jainas, as in Madurai (Venkataswamy 1954, pp. 68–69; my translation).[2] *Tiruvārūr Tirukkolam* is a tank feeding 18 acres. The *Periyapurāṇam* mentions that the *Taṇṭṭiaṭikaḷ (Śaiva)* tank was a small one surrounded by Jaina land and *paḷḷis* [Jaina monastic institutions] on four banks. The *Śaivas* wanted to make it bigger by removing the Jaina settlements. The Jainas protested. *Cēkkiḻār* mentions that *Śiva* appeared in the dream of the king to command destruction of the Jaina settlements at this place. (Ibid., p. 70; my translation)

Thurston, too, records two stories regarding the Śaiva-Jaina conflict:

[1] The Madura District Gazetteer mentions, taking from the Madura Sthalapurana[15] about the origins of Anaimalai - The Jains of Conjeevaram tried to convert the Saivite people of Madurai to the Jain faith. Finding the task difficult, they had recourse of magic. They dug a great pit 10 miles long, performed a sacrifice thereon, and thus causes a huge elephant to rise from it. This beast they sent against Madura. It advanced towards the town, shaking the whole earth at every step, with the Jains marching close behind it. The Pandya king invoked the aid of Siva and the god arose and slew the elephant with his arrow at the spot where it now lies petrified... In connection with the long barren rock near Madura called Nagamali - Local legends declare... it is the remains of a huge a serpent, brought into existence by the magic arts of the Jains which was only prevented by the grace of Siva from devouring the fervently Saivite city it so nearly approaches. (Thurston 1909, p. 434)[2] For the following account thereof, I am indebted to Mr. K.V. Subramani Aiyar.[16] Sri Gnana Sambandar Svami who was an incarnation of Subramanya, the son of Siva... was sent into the world by

---

[15]Mythological place-history of Madurai.
[16]Note that his 'source for the story' is a *brāhmiṇ*.

Siva to put down the growing prevalence of the Jain heresy, and to re-establish the Saivite faith in Southern India… At the time a certain Kun Pandya (hunchback) Pandyan was ruling the Madura country, where as elsewhere Jainism had asserted its influence… The Queen and the prime minister were Saivite, invited Gnana Sambandar (to extirpate the Jains). He came with thousands of followers and took abode in a mutt[17] on the north side of Vaigai river… Jain priests, 8000 in number, found this out… set fire to his residence. But disciples extinguished the flames… Sambandar made flames take the form of a virulent fever to affect one side of the King's body, which he cured… The king became beautiful and was called Sundarapandya thenceforth… Books of Saivites travailed upstream and Jains' books perished; (Post these trials, etc.) many converted to Saivites. The number (of those who converted) was so great that the available supply of sacred ashes was exhausted. (Those who could not be converted) were impaled on stakes resembling sula or trident… The events (are)… gone through at 5 of the 12 annual festivals at Madura temple. On these occasions an image representing a Jain impaled on a stake is carried in procession. (Ibid., pp. 435–438)

The village Tayanur (near Cenji) of Gangeya Udaiyar, who helped the Tamil Jainas at the time of persecution, holds special importance in the memory of the Tamil Jainas. The present-day Tamil Jaina villages—Vilukkam, Cenji, Agalur and Melcittamur (settled by the Tamil Jainas since centuries)—especially recount the story of the *cakkili rājā* of Cenji. These are sacred in relation to the 'revival' of Jaina faith after a period of persecution. The *cakkili rājā* story has many elements of a near-ritual performance of a story, a memory which reiterates the victimization as well as the vindication of the community's honour in being true to its identity.

One of the important aspects to the memory of persecution of the Tamil Jainas is that these constantly refer to the political context of the Tamil country, where the cultural-religious realm of brahminical temple and land nexus played a crucial role in marginalizing religions such as Buddhism and Jainism. However, even these religions were not free from the land and temple paradigm in the medieval period. Initially, the Jaina sacred centres were rock-cut caves and natural caverns with donative inscriptions in *Brāhmi* script and Tamil language. In the medieval period, you find temple structures with Buddhist and Jaina images coming up. In the ultimate contest, however, the *Brāhmiṇ* and *Veḷḷāḷa* landlords of *Śaiva* and *Vaiṣṇava* denominations seem to have captured the political sphere and worked towards establishing a larger idiom where neither Buddhism nor Jainism held any significance.

Aleida Assmann points out that:In three aspects, the political constructions of memory differ clearly from personal and social memory. First, they are not connected to other memories and the memories of others but tend towards homogeneous unity and self-contained closure. Second, political memory is not fragmentary and diverse but emplotted in a narrative that is emotionally charged and conveys a clear and invigorating message. And, third, it is not something volatile and transient, but is anchored in material and visual signs such as sites and monuments as well as in performative action such as commemoration rites, which periodically reactivate individual memories and enhance collective participation. In this way, a political memory is stabilized and can be transmitted from generation to generation. (Assmann 2010, p. 43)

[17]A religious/monastic establishment.

In this sense, the Tamil Jaina memory—of various persecution stories, or epi-sodes, of which I just mentioned two—is a political construction. It must be mentioned in this regard that the village names associated with the story and the 'special respect' granted, even to this day in temple festivals, to members of the village (which is supposed to have re-instated the Jaina religion through the intervention of Gangeya Udaiyar), acts as the ritual act of commemoration. Incidentally, in recent times, two groups of Tamil Jainas have begun what is called 'green walk' and 'ahimsa walk' which retraces, and in that act, 'recovers', ancient Tamil Jaina sites, some of which are no longer Jaina and have other visible non-Jaina appropriations (marks of local cultic traditions).

> According to Pierre Nora:
> Our interest in *lieux de memoire* where memory crystallises and secretes itself has occurred at a particular historical moment, a turning point where consciousness of a break with the past is bound up with the sense that memory has been torn—but torn in such a way as to pose the problem of the embodiment of memory in certain sites of historical continuity persists. There are *lieux de memoire,* sites of memory, because there are no longer *milieux de memoire*, real environments of memory. (Nora 1989, p. 7)

The *sites of memory* in the Tamil Jaina case are also *sites of pain*, located in the *real environments of memory* as well and intrinsically connected to the idea of their identity having been constantly in a state of conflict and contestation. The stories and the historical records—aided by constant efforts by mainstream religious groups to appropriate older Jaina sites and newer economic developments, like stone quarrying from ancient Jaina rock-cut caves—keep the memory of the per-secution alive. In this sense, one tends to agree with Nora when he points out that:

> The defense, by certain minorities, of a privileged memory that has retreated to jealously protected enclaves... intensely illuminates the truth of *lieux de memoire*—that without commemorative vigilance, history would soon sweep them away. We buttress our identities upon such bastions, but if what they defended were not threatened, there would be no need to build them. Conversely, if the memories that they enclosed were to be set free they would be useless; if history did not besiege memory, deforming and transforming it, penetrating and petrifying it, there would be no *lieux de memoire*. Indeed, it is this very push and pull that produces *lieux de memoire*—moments of history torn away from the movement of history, then returned; no longer quite life, not yet death, like shells on the shore when the sea of living memory has receded. (Ibid., p. 12)

12.4   Further Problematising

Elaine Scarry speaks of the "difficulty of expressing physical pain..." and "the political and perceptual complications that arise as a result of that difficulty...and... the nature of both material and verbal expressibility or, more simply, the nature of human creation..." (Scarry 1985, p. 3). She continues:

Physical pain has no voice, but when it at last finds a voice, it begins to tell a story, and the story that it tells is about the inseparability of these three subjects, their embeddedness in one another (Ibid., p. 3).

But physical pain can still be expressed, in words, even if the semantics is insufficient. Being in a constant pain of remembering a past, or thinking of an uncertain future, on account of the present self being in pain, as in the two instances of displacement and permanent dislocation from roots that I have located, is expressed, sometimes very specifically, by people. But of all the things that are recognized in their narration, pain is not. Pain is not something that can be quantified or compensated for. It is not accounted for as a matter for consideration in all these cases. In the Tamil Jaina case, the collective memory of victimhood and persecution is integral to their construction of their Self. In the history of religion, which is a historical fact and something remembered by the community, the Jaina doctrine (along with Buddhist, *Ājīvika*,[18] and others) had once countered the then dominant Vedic religion; but over a period of time, thanks to political change and social constructions, the Vedic (with adoptions from other religious ideas and becoming more overarching, with the brahminical structure) managed to overpower all other religious constructs in India, so much so that the dominant idiom today is the so-called 'Hindu'. In constructing the Self that was persecuted, the Tamil Jainas also refer back to all these pasts which rendered them marginals of the system, which is a reality of their present as well. So in reliving the painful memories of that past, they force us to not forget that history, which so few speak about today.

Scarry uses the word 'weapon' (often) and 'sign of a weapon' (when she looks at 'torture' as a weapon). In our case, then (in the case of the Tamil Jainas and that of the displaced or to-be-displaced adivasis), what would we see or read as a 'weapon' that 'tortures'? For the Tamil Jainas, or any other presently minority community with their history of persecution, their memory itself might be a weapon that tortures; it could be the dominant cultures, traditions, the loudness of it all, the way Hindu prayers and symbols are either the main text or the very visible sub-text in politics, commercial marketing, etc.; the reading out of certain prayers and performance of certain rituals (for instance ritual enactments of events that contain memory or history of a pain of the past, impaling on stakes of Jaina monks used to be ritualized in a temple in Madurai until early twentieth century); or razing to the ground a mosque or the re-enactment of it; or even the sound of music that reminds a community of its present state of marginalization. In the case of the tribal people displaced, the weapon of pain, especially in today's context, could be the structure of a dam built over their homes, now in an ongoing process of ruination. An airport on ruined fields, or, simply, the language and idiom of economic power and middle class wellness advertisements which are devoid of tribal heritage, tribal languages

---

[18]The ascetic *Ājīvika* school (said to have been founded by *Makkali Gośāla*) is said to have emerged alongside the Jaina and Buddhist traditions and remained significant as a contending contemporary to these traditions. The *Ājīvika* believed in the predetermined course of events in life (and hence a kind of acute non-interference in the flow of events, thereby a kind of non-action) and liberation from this through the ascetic way of life. Its founder was *Makkali Gośāla*.

and worldviews; just as for an indigenous American, the presence and over-whelming numbers of white American settler colonies or weekend or seasonal rock climbing 'adventure sports' (in the "pursuit of happiness", which is guaranteed legally in America) over their sacred mountains.[19] The weapon that is constantly flashed, so far as the tribal communities (in Godavari or elsewhere, in Odisha or Chhattisgarh) could be, their soon becoming the 'memory' of a nation, even while they are alive; and the fact is, there isn't any therapy nor a psycho-session for relief of the 'patients' from these kinds of pains. For, the relief must come from a political consciousness of these pains, and their active removal in the form of acknowl-edgments, which only happen in a radical political reconstruct of the system which does not constantly 'exclude.'

In some cases, is 'closure' ever possible? In the Tamil Jaina case, some opt for closure through negotiating with the mainstream or the dominant, by way of either compromise or adjustments in order to survive, but in cases of the displaced tribal communities there is never a closure. Yes, survival happens, but in many ways, displacement is only a starting line and from that point the journeys are often to oblivion. But, in the larger canvas, there appears to be no real 'closure': you just need to witness a site of appropriation, and out comes the story of a past persecution or pain.

12.5   On Cartographies

Finally, I posit the idea of cartography: there is a map, of either sacred sites or sites of everyday settlements, over which new cartographies are raised and forced. There are places remembered in stories; sites from where people did this or did that and where they lay claims for their belonging to a history of their own, which never becomes official history (on account of the politics that goes into making official histories, in a certain time and space; and which is a good since official history puts a stamp, usually, a stamp on the dominant or dominating). Sometimes, its *not becoming* official recorded history pains them; and at others it seems to set them free, in the sense that they are autonomous and free to etch in their memory (a collective memory shared across generations) where people remember what they have not 'seen' but 'heard' from their parents and grandparents; an event or a series of events that reminds them of their loss. Their cartographies are constructed out from sites of loss and pain of that loss, and in 'real', 'mundane' 'this-world' sense, the maps (political maps, usually) give us the evidence of what *was* (which is lost in political sense—of the dominant history) and what *is*, in its place. In the mental maps, retrieved through memory (in great detail) there are sites not yet lost but painfully different from 'what was there before' or 'what was' which is lost: Jaina rock-cut cave with its recorded archival history of visitations by monks and nuns and

---

[19]As shown in a Documentary Film, titled "In the Light of Reverence," produced and directed by Christopher McLeod, which was shared with me by an American environmental activist called Alex.

teachers, which is now a *Murukaṉ*[20] or *Śiva* shrine, where even animal sacrifices are offered by some communities, though to the Tamil Jainas animal sacrifices are offensive to their basic tenet. And sometimes, when these changes occur, they seem to signify the present position of relative insignificance of the Tamil Jains in terms of numbers and as a faith or religion with its own antiquity in Tamil country. At a deeper symbolic level then, it hurts them to find that the rock-cut caves, natural caverns with *Brāhmi* inscriptions and carvings of tirthankaras, who taught the value of *koḷḷāmai* (in Tamil, literally, non-killing), should over time become sites where dominant communities have virtually established their stamp. The silence of the rocks seem quite stark against the din of the quarterly, or weekly or annual sacrificial rites carried out at the base of these rock caves, in some of the places. At times, the Tamil Jaina person accompanying you will show you the icon of their *tīrthankara*, a seated (in meditation posture) *Mahāvīra*, or *Ādinātha*, transformed into a *Muṇiyāṇḍi*, a Hindu deity with Hindu embellishments with Hindu ritual paraphernalia accompanying that image. The icons of *Muṇiyāṇḍi* or a goddess, made from original *tīrthankara* images (with a 'historical' stamp on them, with ample 'evidence'—the Jaina will lay stress on the fact of historical evidence in order to convince you of their very ontological being and presence in Tamil history) can be found in several places in Tamilnadu with a Jaina or Buddhist past. And these will be usually associated with myths of sudden appearance in someone's dream and a temple built for the new deity which will be installed with great fanfare. For the Tamil Jainas, watching these changes and obvious power of the dominant tradition is painful and hurtful, even as they show you these signs to prove their point of how they have been marginalized and cast aside in the course of history of Tamil country. The present—of a *tīrthankara* image dressed up as a Hindu one—and the past atrocities of persecution and violent suppression of their faith to them seem part of one long, nearly unbroken thread, showing them their own insignificance built over time. Even today, in one of the rock-cut cave sites at Kongarpuliyangulam near Madurai, one can spot the *vēl* (spear) associated with *Murukaṉ* placed at the bottom of the hillock, where animal sacrifices are offered during festivals. Against this backdrop, the Tamil Jainas seem to find it simpler to live with their loss of significance and seem to feel it sufficient to narrate the tales of their loss in their own narratives, and when they point to the overt changes. Pain, it seems, will be their constant. The other moments of pain as a community comes out when their naked monks are hurled stones at by other communities who object to seeing a naked man walk past. Hence, there is a police force and a group of Jaina laity that usually walks with a Digambara monk on occasions when they come visiting the Tamil Jaina villages. The visit of a Digambara monk is always accompanied by anxiety and fear of attack from other communities.

---

[20]The original hill-god of the Tamils (worshipped by hunter-gatherers, in early periods), *Murukaṉ* was transformed into the (Hindu) *Purāṇic Subrahmaṇya*, son of *Śiva* in the later periods. He is still considered the quintessential Tamil god.

In the case of the Koyas and Kondareddis of Godavari–Sabari river region, it is the loss of their Tamarind tree and their forest, which becomes a marked site for the government's destruction project. Trees, wherein sometimes inhere sacredness, will be marked with white paint and they metamorphose into boundary markers of destruction, for the construction of a project of expressed/stated 'modernity', a dam. The ancient boulder there or an ancient Tamarind tree (*chinta cheṭṭu*) or a Mango tree (*māmidi cheṭṭu*) or *ippa cheṭṭu* (*Mahuca indica*) assume new forms of meaning as government sites, or markers for government sites, and markers of a newly created 'gate' against the tribal people who now become the 'encroachers', by virtue of a paper or a note or an announcement to that effect under an official ordinance. What were once paths towards last year's annual ritual animal-hunt expedition of the Kondareddis or Koyas, become parking spaces for earth movers and sand crushing machines, which, when they move, slowly, destroy the last signs of *adivasi* histories and cultures creating a new cartography over the old, which will again get etched in memory of the *adivasis* and their future memories will be built from the point of this rupture, a new rupture. And what happened before the dam and after the dam. The earlier histories of their earlier ruptures, with the colonial masters reserving vast tracts of *adivasi* forest land against *adivasis* and calling them "uncivilised tribes… illiterate and ignorant of the ways of the world and yet ready to go out on the warpath if once any of their many peculiar sensibilities are wounded" (Hemingway 1915, pp. 188–189). That rupture, marked by the colonial rulers, will go into deeper recesses of the adivasi social, cultural or community memory, to be recalled with pain and a sense of having suffered injustice and cruelty under the British, a loss they will never speak of in terms of 'future gain'.

So the essence of pain in all these encounters has the element of politics, social construction and emotional upheaval, very much rooted in the ontology of their being. For the fishermen by the Godavari, the pain erupts when they watch dwindling numbers of fish in the same river that has been their traditional fishing zone. There will be expression of nostalgia; the past is always spoken of in terms of plenty of fish; the present is a construction of destruction, which is purposefully meant to terminate their existence. It is seen in terms of a conspiracy by the state.[21] And these are people who have a definite sense of their past and present and their present in the wake of their past. The constant inflow of tourists with their loud film music enjoying a cruise on the river and their enjoyment sharpens the pain within the hearts of the fishermen and the adivasis of Godavari, like an injection on a wound that numbs your senses.

Pain, in these instances, is in fact, visible in their eyes, as they see an entire humanity and an entire polity literally passes them by, cruise through their veins— metaphorically—by the day, as a giant project promises to crush their earth and blind their skies. The pain here is both the pain of these people and the pain of someone who watches, conscious of what is to be lost and what is to be built in its

---

[21]For elaborate discussion on the dislocations of fishworkers/fisher communities of Godavari, see Umamaheshwari (2014, pp. 287–347).

place, at the stake of the loss of histories of entire communities. The impending loss of a home, to be razed to the ground, the fear of it, is very real and very everyday and an abject constant. In some cases, the wounds inflicted for the project are physical, as in the case of Rajanna Dora or Veerasamy when they are beaten up or arrested. Even in these cases, the pain is physical, as it is cultural and political. Of being disembodied from land and forest and river and, finally, history.

References

Note: References to Tamil Jaina stories, etc., are based on my unpublished Doctoral Dissertation, titled *Identities in Conflict: Jainism in Early Tamilakam*, Jawaharlal Nehru University, New Delhi, and on updated research for my current engagement at IIAS, Shimla on "Reading History with the Tamil Jainas: Locating Identity, Memory and Marginalisations in Historiography".

Colonial Archives

Hemingway, F. R. (1915). *Madras district Gazetteers: Godavari district*. Superintendent, Madras: Government Press.
Mackenzie Manuscripts (1837). *Account of the Raja of Gingee who persecuted the Jainas* (D 3796, Vol. I, Section 2). Madras: Government Oriental Manuscripts Library.
Thurston, E. (1909). *Castes and tribes of southern India* (Vol. II). Madras: Government Press.

Others

Assmann, A. (2010). Re-framing memory: Between individual and collective forms of constructing the past. In K. Tilmans, F. Van Vree, & J. Winter (Eds.), *Performing the past: Memory, history, and identity in modern Europe* (pp. 35–50). Amsterdam: University Press.
Connerton, P. (2009). *How modernity forgets*. Cambridge: Cambridge University Press.
Kansteiner, W. (2002). Finding meaning in memory: A methodological critique of collective memory studies. *History and Theory, 41*(2), 179–197.
Nora, P. (1989). Between memory and history: Les Lieux de Mémoire. *Representations, 26* (Special Issue: Memory and Counter-Memory), pp. 7–24.
Petersen, K. (2014). Through the eyes of the dispossessed: Review of *An indigenous people's history of the United States* by Roxanne Dunbar-Ortiz. *Dissident Voice: A Radical Newsletter in the Struggle for Peace and Social Justice*, December 15, 2014. http://dissidentvoice.org/2014/12/through-the-eyes-of-the-dispossessed/.
Ramazani, V. K. (1996). Writing in pain: Baudelaire, Benjamin, Haussmann. *Boundary, 23*(2), 199–224.
Sastry, M. (1995). *Tamilnadu ka Jain Itihas (Hindi)*. Delhi: Kundakunda Bharati.
Scarry, E. (1985). *The body in pain: The making and unmaking of the world*. Oxford: Oxford University Press.
Umamaheshwari, R. (2014). *When Godavari comes: People's history of a river (Journeys in the zone of the dispossessed)*. Delhi: Aakar Books.
Venkataswamy, M. S. (1954). *Samaṇamum Tamiḻum (Tamil)*. Tirunelveli: South India Saiva Siddhanta Publication.

Chapter 13
AFSPA and the Tortured Bodies: The Politics of Pain in Manipur

Malem Ningthouja

Abstract This chapter looks at the controversial Armed Forces Special Powers Act 1958 (AFSPA) in Manipur as a concrete context of the politics of torture and pain. The contentious agencies at play at various levels interpret torture in their respective ways, either in support of AFPSA, or against it, by parading the objectified enemy and the tortured bodies of victims. This chapter analyses the manner in which individual torture becomes social and political phenomena. It highlights the socio-political construction of torture as a means of organized protest, and argues that the narratives of torture at various levels not only objectify bodies as victims but also encourage them to fight against torture. In that sense, torture that is being rendered demonstratively visible and audible enters into a framework of schematization. Schematized pain involves such strategies as embracing a certain pain to avert torture, making pain demonstrably visible, hurting the pained and fragmenting the depiction of pain. The chapter concludes with the observation that the dialectics of the AFSPA and the tortured bodies suggests a dialectical unity of the opposites in the political totality.

Keywords AFSPA · Collective memory · Manipur · Security · Terror · Torture

M. Ningthouja (✉)
Indian Institute of Advanced Study, Shimla, India
e-mail: mningthouja@yahoo.com

© Springer India 2016
S.K. George and P.G. Jung (eds.), *Cultural Ontology
of the Self in Pain*, DOI 10.1007/978-81-322-2601-7_13

13.1 Introduction

Torture signifies pain, intense physical suffering as well as trauma, deliberately inflicted upon embodied subjects. According to the International Convention against Torture and Other Cruel, Inhuman or Degrading Treatment or Punishment, adopted in 1984 (CAT 1984), torture is any act that inflicts severe pain or suffering, whether physical or mental, involving a public official and carried out for a specific purpose.[1] John Heath defines torture as "infliction of physically founded suffering or the threat immediately to inflict it, where such infliction or threat is intended to elicit, or such infliction is incidental to means adopted to elicit, matter of intelligence or forensic proof and the motive is one of military, civil, or ecclesiastical interest" (as quoted in Peters 1985, p. 2). In 2010, the Indian State attempted to define torture as "grievous hurt, danger to life, limb or health, severe mental pain, agony, trauma or suffering caused to any person by cruel, inhuman and degrading treatment"[2] inflicted by public servants or any person with the consent or acquiescence of any public servant in the name of duty.

Within the framework of these definitions, deeper questions may be addressed regarding the nature of torture with reference to concrete political instruments like the Armed Forces Special Powers Act 1958 (henceforth AFSPA)[3] of India. Critical commentary considers that the AFSPA causes torture. This view is widely held by the victims of AFSPA and critics who oppose torture. However, in thinking about the nature of torture, the relation between AFSPA and torture needs to look beyond this commonsensical perception. The understanding that the AFSPA causes torture explains only one side of the contentious views surrounding the Act. The social form this view has taken emerges as a repulsive force to do away with AFSPA so that the torture emanating from it can be averted. The other side of the contentions surrounding the AFSPA projects it as a necessary force to avert the pain that 'tortures the nation'. The AFSPA stands as an objectified schema between the repulsive and attractive forces that represent two different types of pain via 'torture': the first being the pain of the community 'tortured' *by* the 'nation', and the other being the 'pain of the nation' that is tortured through 'terror'.

---

[1]As given in the UNHR Convention against Torture which was ratified by the General Assembly in 1984 and came into force in 1987. Online: http://www.ohchr.org/EN/ProfessionalInterest/Pages/CAT.aspx

[2]As given in the International Commission of Jurists Legal Opinion on the Revised Prevention of Torture Bill currently before India's Parliament, November 2011. Online: http://icj.wpengine.netdna-cdn.com/wp-content/uploads/2012/06/India-opinion-prevention-torture-legal-submission-2012.pdf.

[3]The AFSPA enacted in 1958 is a law that grants sweeping powers to the Indian Armed Forces in areas deemed 'disturbed' in the eye of the Government. The powers thus vested on the army personnel include indiscriminate use of force against persons suspected of acting against the law and entering and searching their premises and arresting them without warrant. For more on the AFSPA, see n. 8 below.

However, the latter rendering of AFSPA has been deliberately silenced or rendered oblivious by the attractive force (agency) that upholds the AFSPA and maintains an ambiguous silence about the implicit assumption of it being tortured. The term torture, or the idea of 'tortured nation', is not being used anywhere by the State in justifying the imposition of AFSPA.[4] This is being done probably to avoid formulating a legal definition of torture, which may become a legal reference in challenging any 'torture' committed by the State and in the development of a discourse that precisely formulates the identity of the people of Manipur along the paradigm of a 'tortured community' within India. Further, a legally enforceable definition of torture may invalidate the instrument of AFSPA which was itself created to eliminate the torture of the 'Indian Nation'. However, without linking up these two types of torture with the AFSPA, the picture of pain and torture, and its connection with the AFSPA remain unclear. The point is that there are volumes of information on the State's discourse on terror that defend the political objectives and functional aspects of AFSPA. These sources can very well be used to bring to light the perspective of the idea of a 'tortured nation' that is in a state of perennial 'terror' experienced by virtue of the rebellion in the region, and to portray the agency as tortured and defenceless without the AFSPA. It can, thus, be pointed out that both the torture emanating from the 'use'[5] of AFSPA and the torture emanating from 'terror' are interconnected in terms of objectifying the AFSPA as the political instrument to justify the respective claims and counter-claims of being tortured. 'Terror' flourishes on the torture instituted by the State's instruments like the AFSPA while State oppression flourishes on the alibi of torturous terror that targets it.

The question is: is AFSPA an instrument of torture to avert terror or activities and situations that are being perceived as torturous? In the totality of the two types of torture, does the AFPSA embody different perceptions of torture on the one hand, and different bodies that are being tortured on the other—bodies of those it protects on the one hand and of those it victimizes in the name of torture on the other? What are the bodies and whose are these bodies that are being tortured by the AFSPA? What are the bodies that hold on to the AFSPA to avert torture? Do these bodies that are attracted towards, or repulsed from the AFSPA, constitute objectified aggregations of living beings or are they schematically animated 'imagined' anthropomorphic bodies constructed by contentious agencies? Are these contentious agencies, in their totality, operating within the framework of the dialectics of the unity of the opposites? While trying to find answers to these questions, don't we

---

[4]The State avoids using the term 'torture'. It uses terms such as 'disturbance', 'threats', 'terrorism' and so on. My argument is that the term 'torture' is not being used so as to avoid formulating a definition of torture.

[5]There are many who talk about the misuse or abuse of AFSPA by the law enforcing agencies. I avoid from using the term 'misuse' or 'abuse' because I believe that AFSPA authorizes the personnel to suspect and act accordingly. Therefore, when military personnel kill or torture someone on the ground of suspicion, there is no abuse of the Act. The personnel are merely acting under the provisions of the Act.

also need to move away from the legal definition of torture and focus on a more holistic understanding of it in order to formulate policy and resistance as well? These issues are taken up below for discussion under the following subheadings: Sect. 13.2 AFSPA as Instrument *Against* Torture, Sect. 13.3 AFSPA as Instrument *for* Torture, Sect. 13.4 Collective Memory of Torture, Commemoration and Protest and Sect. 13.5 Conclusion.

13.2   AFSPA as Instrument *Against* Torture

In his discussion on 'torture' as a form of punitive method, Foucault argues that the latter should be analysed "not simply as consequences of legislation or as indicators of social structures, but as techniques possessing their own specificity in the more general field of other ways of exercising power." (1977, p. 23). Foucault is thus clear that we ought to "regard punishment as a political tactic" (Ibid.). He further argues that the right to punish "is an aspect of the sovereign's right to make war on his enemies" (Ibid., p. 48). In the Indian context, the ideological position and general presumptions that held the Indian State responsible for the institutionalization of torture, however, must not fail to see the other side of the narrative that makes the State see itself threatened and tortured by 'disturbance.'[6] The fact that the State relies on torture and remains powerful enough to be kowtowed by both rebels as well as rights activists doesn't necessarily mean that a peaceful context of enjoying absolute loyalty and freedom from threats to the regime exists. On the contrary, torture is a policy to overcome the fear of losing the regimes' control over territory, resource and governance. Peters, in his historical study of torture argues that "paradoxically, in an age of vast state strength, ability to mobilize resources, and possession of virtually infinite means of coercion, much of state policy has been based upon the concept of extreme state vulnerability to enemies, external or internal" (1985, p. 7). Kelmen substantiates Peters' view and argues that "torture becomes state policy when the authorities perceive an active threat to the security of the state from internal or external sources and decide to use the vast power at their disposal to counter that threat by repressive means" (1995, p. 26).

If fear of external or 'internal' threats is the *raison d'être* of militarization and repressive laws, the question is, can't it be axiomatic that fear also generates insult, humiliation and anger, which in totality inflicts psychological torture and pain to the regime? The Constituent Assembly debates and the subsequent parliamentary debates in India provide substantial amount of evidences related to the deep-rooted and painful anxiety about 'security' that the Indian State bears. The anxiety, which is being negatively termed 'security paranoia' by the critics of AFSPA, consists of manifold and interplaying fear presumptions, such as: (a) threat to the 'integrity' of

---

[6]Indian State uses the term 'disturbance' while referring to rebellion and other forms of social unrest. The AFSPA is imposed in 'disturbed areas'.

the State, (b) security threat to the lives and properties of loyal citizens, (c) threat to the lives of the deployed military and paramilitary forces and (d) threat to the resources, land or territory and 'capitalistic' projects. The rebels are being held responsible for the threat to the State and the 'nation,' for causing injury to the pride of India, for tumultuous disturbances, and physical pain and for psychological torture at various levels. In brief, Indian State projects AFSPA as a counter measure to its 'tortured self' and the pain emanating thereof.

The 'security paranoia' is being addressed by the adoption of the policy of torture to avert torture. The policy must be mandated by the 'people.' For this, 'manufacturing consent'[7] is achieved by the systematic dissemination of the imagination about a 'tortured nation.' The propaganda of the 'tortured nation' becomes receptive to many through the formalized parading of the objectified enemy, which in turn invokes patriotism and moulds public opinion to suppress rebellion. What becomes apparent is the continuous objectification of a 'nation' in the form of an organic 'Mother India', which is an entity formed of the aggregation of the generalized loyal individuals, including those members of the suspect peoples in the disturbed areas, who are shown leniency on the basis of proving their individual innocence and loyalty. Therefore, when there is objectification of a tortured nation, the aggregation of the loyal individuals is automatically pitted against the objectively projected bodies of the 'torturer rebels.' In the schematized subsuming of the individual in the aggregated 'national self,' the depiction of the 'tortured nation' and the power of propaganda for constant repetition gives what Reinhart has phrased "the status of objective truth in millions of consumers" (2003, p. 22). Constant repetition makes the news a real perception at the receiving end (Said 2002, p. 147). The perception of being 'tortured' causes pain and it places the targets of attack outside the perimeter of human rights and democratic safeguarding. The AFSPA, therefore, has been continuously superimposed on the nation in the name of averting torture without effective opposition both in the parliament and in the predominant public domain of India.

---

[7]Herman and Chomsky, in their book *Manufacturing Consent: The Political Economy of the Mass Media*, use the phrase 'manufacturing consent' to refer to the manner in which popular subjective consciences are being manipulated by the propaganda of policy makers which in turn, relies on that consent to justify the adoption of certain legislation or policy (Herman and Chomsky 2008). The argument is that public opinion or consent is important in legislation and policy making. However, public opinion is not independent of the influence of the 'hegemonic' mobilization and campaigns of the policy makers that disseminate ideas and contribute to 'manufacturing' ideas at the receptive end.

13.3   AFSPA as Instrument *For* Torture

Functionally, the AFSPA creates the legal framework for torture.[8] It legitimizes torture through schematising crisscrossing parameters of coercion that Kelman, in a different context, analyses as "authorisation, routinisation and dehumanisation" (1995, p. 28). The Supreme Court of India in 1997, after 10 years of debating on torturous incidents, upheld the Act on the ground that "deployment of the armed forces of the Union shall be for the purpose of enabling the civil power in the state to deal with the situation affecting maintenance of public order which has necessitated the deployment of the armed forces in the State".[9] The Court acknowledged tortures under AFSPA and prescribed a set of 'dos and don'ts' for those acting under the Act to ensure protection of human rights. Many had hoped and believed that this prescriptive directive of the Supreme Court would do away with the 'misuse of power' under AFSPA. The prescription, however, did not do away with torture with impunity under the provisions of the Act as hoped. Those forces acting under the AFPSA continue to indulge in creating a torturous situation that is being generally referred to as the 'culture of impunity.'

Killing and torture of civilians, which, in the perspective of the local community members there, has nothing to do with suppression of rebellion, continues without restraint. Many suspect that the primary motive of killing and torture is to fulfil vested personal interests, such as: (i) to score more 'points' for the personnel for promotion and pride, (ii) to extract money from the local community members on flimsy grounds, (iii) to settle personal grudges, (iv) to fulfil malicious intentions such as sexual violence, jealousy and hatred and (v) to enjoy fun, gaming and virile domination. The prevalent culture of impunity thus promotes the growth of a category of thugs and ruffians, who indulge in crimes and hooliganism without fear because of their connection with military or paramilitary personnel. It is also

---

[8]Section 1 of the AFSPA empowers the Governor of a State or the Government of India to construe any area or territory as disturbed or dangerous, thereby empowering any commissioned officer, warrant officer, non-commissioned officer or any other person of equivalent rank in the Armed Forces to exercise powers prescribed by the AFSPA. Section 4 of the Act empowers the concerned officer to 'suspect' and consequently act on 'his' suspicion to arrest anyone without warrant, to search any premise without warrant, destroy, and "fire upon or otherwise use force, even to the causing of death, against any person who is acting in contravention of any law or order for the time being in the disturbed area prohibiting the assembly of five or more persons or the carrying of weapons or of things capable of being used as weapons or firearms, ammunition or explosive substances." Section 5 of the Act empowers the concerned officer to detain any arrested person with the least possible delay and does not stipulate any time frame of the detention. Section 6 of the Act defends guilty personnel as "no prosecution, suit or legal proceeding shall be instituted, except with the previous sanction of the Government of India against any person in respect of anything done or purported to be done in exercise of the powers conferred by this Act" (Ningthouja 2011, pp. 145–155).

[9]Supreme Court of India Judgment on Naga People's Movement for Human Rights versus Union of India, dated 27 November, 1997. Online: http://indiankanoon.org/doc/1072165/ and http://judis.nic.in/supremecourt/imgst.aspx?filename=13628.

suspected that gangs, who indulge in extortion and criminal activities in the guise of rebellion, are operating under the patronage of the military and paramilitary forces. The level of impunity is deeply rooted in society to the extent that much of the youth population of the community there wants to join the army, not for the cause of defending India, but for money and for the perceived possibility of fulfilling one's personal and/or malicious goals.[10]

The AFSPA bypasses the expectation of aiding civil administration and creates a coterie of personnel, who, at their own discretion, exceed the limits of what Kelman paraphrases as the "crime of obedience" (1995, p. 21). There are several such reported interferences by the armed forces in the civil administration, politics and judiciary in the region. In summary, the nature of torture experienced by the people in the region under the AFSPA include cold-blooded fake encounters, massacre, harassment, illegal detention, forced disappearance, killing as a result of mistaken identity, rape, molestation, sodomy, post-traumatic stress disorder and destruction of property. The United Nations in 1991 acknowledged the scale of torture under the AFSPA. Individuals and organizations published accounts of torture, viz., "Mini-Emergencies to Suppress the Poor" (Ram 1978, 1880), "Use of Coercive Power" (Mathur 1992, pp. 337–349), "Obstructing Justice" (Bose 1989, p. 214), "Official Sanction for Killings" (Amnesty International 1997), "National Security Tyranny" (SAHRDC 2008), "Hard Option" (EPW Editorial 1990, p. 2225), "Where Peacekeepers Have Declared War" (NCC 1997), etc. In 2005, the Report of the Committee to Review the AFSPA noted that the AFSPA had promoted violence. The recommendations of the Second Administrative Reform Commission and the United Nations Universal Period Review 2012 advocated repealing of the Act. On 20 November 2012, the National Security Advisory Board (NSAB) of India stated that the recommendation for 'repealing' or 'amending' of the AFSPA will be part of its report to the Government of India (*Hueiyen News Service*, November 20, 2012). On 23rd November 2012, the Supreme Court of India expressed shock over the attitude and orientation of the affidavit filed by the Government of Manipur on the case of extrajudicial executions by the government forces. Questioning the very legitimacy of implementing the AFSPA, a two-member bench constituted by the Supreme Court of India, asked the Counsel of Manipur Government: "How can a State Government file an affidavit stating that they are killing 'us' and so we are killing 'them'. … Are we in a state of war? Are you trying to make the National Human Rights Commission an alibi to all the killing?" (*Hueiyen News Service*, November 23, 2012). Torture, over the decades, has rendered the AFPSA "a symbol of oppression, an object of hate and an instrument of discrimination and highhandedness" (Report of the Committee to Review, the Armed Forces [Special Powers] Act, 1958, 2005, p. 75).

---

[10]This is based on my interactions with young people. For instance, my nephew wanted to join the Army for money, pride and to avenge humiliations that he was subjected to by various agencies and individuals, both working for State such as the army and the police or ordinary members of the local community. In other words, the legitimate possession of a gun under the projection of the AFSPA opens up an enormous avenue of wielding power.

13.4   Collective Memory of Torture and Commemoration

Institutionalization of coercive corporal torture that causes casualty and trauma inflicts unimaginable pain on the tortured body that becomes the immediate victim. When the particular physical pain of an individual body subject or a 'body corporate' is expressed in speech or body-manifestation or through any other means in public, such act "enables pain to enter into a realm of shared discourse that is wider, more social, than that which characterizes the relatively intimate" sharing of pain (Scarry 1985, p. 9). Although the intensity of pain cannot be confirmed by others and differs from person to person, when narratives of torture enter into the midst of others who are in the realm of the shared discourse of pain, there is then no denial of the body being tortured and the intensely private experience of pain becomes public and sharable. This is why the classic work of Elaine Scarry on pain insists that "to bring pain into the world by objectifying it in language" means to destroy it "as in the case of Amnesty International and parallel efforts in other areas" whereby "the pain is objectified, articulated, brought into the world in such a way that the pain itself is diminished and destroyed" (1985, p. 51).

Instantly killed bodies are silent as they no longer speak, but the survivor families, dear ones and those who outlive torture objectify the felt-attributes of pain verbally for the sake of bringing out the secret pangs of pain into the world in its magnified scope for everyone to sense and identify with its deep, lonely privacy and to enable the reported pain to become a reference point for others so that the victim may receive immediate relief through the human magic of the social and the sharable, and more importantly, to avenge the unjustly inflicted pain. Thus the pain-experience of an individual assumes the form of a pain that is collectively felt. Even the instantly killed bodies have something to show like certain signs of pain felt before dying, which too can become a narratively objectifiable public experience and shape the contours of the collective memory of the community. Even the individuals who have 'disappeared', technically labelled as 'forced disappearance', with no visible physical and audible evidences of torture and pain to show, in their strict speechlessness and 'visual blackout', generate certain perception of being tortured and pained, ambiguous and unconfirmed, but nevertheless sensed by the social body in the absence of their individual bodies. When Rose,[11] Sanjita[12] and Manorama[13]

---

[11]Miss Rose Ningshen (born on February 2, 1954), a Tangkhul Naga tribal woman of the Ngaprum Khullen village in the East District (now Ukhrul) of Manipur was gang raped during the night of 4 March 1974 by Major Pundir and Captain Negy of the 95 Border Security Force. She committed suicide on 6 March 1974 (Haksar and Luithui 1984, pp. 205–208).

[12]Miss Nandeibam Sanjita (15) of Jiribam sub-division, Imphal East District of Manipur, was raped by 2 Grenadiers inside a farmhouse at Jiribam on October 4, 2003. She instantly consumed poison and died (*The Sangai Express*, October 05, 2003). Also see: (*The Times of India*, January 17, 2005).

[13]Thangjam Manorama Chanu alias Henthoi (born on 25 December 1971), daughter of late Thangjam Bihari and Thangjam Ongbi Khuman Leima of Bamon Kampu Mayai Leikai, Imphal East, was 'sexually' tortured in front of her family and arrested from her home by a team of the

were raped, the pain was more about the illegitimate encroachment on privacy, humiliation and pervert objectification of the woman's body and the loss of socially prescribed chastity. Rape of one woman became social torture and the pain of the victim transformed into a shared pain felt by the community as a whole. Such torture never confines itself in the body of the immediate victim. According to Olick, "[w] hether inscribed physically on the brain or cognitively on the mind, of course, such thorns in the spirit have profound implications at the personal and aggregate levels. The burdens of trauma, of course, do not reside purely at the personal level" (1999, pp. 333–348). On the contrary, social cognition of torture and pain of a victim generates traumatic torture at various levels amongst the victims' families and community at large. Torture, thus, becomes social and transcends the confines of the personal, metamorphosing into the pain-experience that is shared by the community.

The experience of being tortured entails the experience of being acted upon, thereby, the identity or the agency that inflicts the pain becomes demonstrable and the target of protests and resistance. Thus, pain creates a perceptual shift in identifying the agency, depending on political interpretations, and produces the visibility of the torturer and the political regime he represents. In the words of Scarry, "what assists the conversion of absolute pain into the fiction of absolute power is an obsessive, self-conscious display of agency.: torture is a process which not only converts but announces the conversion of every conceivable aspect of the event and the environment" (1985, p. 27). When torture perpetrated by the agencies representing the political regime is neither devoid of political purpose, nor is occurring in a situation of absolute political vacuum, rebels who are ever ready to disgrace the regime, necessarily objectify torture as instruments of subjugation and coercion. The rebels' organic theory of the nation compresses all objectified and ethnically affiliated individual segments into an imagined nation. Torture of any individual by the 'national enemy' would be symbolically transferred to the most visible forum to substantiate the polemics of 'tortured nation' and painful 'colonial coercion.'

Therefore, when the Indian State and the tortured bodies are juxtaposed with differently ascribed national tagging, and when an individual is objectified with an imagined nation that is believed to be in the quest for liberation, torture comes to be shaded through political interpretation. Of course, torture is always political even if it is confined to the four walls of the patriarchal family. But torture becomes manifestly political and symbolic of the nation in pain in such a scenario as in Manipur, where a nation is being imagined through armed rebellion and also through various forms of 'democratic' assertions. What is being discovered in totality is the persistence of a political culture where propaganda and exhibition of torture and pain is competitively articulated by the contentious agencies, the State and the rebels, who have common aspirations in armed conflict to wipe out one

---

(Footnote 13 continued)

17th Assam Rifles in the intervening night of 10 and 11 July, 2004. Manorama's body was found abandoned with multiple gunshots and other injuries on various parts of her body, including on her genitals and thighs, on the roadside land of Ngariyan Yairipok Road near Imphal, Manipur.

another. As Kosicki asserts, "[p]arties to a conflict tend to perceive themselves as victims and each other as aggressors, independently of the objective question of agency, that is, who perpetrated aggression against whom" (Kosicki and Akania 2007, pp. 3–9). Torture, in this context, is socially perceptible and politically audible. In this sense, torture and pain become manifestly political.

However, since the actions of physical torture occurs intermittently with the passage of time, and although there is variation in the actual time of the incidents of torture and the corresponding social cognition, individual trauma and social or political pain are posterior objectifications of aggregated pain within the framework of social construction of collective memories. In other words, time passes; every second moment is a second to the one it supersedes, leaving behind itself, as it too fades away, leaving behind only intangible past in the form of inaccurate memories. Every moment of infliction of torture and pain on a body is a passing moment. What are being demonstrably expressed as pain are the objectified narratives of the subjective characteristics of those pains, or the conflated memories of aggregated physical pains of the body. This by itself can stimulate certain passing courses of pain to the self and the sympathetic others. At the same time, the pains that are being demonstrated or documented or conveyed to others pass through times across different spaces and 'consumers'. Those pains constitute a 'narrative memory' at the receiving end, which may or may not, stimulate levels of momentarily subjective pain.

However, when there is an aggregation of objective injuries and subjective pains —like (a) all individual aggregates of immediate physical pains and trauma that have occurred in non-contiguous times and spaces, (b) all aggregates of social pains centred on those individual pains and trauma, (c) aggregates of latent paranoia that is developed around the fear created by the presence of 'forces' that are operating with impunity under the provision of repressive laws such as AFSPA and (d) when such pains are located in the totality of duration of a historical timeframe to connote an ongoing 'present' epoch that identifies it with a living moment of the tortured nation's life that inhabits a 'coerced territory'—the objectified aggregation of pain becomes the living moment of the 'tortured nation' and demonstrates the lived experiences of pain. This aggregation does not contradict but rather explains the concomitance of the overlapping memories of recent and distant tortures and pains. The latent subjective paranoia or fear itself, which necessarily prompts or exem-plifies reverberation of the memories of torture and pain, along with the latent agenda of demanding the repeal of AFSPA to avert torture and pain, is founded on the persistent memories of torture. Halbwachs contends:

> …what makes recent memories hang together is not that they are contiguous in time: it is rather that they are part of a totality in thoughts common to a group, the group of people with whom we have a relation at this moment, or with whom we have had a relation on the preceding day or days. To recall them it is hence sufficient that we place ourselves in the perspective of this group, that we adopt its interests and follow the slant of its reflections. (1992, p. 52)

The point is that while the State and its agencies indulge in objective torture and subjective threat in an attempt to quell rebellion and to justify excesses committed under the provisions of repressive laws, individual recollections of torture in this context are shared and become operational within the strategic framework of the politics that provides functional spaces for those recollections at the hands of the 'rebels'. In this, the torture that many presume to be 'collectively' experiencing is largely the subjective embodiment of the social schema of converting aggregated recollections into 'collective memory'.

The perception is that collective memory is crucial in schematising protest or agitation to avert torture. This understanding raises a few other issues. To what extent torture—whether real or 'construed'[14] at the individual, social or political levels—interplays with (a) instant or posterior protests and (b) organization of protests, which contribute to the construction of collective memory and vice versa? To what extent is such collective memory, not only bent on premeditated screening and censoring of recollections to ensure pedagogical objectives of motivating group unity and collective action, but also embodies in its symbolic anchoring a protest course marked by objectified expressions of pain and resistance to torture? To respond to these, one needs to look into some interplaying social indicators of collective memory: (i) protests, (ii) objectives and (iii) forms and means.

(i) Protest: A protest or resistance is a course of action that may begin somewhere and occur at various levels such as individual, family, village, locality, group or party, tribe or community, ethnic or 'national'. Or, the course may stop at one of these levels. The magnitude of different episodic protests in their totality may vary in time, length, nature of demand, geographical spread, crowd composition and number, and the level of solidarity with others. But every protest, in the era of widespread and well-networked human rights movement, is marked by the dialectics of spontaneity and organisation. An individual or a family or a small group may launch an immediate protest and resistance, but the consciousness of the right to resist, the courage to do it, and the larger socio-political base are structured in the overarching framework of resistance informed by collective memory. A protest itself, in its posterity, could add to the constituency of collective memory.

(ii) Objective: Gabel argues that "collective memory is a product of ideological construction that can be used as a key element in the elaboration of collective identity" (2013, p. 250). Referring to the works of Gongaware, he points out that "collective memory is the result of an interactive process of selecting, processing and organizing past events or periods within a framework that grants them political and social significance" (2013, p. 251). Collective memory, according to Misztal, "enacts and gives substance to the group's identity, its present conditions and its vision of the future" (2003, p. 25). It can connect memory and the present circumstances and mould perception that can serve as an instrument of confrontation with its opponents. Gabel believes that collective memory can bestow the legitimacy on the political demands of the movement (2013, p. 250). The objective of creating a horizontal comradeship or imagining as phrased by Anderson (1995) persists to encourage or contribute to individual actions that are socially carried out so that they can have a certain political meaning and orientation.

(iii) Forms and means: According to Halbwachs, "we preserve memories of each epoch in our lives, and these are continually reproduced; through them, as by a continual relationship, a sense of our identity is perpetuated" (1992, p. 47). The collective memory is constructed and continuously maintained through commemorative programs, memorial

---

[14]Construed, if it is subjectively disseminated through manipulative propaganda, but creating a form of pain to those who consume it.

tombs or pillars or columns, parades or light vigils, propaganda literatures, photo exhibitions, awareness campaigns, public gatherings, songs and poems. The preservation and reproduction of memory involve a certain formalised process that can be fitted into what Hobsbawm and Ranger term the 'invention of tradition' (1996). Gongaware believes that collective memory is constructed and maintained through mnemonic practices and narrative commemorations. He further contends that "[m]nemonic practices are those activities, such as celebrations, monument building, and myths, which relate to the memory … (and which) … serve as mechanisms for establishing and maintaining movement unity". (2003, p. 488)

In short, collective memory involves formalized selection, invention, reproduction, maintenance and ritualization of objectified mnemonic artefacts that become the essential tools of resisting torture and pain. The concurrent discourses of protests, documentation and circulation of tortured narratives, annual commemorations, constructions of memorials and tombs, and such other practices keep collective memory alive. Some of the memorial constructions are: the memorial tombs of Miss Rose Ningshen and Miss Nandeibam Sanjita who committed suicide in 1974 and 2003, respectively, after being 'raped' by the paramilitary personnel; memorial tomb of Miss Luingamla Muinao, killed in 1986 for resisting sexual assault; Heirangoithong Massacre Memorial Column; RIMS Firing Victims Memorial Square; Operation Blue Bird Memorial Pillar at Oinam Village; Ten Innocent's Memorial Park, Malom; Meira Paibee Square at Tharo Devi Lampak; and Meira Paibee Martyrs Memorial Square. There are also annual commemorative observances such as: the International Human Rights Day since 1988; Death Anniversary of Thangjam Monorama; Student's Martyrdom or Death Anniversary of Chittaranjan; Hunger Marchers' Day; and Meira Paibee Day. The rebels also commemorate their martyrs' day[15] and keep alive the memory of 'their' nation as opposed to the Indian 'nation' and language through such acts as banning Hindi films and Hindi songs, boycott of Republic and Independence Days and commemoration of their 'foundation' and 'raising' days.

13.5   Protest: Memorializing Pain

The pain of torture at the individual, social and political levels interplays with anger and frustration. It is inflamed when the demand for justice is either delayed or not fulfilled. Therefore, protests or agitations are natural outcomes of what is interpreted as injustice. On the other hand, torturous repression of protest causes casualties and arrests, and adds to the narrative of torture in various forms. It also promotes further protest and agitation, which are aimed at averting torture. What is apparent in the course of an agitation, however, is the typical course of inviting further torture. In that sense, the vicious cycle of embracing torture to avert torture

---

[15]Kept on 13 April, to commemorate the fallen 'heroes' at the battle of Kodompokpi, fought by the People's Liberation Army, a prominent rebel group of Manipur.

becomes evident. This tendency of embracing pain usually occurs in two broad ways.

(a) The first course of action constitutes the primary instance. It often occurs during the time of arrest, or combing operations or torture in the victim's house and in public view. In this case the targeted individuals and the families or the groups who are present at the scene of torture, if they have the will to embrace pain, knowing that they would be targeted for any obstruction vis-à-vis the agency of torture, confront to prevent the arrest to save the target. This variable of embracing pain occurs while carrying out the instant expression of anger in the immediate aftermath of killing or atrocities. These are spontaneous acts of confrontation that invite reprisal and repression, thereby, knowingly embracing pain out of exigency and anger.

(b) The second course of action is schematized forms of agitation—fitting spontaneous protests into the schema of a course of agitation—directed against the immediate 'torturer' and the State, which usually happen as follow-up action to the primary reaction. The schematized agitation raise demands that may vary depending on the nature of the immediate issue: release of the arrestee if he/she is in the custody of the torturers, punishment for torturers and compensation to victims if they were seriously disgraced or injured or killed, shifting the entire post or battalion if it is the issue of perpetual threat and harassment to the 'public', repealing of the AFSPA, and so on. There were instances when agitators attempted storming of the concerned post or battalion, obstruction of their route, imposition of blockades and general strike, destruction of public properties or government buildings, defiance of curfew, fighting pitch battle with the repressive forces, and so on. In such cases, the organizers and agitators anticipate brutal repression and are always ready to embrace pain to register their protest-agenda successfully. Three examples can be given to substantiate it: (i) agitators preparing themselves with onion and toothpaste as pain reliefs, (ii) schematization of nude protest, and (iii) schematization of self-immolation.

(i) In most of the urban centred agitations, where the numbers are strong enough to confront, many who take part in the agitation expect brutal repression. The protest organisers might even wish for some form of torture to take place, anticipating that it would ignite public fury and consequently accelerate the tempo of their agitation. In other words, in such cases there is an evident schematized intertwining of protest and torture. Presuming repression, many prepare themselves with onion peels and toothpaste to be applied on the faces in order to relieve the pain that would be caused by the smoke of tear gas in the case of its use by the 'repressive forces'. Many defy prohibitory orders, break police barricades if their number is strong enough, retaliate with sling shots (mostly by men) and engage in 'pitch battles' with the 'repressive forces'. Agitators know that repression can cause killing, injury, arrest and torture. But the protestors perceive repression as either a normal course or *fait accompli* or the inevitable to achieve their immediate demands. But they rise in agitation by willingly embracing some form of pain for a bigger cause. (ii) When the nude protest of Manipuri women was schematized on 15 July 2004, demanding justice for Manorama and a demand to repeal the AFSPA, the activists indulged in what may be characterized as the 'politics of the body' (*The Sangai Express*, July 15, 2004). They involved in self-exposing of what was considered within the community as sacred and intimate, namely the body of women. They voluntarily embraced some form of self-inflicted pain by disgracing the honour that was culturally embodied in the privacy of the woman's body in order to protest against, and rectify, something that they considered to be more torturous than the torture of self-exposing their nakedness. It was considered to be a novel and qualitatively higher form of self-infliction of pain that aimed to expose the utter helplessness of women under the objectified military regime. 'Indian Army Rape Us,' they cried, which in the rhetorical context of the protest was an effective hyperbole to say the opposite of the literal meaning of the words. The media visually magnified the nudity of the protesting women, thereby ensuring with certainly, an obscene pictorial representation, which pained them, their family and the community continuously by reminding them of the 'inflicted torture upon these bodies' every time the images were invoked. But they nevertheless accepted the outcome and embraced the pain as a form of protest.(iii) On 24 July 2004, five male volunteers of Manipur Forward Youth Front (MFYF)[16]set themselves on fire after soaking themselves with petrol and marched towards the gate of the Chief Minister's Office shouting slogans to withdraw Manipur's status as a 'disturbed area'. They rolled on the ground in extreme pain, sustained serious burn injuries and were hospitalized; one of them for several months at the All India Institute of Medical Sciences, New Delhi. Thereafter, occurred on 15 August 2004, the controversial self-immolation of Pebam Chittaranjan. Although schematised, the MFYF volunteers and Chittaranjan knew that burning themselves would be an extremely painful and life-threatening act. They voluntarily embraced the extreme pain to become martyrs of the movement against the AFSPA. Chittaranjan confessed: "It is my own conscience [to commit self-immolation] against the black law and the consistent tortures on this land by the Government of India. I am disheartened by the situation of retreat in our movement and in order to give courage to it I have willingly decided to become a human torch so as to become a pioneer of the people."[17] These instances are premeditated and there are many who encourage such embracing of pain so that they can stimulate the spirit in others to fight against the AFSPA.

The second type of schematized form of protest narrated above adopts a voluntary embracing of some form of symbolic and demonstrative pain, and fetch media coverage, photographic shots and video footages which are premeditated within the schematic framework of protest. Therefore, these can be fitted into the rubric of demonstrative pain, which can then subsequently become the rallying point of the mnemonic techniques of recreating and maintaining collective memory. But the schematization of demonstrative pain, in trying to either encourage victim families to recollect pain or parade the victims to serve as living testimonies or martyrs of torture, can have the untoward impact of inflicting fresh pain on the 'victims.' It further pains the already pained, thus hurting the pained 'twice'. In other words, pain that could have been comparatively forgotten or reconciled with is being continuously brought into display, thereby keeping it alive. This schema can add pain to the victim families due to repeated enquiries, fact findings, narrative tellings, reporting, and parading victims as martyrs on ceremonial occasions. There are evidences to substantiate this point. (i) Ms Lata cried a lot while recollecting the death of her son Orsonjit. She lamented, "as I stand here today, my heart is filled with mixed emotions. On the other hand it is a victorious moment for me because

---

[16]They were: Lalit Chandra Oinam, Moirangthem Ranjan, Sanjoy Khaidem, Thangjam Ibotombi and Vicky Yambem.

[17]The text is an excerpt from a transcription of the video statement delivered by Chittaranjan before committing self-immolation.

my son finally gets justice, years after he had passed away. On the other hand, it reminds me that he will never come back. Even this moment of victory cannot fill the vacuum that he left in my heart.[18]" (ii) The brother of Rose Nighsen,[19] Mr. Prangam Ningshen, did not want any interview as it would be a recollection of the torturous event and inflict long lasting mnemonic pain on him. (iii) Mother of Thangjam Manorama[20] is pained by the injustice done to her and the repeated recollection caused by the interviews of the fact finding teams and journalists, and the annual commemorations. (iv) Brother of Irom Sharmila,[21] Mr. Irom Singhajit, felt that he was repeatedly subjected to pain by the interviews and statements he was to make about the hunger strike of his sister. (v) The husband of Rabina,[22] Mr. Thokchom Chinglen,

> appealed to the public for seeking his prior permission before reproducing any of the photographs or the video footages involving his wife in the future (since) reproduction of the photographs and video footages over and over again in music video album, journal, article, magazine, etcetera have only increased the burden and the pang of separation being experienced by his son Russel and other family members. (*The Sangai Express*, March 27, 2010)

There is, of course, torture and pain centred on the AFSPA. But then, although what is being displayed as torture and pain in the form of collective memory, gives us a general picture of torture and pain, it also simultaneously suggests a fragmented picture of pain. The picture of pain in this context is fragmented because, while the depiction of social pain with respect to Manipur is authentic in its totality, the political commemorations of pain lacks contiguity in time and space, coordination among organizations and collective community orientations. The picture of pain is also fragmented because there are many tortuous incidents and painful experiences that are being left out from the commemorations and the shared discourse of collective memories. There can be various reasons for this: (i) the venues and people involved in those incidents are too remote from the main organizers in terms of distance and communications facilities, (ii) lack of initiative from the concerned victims and their families and (iii) the issues are considered to be settled, and so recollecting and commemorating them would be meaningless. Therefore, what are being displayed in totality in the form of collective memory are in fact recollections of a fragment of the totality of reality. In other words, silencing of pain also contributes to this fragmentation.

---

[18]Statement delivered by Ms. Kh. Lata, mother of Khumgbongmayum Orsonjit, a 19 year old boy killed in a fake encounter on 16 March 2010 (Ningthouja and Hidam 2014, 147–8).

[19]See n. 11 above.

[20]See n. 13 above.

[21]Irom Sharmila is a Civil Rights Activist from Manipur, India, who has been on the world's longest hunger strike since the year 2000 and still continuing without break. Her main demand is the repeal of the AFSPA.

[22]Rabina Devi was killed by a stray bullet during an indiscriminate firing session of the police to cover up a fake encounter on 23 July 2009 in Imphal.

Silencing of pain occurs when the tortured reconcile with the torturers and impose self-silencing of pain, thereby discouraging any intervention or support for justice from others. This is substantiated by four case studies that had occurred in different temporal and spatial locations.

(a) On May 5, 2005, a team of the 14 Assam Rifles Battalion indulged in cold blooded killing of three women of a family in broad day light at Saitu Village in Senapati District, Manipur.[23] Immediately there was uproar against the mayhem, but the Assam Rifles suppressed it (*The Sangai Express*, May 5, 2005). In the meanwhile, the Assam Rifles summoned the chiefs of thirty one villages and entered into a negotiation. On the following day, they paid what was called customary fine amounting to Rs. 1.4 lakhs to the family, organised a community feast and the matter was silenced (*The Sangai Express*, May 6, 2005). Many organisations visited Saitu Village to investigate into the matter and to help the families if they were willing to fight for 'justice.' The families, probably under the pressure from the Assam Rifles and the chiefs, had reconciled with the loss and were reluctant to raise the issue since it was considered to have been settled.

(b) On January 29, 2015 the people of Tengnoupal village launched a week long agitation against the 24 Assam Rifles Battalion at Sita Lamkhai by blocking the National Highway 102.[24] The agitation went on for weeks and was supported by organisations across communities and regions.[25] However, it came to an abrupt end at the discretion of the Tengnoupal people, without achieving their main demands such as punishment of the personnel responsible for harassment and shifting of the Assam Rifles post. When a delegation of Coordination for Democratic Rights and Organisations from several parts of India visited the village, the leaders of the Tengnoupal village refused to openly discuss the issue due to the following reasons: (i) an army Deputy Inspector General had collected money from the soldiers and had organised a grand customary compromise feast on February 8 to settle the matter, (ii) raising the issue of torture would hold people of the area accountable for the violation of the 'truce' or customary compromise, which they feared would anger the Assam Rifles and justify future reprisals and harassment, and (iii) the people did not want to entertain 'outsider' rights activists into their village, as it would arouse the suspicion of the Assam Rifles. There was no one to come out and testify of being tortured or harassed. There was only a copy of the draft memorandum that was leaked out by someone. The villagers had reconciled with torture and pain, and the matter was silenced.

(c) The Sadar Hills Rally in support of the AFSPA in August 2004 was allegedly carried out under the instigation of the 14 Assam Rifles to discredit the agitation against the AFSPA. The objective was to cover up torture, to silence pain inflicted under the AFSPA and to justify continuous imposition of the Act (*The Sangai Express*, August 21, 2004).

(d) Individual pain is being silenced for fear of reprisal. For instance, on May 7, 2014, Ahanthem Nandakishor of Lei-Ingkhol, Imphal, a retired cadre of a rebel party, leading a normal life, was abducted at gun point from his house by the personnel of the Assam Rifles. He had no criminal record. The purported reason was that Naoba had a heated argument over business with someone, who was connected to the Assam Rifles. Naoba was tortured

---

[23]Those killed were: (i) Linkholane Haokip (50), (ii) Lalneithen Haokip (25) and (iii) Hoineichoung (*The Sangai Express*, May 5, 2005).

[24]The charge against the 24 Assam Rifles was regular harassment of people. I conducted an interview with the President of the All Tribal Women's Organisation, Chandel District, Lalam Mate, and Chief of Tengnoupal Village, John Thangkholen Mate, on 14 February 2015 at Tengnoupal Village.

[25]For several years the paramilitary check post at Khudengthabi and other areas had been unpopular on account of inconveniencing and harassment of the travellers.

but released due to pressure from political leaders. He was released on condition that he would neither go to a hospital for medical treatment nor inform the media and police to expose the incident. The trauma and stress suffered by him was so severe that he neither went to the hospital nor disclosed the matter to the human rights activists who approached him. He wanted to remain silent as he feared disclosing the matter to others would have worse consequences. He continued to live in a state of trauma.[26]

This highlights, though enigmatically, the fact that the discourse of pain must sometimes be laced with a deliberate silencing of some pains, so that the discourse of pain as such might continue.

13.6 Conclusion

The Indian State has the priority to defend its idea of the 'nation' and the 'prescribed' rule of law. By asserting the sovereignty of the 'nation' and outlawing rebellion, the State holds the responsibility to protect the rights and security of the people. Therefore, the onus of the charges against 'torture' has been directed against the State. The charges have been substantiated by the fact that militarization, repressive laws, and certain counter-rebellion tactics have contributed to torture. Regarding counter-rebellion tactics, many in Manipur suspect that the State is in collusion with some 'rebel' parties—particularly with those that are under Ceasefire, Suspension of Operation, and Memorandum of Understanding—for two basic reasons: (a) to create conflict among the rebel parties to weaken them and (b) to create a torturous situation in order to justify continuous imposition of the AFSPA. What adds to this suspicion is the recent statement of the Union Defence Minister Manohar Parrik that "you have to neutralize terrorists through terrorist only" (Kulkarni, May 22, 2015). The question is: should 'terrorism' be either encouraged or sponsored to defend the State without taking into consideration the security concern of the people who will be affected by it? For several decades, the AFSPA has neither been successful in wiping out the rebels nor in undoing torture. The supposedly 'responsible' State has failed to keep the promise of the former Prime Minister Dr. Manmohan Singh, who, on November 1, 2014, assured to replace the AFSPA "with a more humane law" (*The Hindu*, November 1, 2004).

There has been a dialectics of the AFSPA and the tortured bodies, which also suggests dialectical unity of the opposites in the totality of the polity. The Act does not merely torture some 'bodies' and inflict pain on them, but is used as an instrument to avert the torture suffered by some other 'bodies', purportedly emanating from certain historical conditions that are being politically interpreted as

---

[26]The incident occurred when I was present in the village.

disturbing. For more than six decades, the contentious postulations of two different agencies, the Indian state on the one hand and the 'projected independent nation' of the rebels on the other, wedded to two different political polemics have, respectively, demanded the retaining or repealing of the AFSPA, largely by parading the, respectively, schematized statistics of 'tortured bodies.' However, the representation of the meaning of the effects of the AFSPA, have been differently formulated. Although the two contentious postulations are often seen as conjectural courses of negation, adopted by diametrically opposed agencies, there is nonetheless the dialectics of the two in constituting an overarching unity of the opposites, marked by the schematized representations of torture. Both contribute to sustain the dialectics of the discourse of torture; without the one, the other discourse dissolves itself. While both representations objectify the other as 'enemy' and as the agency of inflicting torture, their commonality lies in the politics of negation, marked by the articulation of emasculated victimhood, the suffering 'self', the being of which embodies involuntary torture and pain inflicted by the 'other'.

Therefore, on the one hand there is a phenomenological unity of the negating agencies as two opposing ends of a pole that depend on each other for the purposeful existence of the two different 'selves'; and, on the other hand, within the objectified 'self' of the negating agency, there is a relative unity of torture and pain as the relative cause and effect of the enduring conflict with the 'other' as the construed enemy. But these are not the only two sets of agencies on the two extremely opposite poles, correspondingly representing the State that upholds AFSPA and the opposing agencies that spearhead the movement against it. The two poles, which operate in the name of 'public security,' are connected to and rest on the supposedly insecure masses, amongst whom, choices to temporarily co-opt with either of the poles in relation to certain instances of immediate or prolonged torture are marked by ambiguity and indeterminacy. In other words, while the agencies and their respective policies and propaganda are marked by constancy and homogeneity, the impact and response of the people are marked by ambiguity and heterogeneity. They do not comply with uniplanar cohesiveness and progression; they rather respond sporadically and intermittently through unrests that emerge differently in different times and spaces, and against different targets. At the same time, however, there is the persistence of an encompassing social context of torture and pain, where everyone is a victim in a way and someone is always held responsible for it. The politics of torture, which showcases deliberate attribution of victimhood to objectified 'bodies,' is carried forth through the promotion of commemorative memorials and rituals that take place as a form of organization and protest against the AFSPA. The dialectic continues.

References

Newspapers and Magazines

Disturbing Option: (1990). *Economic and Political Weekly* (henceforth *EPW*) 25(40): 2225.
Where peacekeepers have declared war: (1997). *Report on violations of democratic rights by security forces and the impact of the Armed Forces Special Powers Act on civilian life in the seven states of the northeast.* Delhi: National Campaign Committee against Militarisation and Repeal of Armed Forces Special Powers Act (NCC).
Girl commits suicide after being frisked by armymen at Jiribam: (2003, October 5). Family refuse to take back body. Imphal: *The Sangai Express.*
Sadar Hills rallies to endorse AFSPA: (2004, August 21). Imphal: *The Sangai Express.*
Women give vent to naked fury in front of 17 AR at Kangla: (2004, July 15). Imphal: *The Sangai Express.*
Review of Armed Forces Act will be considered: (2004, November 1). Manmohan. New Delhi: *The Hindu.* Online: http://www.thehindu.com/2004/11/02/stories/2004110209670100.htm.
Report of the Committee to Review the Armed Forces (Special Powers) Act, 1958: (2005). Delhi: Ministry of Home Affairs. Unpublished.
Nandeibam Sanjita Report confirms rape by another Jawan: (2005, January 17). *The Times of India.* Online: http://timesofindia.indiatimes.com/india/Report-confirms-rape-by-another-jawan/articleshow/993207.cms.
AR man goes berserk, two women, one child killed in indiscriminate firing, KSO demands capital punishment: (2005, May 5). Imphal: *The Sangai Express.*
AR pays customary fines for Saitu victims: (2005, May 6). Imphal: *The Sangai Express.*
A study in national security tyranny: (2008). *Armed Forces Special Powers Act.* Delhi: South Asia Human Rights Documentation Centre (SAHRDC).
Husband pleas: (2010, March 27). Imphal: *The Sangai Express.*
National Security Advisory Board (NSAB) for repealing AFSPA: (2012, November 20). Imphal: *Hueiyen News Service.*
Is there a war going on? SC asks Manipur Govt: (2012, November 23). Imphal: *Hueiyen News Service.*

Reports, Books and Articles

Amnesty International. (1997). *Official sanction for killings in Manipur.* AI INDEX: ASA 20/014/1997. Online: http://lib.ohchr.org.
Anderson, B. (1995). *Imagined communities: Reflections on the origin and spread of nationalism.* London: Verso.
Bose, T. (1989). *Obstructing justice. EPW, 24*(5), 214.
Foucault, M. (1977). *Discipline and punish: The birth of the prison* (A. Sheridan, Trans.). New York: Vintage Books.
Gabel, I. (2013). Historical memory and collective identity: West bank settlers reconstruct the past. *Media Culture Society, 35*(2), 250–259.
Gongaware, T. B. (2003). Collective memories and collective identities: Maintaining unity in Native American educational social movements. *Journal of Contemporary Ethnography, 32*(5), 483–520.
Haksar, N., & Luithui, L. (1984). *The Nagaland file.* New Delhi: Lancer International.

Halbwachs, M. (1992). *On collective memory* (L. A. Coser, Ed., & Trans.). Chicago, IL: University of Chicago Press.

Herman, E. S., & Chomsky, N. (2008). *Manufacturing consent: The political economy of the mass media*. London: The Bodley Head.

Hobsbawm, E., & Ranger, T. (Eds.). (1996). *The invention of tradition*. Cambridge: Cambridge University Press.

Kelman, H. C. (1995). The social context of torture: Policy process and authority structure. In R. D. Crelinsten & A. P. Schmid (Eds.), *The politics of pain: Torturers and their masters*. Oxford: Westview Press.

Kosicki, P. H., & Jasińska-Kania, A. (2007). Guest editors' introduction: Aggressors, victims, and trauma in collective memory. *International Journal of Sociology, 37*(1), 3–9.

Kulkarni, P. (2015 May 22). Kill terrorists by using terrorists. Kolkatta: *The Indian Express*. Online: http://indianexpress.com/article/india/india-others/kill-terrorist-with-terrorist-defence-minister-manohar-parrikars-idea-2/99/.

Mathur, K. (1992). The state and the use of coercive power in India. *Asian Survey, 32*(4), 337–349.

Misztal, B. A. (2003). *Theories of social remembering*. Berkshire: Open University Press.

Ningthouja, M., & Hidam, P. (Eds.). (2014). *Maheiroi 2014*. New Delhi: Manipur Students' Association Delhi.

Ningthouja, M. (2011). Violence as AFSPA 1958 and people's movement against it. *Eastern Quarterly* 6(IV), 145– 55.

Olick, J. K. (1999 Nov). Collective memory: The two cultures. *Sociological Theory, 17*(3), 333–348.

Peters, E. (1985). *Torture*. New York: Basil Blackwell.

Ram, M. (1978). *Mini-emergencies to suppress the poor*. EPW, *13*(46), 1880.

Reinhart, T. (2003). *Israel/Palestine: How to end the war of 1948*. New Delhi: Left World Books.

Said, E. W. (2002). *The end of the peace process*. New Delhi: Penguin.

Scarry, E. (1985). *The body in pain: The making and unmaking of the world*. Oxford: Oxford University Press.

Chapter 14
Medical Mission and the Interpretation of Pain

Parinitha Shetty

Abstract It is at the intersection of the corporeal experience and the cultural interpretation of pain, that slippery tenuous site where knowing and being are constantly confronting and dismantling each other, that new cultural recognitions of pain are produced as well as inscribed on bodies. These new recognitions are simultaneously personal as well as social. They are historically specific and culturally rooted and they restructure existing cultural practices of the body. Very often, such transformations have taken place in the context of interactions and confrontations between people of different cultures, religions, and nations. In this chapter is attempted a 'cultural ontology of pain' through the exploration of a historically specific recognition of pain that emerged in the context of the confrontation of European Protestantism with the indigenous faith traditions of India.

Keywords Pain · Basel mission · Medical mission · Heathen · European protestantism

Modern knowledges and treatments of pain have been structured through the discourse of medicine and the institution of the hospital. For the medical gaze, pain as a corporeal dis-ease is the symptom of the pathological body. It is the locus of the medicalized body around which an entire regime of care and cure is structured. However, as an experience of intense corporeal dis-ease, pain not only disaggregates familiar practices of being, but also makes it necessary to seek alternative ways of recognizing it. It makes the body amenable to alternative disciplines of embodiment in an attempt to manage the unbearable presence of pain.

This chapter attempts to reconstruct one strand in the social history of pain. It examines how pain became central to a historically specific technology of subjectivity that emerged at the juncture of social, religious, and cultural confrontations in the nineteenth and early twentieth century colonial India. The paper delineates how a treatment and interpretation of pain was practiced and preached in the Basel Mission hospital under the authority of the science of medicine and the theology of

P. Shetty (✉)
Department of English, Mangalore University, Karnataka, India
e-mail: parinith007@yahoo.com

© Springer India 2016   269
S.K. George and P.G. Jung (eds.), *Cultural Ontology*
of the Self in Pain, DOI 10.1007/978-81-322-2601-7_14

the one true Christian God. It explores how the medical mission attempted to make Christians out of its heathen patients through the event of pain and dis-ease. The paper argues that despite the missionary intentions, pain became a polysemous sign within the Mission hospital. While it disciplined some of its heathen patients into a belief in the soul and the ethics of embodiment that that belief mandated, it also disaggregated the normative practices of embodiment for others and brought them in conflict with the Mission. The chapter places pain at the juncture of socio/cultural confrontations and attempts to understand the ways in which pain became central to a historically specific technology of subjectivity and a bio-politics of the body.

14.1 Pain, Subjectivity, and Culture

The experience of pain, especially when intense and sudden, catapults us for a moment outside all systems of intelligibility through which we make sense of, and live our bodies. It dismantles the temporal/spatial routines and habits of corporeal maintenance that go into the making of our quotidian life, and collapses the whole of being into an intense point of pain. Pain, for a startling moment, decouples the enigmatic, recalcitrant corporeality of our bodies from the cultural meanings and practices through which we live and recognize our bodies. According to David Morris, literary expressions of pain are significant because they encapsulate the complexity of pain. He writes:

> Writers in fact express a range of knowledge and experience for which the person struggling with pain quite often cannot find the words. Most important, they tell a story about pain that differs significantly from the traditional medical account and helps to reveal its limitations. Such voices suggest that pain is never the sole creation of our anatomy and physiology. It emerges only at the intersection of bodies, minds, and cultures. (Morris 1993, p. 3)

Pain exists at the cusp of the body, mind, and culture, always threatening to disrupt and disarray the bounded normative structures of being. And yet, if we have to live with pain we have to negotiate with it, and make sense of it in order to adapt to its unbearable persistence. We have to learn to confront it so that it does not delete all the meanings through which we shape our existence. We struggle to accommodate pain into our existence by giving it a purpose and meaning, an aetiology and a prescription, a classification and a name, so that it does not become a formless scream that cannot be heard or named. When we accommodate pain in all its enigmatic unbearable otherness, the existence into which it is accommodated, itself, becomes unfamiliar and unpredictable. In order to avert this radical uncertainty which pain brings along with it, we recognize it through narratives which gloss over the discomfort, meaninglessness, and unpredictability of pain and provide it with closure. Thus, we recuperate pain into the cultural intelligibilities through which our being in the world is constituted and understood.

However, pain need not always emanate from bodies; it may also be inflicted on bodies or seen to be inflicted on bodies. The infliction of pain may be a part of the disciplinary regime through which power marks itself on bodies. It may also be the instrument through which power subjects bodies through historically specific technologies of subject formation. Hence, pain has been both a radically enigmatic experience of the dis-ease of the flesh, capable of disrupting and disorienting the cultural intelligibilities and practices of human corporeality, as well as the instrument through which power subjects bodies through its disciplinary regimes. Pain has been read as a sign of the body as well as a sign on the body. Pain has been inflicted and explained in the legitimization of structures and stratifications of power. In *Discipline and Punish*, Foucault writes of penal torture thus:

> The term 'penal torture' does not cover any corporal punishment: it is a differentiated production of pain, an organized ritual for the marking of victims and the expression of the power that punishes; not the expression of a legal system driven to exasperation and, forgetting its principles, losing all restraint. In the 'excesses' of torture, a whole economy of power is invested. (Foucault 1995, pp. 34–5)

According to Foucault, the 'spectacle of the scaffold' which displayed the infliction of pain on the body of the criminal was part of a political ritual. Through this ceremony of physical torture, the power of the sovereign was inscribed and displayed on subject bodies.

14.2 The Basel Mission and the Meaning of Pain

While pain has been powerfully deployed in the organizing and disciplining of bodies into docility it has also fomented secret and open revolts in subject bodies. The corporeal experience of pain is always in excess of its cultural legibilities and this excess of the flesh has led to a radical undermining of the disciplinary regimes through which bodies are subjected to docility. Very often, it is this site of excess of the flesh that has enabled the instituting of new practices of the body. Recontourings of the body and its practices of embodiment through new recognitions of pain have been especially fertile and complex at moments of confrontation and contact between people of different cultures, religions, and nations. In the context of India, Colonial Christianity and its proselytizing encounters with the indigenous people, is a site rich in such complex and creative processes of reforming the body and its social embodiments. This was attempted through propagating the metaphysics of the body in pain and instituting a science of treating the body in pain.

In the rest of my chapter, I will attempt a "cultural ontology of pain"[1] through exploring a historically specific recognition of pain that emerged in the context of

---

[1]This is a phrase that I take from the Note circulated by Siby K. George and Pravesh G. Jung among the contributors to this volume. In their words, by this phrase they "refer to the idea that the mode of being of the self in pain, whether intense bodily pain, or trauma or even humiliation, is in a significant sense affected by social and cultural forces that help form the self."

the confrontation of European Protestantism with the indigenous faith traditions of India. My focus will be on nineteenth century India, when a proselytizing religion, namely Protestant Christianity, appropriated pain into its evangelizing agenda and through its medical mission simultaneously medicalized pain, as well as co-opted it into the missionary regime of the maintenance, care, and disciplining of the body. Through its regime of care and cure of bodies instituted through the Mission hospital, heathen bodies were disciplined and inscribed with a Protestant Christian meaning. The missionary organization that I speak of is the Basel Mission,[2] and I shall explore how its missionaries and missionary doctors reinterpreted the meaning of pain for the converted Christians and the heathen patients who came under their care.

The Basel Mission set up its medical mission more than half a century after it had established its first mission station in Mangalore in 1834. The first missionary doctor of the Basel Mission was Dr. Eugene Liebendoerfer from Wuerttemberg. He established a small hospital in Kodakal, in what was then known as the Malabar region, in 1893. Prior to this, he had renovated and furnished a hospital in Calicut in the year 1887. Next to the schools, the hospitals of the Mission were seen as effective sites for the evangelization of the heathens. Like the Mission schools, the Mission hospitals represented the new contouring of spaces, introduced and necessitated by colonial modernity and colonial rule, within which bodies were organized and habituated to new hierarchies and routines of being. Western medicine had been introduced into India through the colonial administrative and institutional structures even before the Basel missionaries set up their first hospitals. 'The Bengal Medical Service' which later became the 'Indian Medical Service', had been set up by the East India Company in 1763 to cater to the military and medical needs of colonial rule (Arnold 2000, p. 58). In *The Birth of the Clinic*, Foucault writes that modern medicine sees itself as originating in the last years of the eighteenth century when "a new alliance was forged between words and things, enabling one to *see* and to say" (Foucault 1994, p. xii). The pathological body was now opened to the authority of the 'clinical gaze'. Describing what he calls the great myth of a pure gaze that would be a pure language, a speaking eye, Foucault writes:

> The observing gaze refrains from intervening: it is silent and gestureless. Observation leaves things as they are; there is nothing hidden to it in what is given. The correlative of observation is never the invisible, but always the immediately visible, once one has removed the obstacles erected to reason by theories and to the senses by the imagination. In the clinician's catalogue, the purity of the gaze is bound up with a certain silence that enables him to listen. (Foucault 1994, p. 107)

---

[2]The Basel Mission was founded in 1815 in the Swiss city of Basel and sent its first missionaries to Ghana in 1828, and later to India in 1834. It was part of the Pietist missionary movement and had close links with Pietist circles in Würtemberg. Most of the missionaries of the Basel Mission came from this circle. It established its first station in Mangalore in India and later established a number of stations in Coorg, Nilgiris, and what was then known as the Canarese and Malabar regions of south west India.

Through this myth of the 'Pure Gaze', western medicine assigned to itself the status of a neutral science of the body and its pathologies. It privileged the speech which spoke the truth that was outlined under this gaze and asserted that this speech could be understood only by those initiated into it. Hence, a doctor trained in western medicine was vested with a skill and ability that gave him the authority to recognize the pathology of the body and heal it. In the colonial context, western medicine came to be seen as one of the markers of European superiority. Thus under colonial rule, western medicine "was taken as the hallmark of a superior civilization, a sign of the progressive intentions and moral legitimacy of colonial rule in India and the corresponding backwardness and barbarity of indigenous practice" (Arnold 2000, p. 63). Through instituting and privileging a science of the body and its cure, colonial rule sought to introduce and normalise a repertoire of corporeal embodiments through which bodies in general could be evaluated and hierarchically placed. According to David Arnold "…to a degree unparalleled in other scientific fields and matched by few aspects of technological change, medicine represented direct intervention in, and interaction with, the social, cultural material lives of the Indian people" (Arnold 2000, p. 57).

The Basel Mission's medical mission, by appointing doctors trained in western medicine and by organizing itself and functioning through the institutional space of the hospital, introduced by the colonial government, appropriated for itself the privileges and powers vested in this institution. However, as a proselytizing mission it had to accommodate its evangelical agenda into this space where the medical gaze had the sole right to prevail. A science of the body had to be appropriated for propagating the metaphysics of the soul. The missionary reports do not give any indication that this duality gave rise to contradictions or conflicts in the functioning of the medical mission… The Basel Mission Report[3] of 1909 describes its medical work in the following manner:

> The blessings of our hospitals and dispensaries consist in the first place in the indirect influence of the relief afforded to suffering men and women, and secondly in the direct preaching of salvation, for which the hospital offers so favourable an opportunity. Each day a catechist meets the patients and reads and explains the Bible to those who are waiting for their turn to see the doctor. (RGEM 1909, p. 71)

In the Mission hospital pain and disease were diagnosed as symptoms of the sinful soul. The reading and preaching of the Bible by the Catechist legibilized the body through a new coprography, to the heathen patients. This corpography was reaffirmed and naturalized through the therapeutic and corporeal regimes by which the pathological body was medically treated and cared for, in the Mission hospital. Through its regimen of cure and care, the Mission hospital attempted to discipline heathen bodies into the routines and repertoires of embodiment that were commensurate with the requirements of the Christian soul destined for salvation. In *Discipline and Punishment* Foucault says:

---

[3]These were the annual reports of the Basel Mission that were published and circulated to the English patrons of the Mission in India. Henceforth, I refer to them as "RGEM" (Report Of The German Evangelical Mission).

It would be wrong to say that the soul is an illusion, or an ideological effect. On the contrary, it exists, it has a reality, it is produced permanently, around, on, within the body by the functioning of a power that is exercised on those punished—and, in a more general way, on those one supervises, trains and corrects, over madmen, children at home and at school, the colonized, over those who are stuck at a machine and supervised for the rest of their lives. (Foucault 1995, p. 29)

In the Mission hospital, the science of the body converged with the metaphysics of the soul, on and through the site of corporeal pain and disease. The Mission doctor attempted an epistemological and disciplinary control over the heathen body through the institutional space of the hospital where the science of western medicine was practised and the efficacy of the clinical gaze displayed. However, this attempt was not always met with success, and the dis-ease of pain within the Mission hospital generated a whole range of interpretations of pain which contested and confronted each other. The complex semiotics of pain within the Mission hospital emerged at the cusp of pain as a radical corporeal dis-ease of bodies and the attempts at translating, legibilizing, and managing pain at the juncture of cultural confrontations and contestations.

The Basel Mission read the corporeal pain and suffering of its heathen patients as the markers of sin writ large on bodies. At the same time, heathen disease and suffering were seen to originate in the social and cultural practices within which the pathological body was embedded and embodied. Pain was a polysemous sign simultaneously signifying the disease of bodies, the immorality of heathen socio-religious practices, the insanitary environment in which heathens lived and the sinfulness of their souls. Its cure necessitated a belief in the one true God and the protocols of embodiment legitimized by this God, medical treatment by the Euro-Christian doctor trained in western medicine, the reform of heathen practices of embodied being, and the restructuring of the material conditions within which the heathens were located and sustained. In the Basel Mission report of 1887 Dr. Liebendorfer writes:

We have no hospital for in-patients, but every morning from 30 to 60 patients present themselves when not only their diseased limbs or bodies are attended to, but also as the true panacea, the Gospel is preached for the healing of their souls. What a picture of suffering offers itself to my view every morning! The blind, lame, dumb and deaf, lepers in different states of disease, poor children whining in the arms of their mothers from sufferings, the result of the lasciviousness of their great-grand-fathers, not to speak of persons bitten by snakes, jackals, dogs etc., and persons with internal injuries, men, women and children, old and young, nay even persons on the point of death are brought on miserable litters before our door...Nobody but a medical man gets such an insight into the sad havoc caused by sin and the miseries attending it. I will not speak of the victims of bad sanitation, bad water, deficient and unwholesome food, and so on. I turn with a sore heart to the sad consequences of the transgressions of the seventh Commandment[4] and to that from excessive drink. How many are the cases of consumption, mental derangement and other sufferings consequent on these sins! Heathenism is simply an abyss of wickedness and misery. I have witnessed the

---

[4]The seventh commandment states, "You shall love thy neighbour as thyself."

most dejected hopelessness of heathen death-beds which baffles description, and yet people venture to speak of the innocence and bliss of the Heathen. (RGEM 1887, pp. 30–31)

The soul was constituted as an inner depth, the essential truth of the body which revealed itself through signs on the body. It was as an interpreter of souls that the Mission doctor treated pain ridden bodies through the knowledge and regimen of European medical science. Through a knowledge, a routine, a spatialization, a care, a cure and an interpretation of the corporeal, put into practice through the institutional space of the Mission hospital the missionary doctor attempted at contouring a Protestant subjectivity for his heathen patients. Through medicalising pain and treating it, the Mission doctor reaffirmed the ontology of the soul. His knowledge of treating ailing bodies was in the service of setting the heathen soul on the path to salvation. He saw himself as following in the footsteps of Christ, the 'true physician'.

The Mission hospital sought to contour a new subjectivity for its heathen patients through framing the meaning of pain through a new grammar of the body. It administered a service of care and a programme of recuperation on this body, thus locating it within new relational networks and hierarchies of authority. The Christian commandments framed the allowed pleasures of the body which in turn shaped the disallowed possibilities of transgressive desires. In the Mission hospital, the provenance of pain was located simultaneously in the pathologies of the culturally contoured body and the spiritual distance between the heathen soul and the true God. Hence, pain could be eliminated through a new regimen of the body which was concomitant with a new faith practice. As a medical doctor, Dr. Liebendorfer's work not only involved the diagnosis of physical ailments but the cure of its spiritual source by replacing the heathen patient's unfamiliar and culturally alien regime of bodily care with a Christian regimen of the body. In fact, heathenism was seen to instantiate itself through a lack of understanding of the body and its proper care, which was understood to have a devastating and debilitating effect on the body and soul of the heathen.

This ignorance was seen to reach its apotheosis in the heathen's attitude to his own and other people's deaths. The missionaries felt that the heathens were mired in their bodies and hence experienced and interpreted death, purely as a bodily phenomenon. In the RGEM of 1899, Dr. Stokes, the successor of Dr. Liebendorfer, describes the heathens' attitude to death as follows:

One cannot help noticing how sadly indifferent the non-Christians behave when they are about to die. To many not even the thought of passing into a complete unknown state will rouse their attention and direct their thoughts to the future. The relatives are just as callous: 'We are still living, let us eat and drink, and when it is our fate may we too so die'. (RGEM 1899, p. 121)

Pain as a sign of the spiritual health or sickness of the soul was read very differently by the missionaries when it manifested itself on the bodies of Christians. The Basel Mission reports are replete with descriptions of deathbed scenes and for the missionaries the deathbed scene was the final confirmation of the authenticity of Christian conversion. For a true Christian, death was a welcome event which was anticipated with joy, while the heathen deathbed was seen to be marked by hysterical grieving. In the RGEM of 1898, Dr. Stokes describes the manner in which a fatal illness led a young man into accepting Christianity and confronting his imminent death calmly:

> A young man came to the Hospital having heard in his native place of a "third religion". He was very ill indeed, and we could not save him, but he found salvation in Christ. Although too weak to walk alone, he wished to be baptised in the church; so we had him helped in, and he received the name of *Simon*. Five days later he passed away peacefully. These few instances show that the Medical Mission is not only philanthropic, but affords almost more opportunities than in any other sphere of Mission-work, of pointing people to the true Physician, who has prepared for them a future, where there will be no sickness and no suffering. Laid aside by sickness they are more willing to hear, and the Word of God falls like healing balm on their weary souls. (RGEM 1898, p. 108)

The missionaries sublimated pain into the great capacity for suffering that a true Christian was believed to have. On the body of a true Christian, pain was the stigmata of the redeemed soul and bore witness to the redemptive suffering of the god-man Christ. The true physician was Christ since only he could release the soul from the pain infested body, and for those who placed complete faith in this promise of liberation, death was a peaceful and blessed release from the pain infested body. Pain was also that intolerable dis-ease of the flesh which breached the cultural boundaries of the body and made it accessible to the recontouring of the corporeal through the conversion of the soul. In the RGEM of 1898 Dr. Stokes describes the patients who came to the Calicut hospital thus:

> Patients come into the Hospital, worn out by pain and suffering, depraved by sin, with despair written on their faces and as God's word works silently in their hearts, we have observed their expressions gradually change to one of peace and happiness, indicating the change within, although in many cases the bodily suffering could not be removed. (RGEM 1898, p. 107)

Thus, within the Mission hospital, the pain suffered by a Christian was read as the means to and manifestation of the redeemed soul. As suffered by a heathen, it was read as signifying both spiritual and corporeal dis-ease. The missionary doctor's training in western medical science and Christian theology was seen to give him the expertise to diagnose the ailments of the soul through the signs of the body. Through the process of healing bodies, the Mission hospital structured a system of legibility for the soul and its mutually reciprocal and causal connections with the body.

14.3   Spaces, Bodies, Caste, Meanings, and Pain

The Mission's interpretation and treatment of pain while attempting to discipline bodies into docility also opened up new and more enabling possibilities of corporeal being. For the indigenous society, the Mission hospital was a radically new contouring of space. Entry into this space and its systems of medical treatment and care of the body required them to temporarily relinquish their own belief and understanding regarding the nature of the body and the cosmology within which it was made sense of. This was very difficult especially for members of the upper caste. Reporting on the hospital at Vaniyankulam in the RGEM of 1898, Dr. Stokes, the medical missionary at Calicut, narrates this incident:

> I was called to attend one very severe labour case of a Nambudri woman. I arrived just in time to perform the operation, but the woman was in a very hopeless condition. I told them the only thing that might save her life would be to bring her to the Hospital for nursing and treatment. Much to my surprise they did, and she recovered. This case is an exception, the majority would rather die than lose caste by coming into Hospital. (RGEM 1898, p. 111)

Hence, for many of those belonging to the upper caste the Mission hospital was a last and desperate recourse when indigenous systems of medical treatment had failed.

The missionaries considered indigenous systems of corporeal legibility as superstitious. In the RGEM of 1893, Dr. Liebendorfer reports on the indigenous belief regarding the cure for snake bites: "The people imagine that after a fatal snake-bite life simply hides itself in a certain corner of the brain, and refusing to believe in death, take the corpse away to the astrologer or sorcerer, who performs certain mantras, to restore life, but of course in vain" (RGEM 1893, p. 84). Indigenous systems of treatment were seen as unscientific and superstitious having a deleterious effect on the body and exacerbating its pain rather than providing relief from pain. In the RGEM of 1904 it is reported: "Everyone who wishes to be treated, has to take off his amulets. The doctor has quite a collection of these foolish and abominable charms" (RGEM 1904, p. 76). Describing the shift to a scientific explanation of pain in the West, Morris writes:

> The vast cultural shift that gives the story of pain its hidden plot centers on the eradication of meaning by late nineteenth-century science. The great breakthroughs in anatomy and physiology by Bell, Magendie, Muller, Weber, Von Frey, Shiff, and other nineteenth-century researchers created the scientific basis for believing that pain was owing simply to the stimulation of specific nerve pathways. (1991, p. 4)

For the Mission doctors their own understanding and treatment of the body was scientific in comparison with the indigenous systems of treatment and care and cure of the body.

From the reports of the Basel Mission it would seem that the Christian narrative of the suffering of Christ and its promise of salvation offered the indigenous patients who came to believe in it an effective means of negotiating with their pain. It invested their pain with a purpose and meaning that enabled them to manage it. It established an analogy between their pain and the sacrificial pain of the man-god Christ, thus ennobling their pain. The memory of Christ who had suffered the intolerable pain of crucifixion and the great redemptive power of that suffering was also continually present before the patients within the institutional space of the Mission hospital through the preaching of the Catechists and the Bible women[5] and

---

[5]These were men and women from the converted Christian community who evangelized the indigenous people. They distributed tracts, preached and accompanied the missionaries on their missionary tours. The Bible women went from house to house narrating bible stories and spreading the message of the Bible to the indigenous women.

the pictures that decorated the walls of the hospital. Hence, pain was valorised within the Mission hospital even as it was medically treated. The vanquishing of pain through a combination of medicine and faith in Christ was ultimately seen to be the work of the true physician Christ.

Entering the Mission hospital was a radically new experience of space for its indigenous patients because the hospital did not map itself out through the architecture of caste. Through the obliteration of caste rules and caste distinctions in its treatment of patients, the Mission hospital also offered a radically new understanding of the body and its pain. Pain was seen as the great equaliser, the common factor of the corporeal which was indifferent to the social distinctions that validated a hierarchy of bodies. Within the Mission hospital, pain and disease were treated without taking into consideration the distinctions inscribed on bodies by indigenous caste practices. For those of the lower caste this would be a radical display of the solidarity of human beings propagated by Christianity which gave their body and its pain a new significance and importance and the right to concern and care. The analogy between the pain of their bodies and the suffering of the man-god Christ would have further privileged their bodies and given it a new visibility and importance that would be lacking in the indigenous communities to which they belonged. The RGEM of 1907 gives this description of the mission hospital at Bettigeri (South Mahratta District):

> The hospital is also making inroads in the bulwark of caste by the very manner of treatment, afforded to the patients. 'It is, indeed, a new world', Dr. Zerweck remarks, 'into which such a poor, oppressed Hindoo is transferred, when he enters the hospital. The first time in his life he gets into conditions which are nothing less than adapted to caste. He here meets with men who are not deterred by caste-restrictions ever so scrupulously prescribed, not even by the threats of all-powerful priests; men who with exactly the same care, love, and attention treat the rich and the poor, the man of substance as well as the beggar, men who entertain no fear of polluting themselves by touching the sick and the dying ones, who not only preach a new way of salvation, but confirm it by actively demonstrating the Christian love to the neighbour'. (RGEM 1907, p. 33)

14.4   Pain and Female Bodies

Pain and disease were also appropriated into the disciplinary regimes of the other institutions of the Basel Mission like the girls orphanages, where destitute children were housed and reared into the Christian way of life. The girls' orphanages, like the boys' orphanages, originally provided an institutional space where destitute indigenous children, as well as children of new converts could be protected from all heathen influences and moulded into a Christian model of femininity. The children of new converts had to be protected, according to the missionaries, from the heathen influences of their home and their almost heathen parents. In later years, the orphanage also included children of inquirers and of poor Christian parents. The working of the Christian influence on the girls of the orphanage was manifested in a renewed idea of community that they came to hold. This was the larger community of human beings who had mutual responsibility toward each other's survival and wellbeing. This idea of a community that transcended the smaller unit of the biological family and the larger unit of the caste group, also recast what had been considered as feminine duties, into Christian virtues. The skill and responsibility of nurture expected as the duty of a wife and mother was recast into the much valorized Christian virtues of sacrifice and selflessness. Within the orphanage it was seen to function in the transformation of the sickly, sore ridden, malnourished destitute who entered the orphanage, into a clean, healthy, and cheerful inmate of the orphanage, through the nurture given to her by her fellow inmates. It was in their confrontation with death that the inmates of the orphanage were seen to truly manifest the signs of their conversion and these deathbed scenes are described in detail in many of the Mission reports. The calm and almost joyful acceptance of death on the part of the dying and its transforming effect on those who watch over them are seen as the most authentic signs of the spiritual transformation brought about by the acceptance of Christianity. The death of an inmate of the girls' orphanage of Mangalore is described in the following manner in the RGEM of 1856: "One manifested only in her last days how truly she loved the Lord. Her repeated prayer was, 'Oh Jesus, when wilt thou take me home? I long only after Thee, Oh my Redeemer'" (RGEM 1856, p. 9).

The girls were also taught to read death and disease as retributions for the sins committed by them and as an intimation to repent for these sins. Since the orphanage was regularly struck with disease and death they were used, with great efficacy, in the service of disciplining those who survived these attacks of sickness. Pain was seen as a corporeal marker of sin and patient suffering as a sign of redemption. Reporting on 'the severe fall of the catechist' employed in the girls' hostel at Mulki, the RGEM of 1867 tells its readers:

> The superintendence of the Girls' Orphanage passed from Mr. *Traub* into the hands of Mr. *Manner* and afterwards Mr. *Mack*. These changes could not but tell disadvantageously upon the institution; but it was brought into jeopardy much more by the severe fall of the catechist employed in it, who was dismissed immediately and his place supplied by another to advantage. And now came the chastising and purifying hand of the Lord, in severely visiting our little flock with diverse maladies and producing deep impressions for good on many of them. (RGEM 1867, pp. 29–30)

14.5 Making of the Christian Subject

> What an excellent opportunity to do good and witness for Christ by word and deed is offered in a Mission Hospital! We have not to go and seek people, they come to us. With many people the bodily sickness is often the first and only opportunity they get for repentance and a stimulus for spiritual and moral health. Their hearts have become susceptible to earnest warning and advice, and the way is paved for a moral and spiritual cure. Many bear in their own bodies the evidence that "sin is the ruin of mankind", and that without renouncing sin bodily cure is not attainable. It is the privilege of the Medical

Missionary to impress on the minds of his patients the connection between sin and sickness
and point out to them the only true remedy. The fulfillment of this missionary duty in no
wise interferes with medical work. Many patients are glad to be offered something more
than pills and tinctures, and after their treatment is over, still keep up a friendly intercourse
with their doctor and visit him or his assistants of their own accord for religious conversation. Religious and moral advice is not forced on anybody; it is the influence of Christian
love in word and deed with consolation and earnest warning that proves attractive. The
result of such work is far more beneficial than any statistics can show. (RGEM 1905,
pp. 32–33)

The diagnosis and treatment of pain and disease were central to the making of a
Christian subject within the Mission hospital. By tracing the pathologies of the
body to the sinfulness of the soul and vesting the authority of both corporeal and
spiritual cure in the Mission doctor/priest the Mission hospital attempted to contour
a Protestant Christian subjectivity for its heathen patients centered around a
spiritual/medical regimen of care and cure. The soul was constituted as the essence
of the body marking its existence and its spiritual condition through the corporeal.
The corporeal in turn was seen as the effect of its religious/cultural embodiments
and the conditions of its social and material embeddedness. Hence, for the Mission,
the soul's spiritual state was simultaneously the cause and consequence of heathenism. This allowed for the ascription of a powerful regulative force to the soul
through which the material structures of heathen embodiment could be changed.
The spatial display and structuring of the hospital further reaffirmed the Christian
truth of the soul as the inner depth of the body and of Christ as the True Physician
as only he could heal the soul. In the RGEM of 1894 Dr. Liebendoerfer gives the
following description of the leper asylum at Calicut:

Through the kindness of the "Society for Illuminated Wall-Texts" in London, and the
generosity of certain Ladies in Calicut, we were enabled to adorn the otherwise bare walls
with Biblical texts and pictures. A Catechist in charge of the asylum conducts Reading- and
Bible Classes, in order to relieve the dreary monotony of the daily life of the in patients, and
to raise their thoughts to something higher. This, added to the necessary sanitary
improvements, has already produced good results both with respect to the moral condition
and the bodily health of the inmates. (RGEM 1894, p. 98).

In the Mission hospital the heathen patients were inducted into a discipline of the
body, a socio/moral code of being and an ontology and epistemology of the soul.
The Basel Mission reports indicate the complex imbrication of religious and cultural beliefs, culturally specific practices of embodiment, and medical/scientific
knowledges of bodies, in the understanding and treatment of pain in the Mission
hospital.

The Mission hospital was peculiarly amenable to the proselytizing enterprise of
the missionaries, for several reasons. The Mission reports indicate to us that in some
cases at least the Mission hospital proved its efficacy over indigenous systems of
healing. Though the Mission hospital explained this efficacy in terms of the scientific and rational basis of its system of medical treatment, it located the ultimate

and true origins of the pathologies of bodies in the spiritual condition of the soul and the efficacy of its cure in the saving grace of Christ. Since indigenous systems of medicine were based on distinct cosmologies of the body in which disease could be the result of planetary influences or malevolent forces like ghosts and spirits, it was not difficult for the heathen patients of the Mission hospital to accept the transcendental basis of the Christian cosmology of the pathological body. While the Christian missionaries in the hospital preached the truth of the one true God and tried to prove his superiority over the false gods of the heathens, for the indigenous people this new God could be easily appropriated into their own pantheon of gods and spirits as an additional resource in understanding and managing their pain. The RGEM of 1896 reports, "Many come to us when every treatment has failed and the disease so aggravated by native medicines, that death seems imminent,— because they say we can intercede on their behalf with our God" (RGEM 1896, p. 59). The Mission reports also indicate to us the strategic ways in which the indigenous patients of the hospital appropriated the Christian cosmology of pain in order to make sense of their particular experience of pain and disease. This resulted in hybrid practices of faith and healing. We have this description of one such hybrid practice of the heathens, by Rev. G. Wuerth from the Bettigherry station:

> A heathen in our neighbourhood daily smeared his sick child with ashes in the name of Jesus Christ, saying the words "Let this child be Thine in life and death". Upon farther [sic.] enquiry we found that these ashes had been given to the man by a Lingayet priest who is said to have cured some cases of Cholera by the same application. Others are said to have been healed of snakebites by calling on the name of Jesus. Nevertheless these people who believe the name of Christ to be so efficacious, will not hear of confessing him openly, although they admit the necessity of so doing. (RGEM 1855, p. 12)

Evangelization through medical mission was not simply a process of disciplining bodies into docilely accepting a new faith through the agency of the missionary doctor and his adjuncts who represented the power of a superior religion and superior knowledge. It was also a process that enabled new possibilities of subject formation for the indigenous people. In the case of the lower caste patients, the Mission hospital offered an enabling subjectivity. In the RGEM of 1899, Dr. Stokes describes the sufferings of a fisher woman thus:

> One of the in-patients was a Hindu woman of the fisher-caste, suffering with a tubercular spine. This woman really made us all wonder at her patience in suffering, and though often in great pain, she hardly ever complained. She was anxious to be baptised and become a follower of Christ. This desire was begotten through hearing in the daily prayers, how much 'The Man of Sorrows' suffered for all mankind. (RGEM 1899, p. 121)

Through their Christian theological narrativization of pain, the Mission doctors seem to have offered relief to at least some of their heathen patients. The Christian valorisation of pain, as the replication of the pain of Christ and its redemptive power seems to have offered a new significance to the bodies of, especially, the lower caste and class. This was in radical contrast to the denigration of their bodies and denial of agency regarding their practices of the body in the indigenous communities. The care given to these bodies within the Mission hospital gave them a new significance and importance.

For the upper caste patients, pain and its treatment had to be regulated by the rules of purity and pollution through which the hierarchies of caste were inscribed on their bodies. The Mission hospital's categorization of human beings on the basis of the spiritual condition of the soul, though it intersected with the hierarchies of race, opened the hospital to all who were in need of a therapeutics of the soul and the body, irrespective of their caste. Its regime of care and cure denied as well as defied the maintenance of caste rules. For the upper caste patients who sought recourse to the Mission hospital, as a last desperate resort, the spatial organization of the Mission hospital and its regime of care and cure led to difficult negotiations. If some of them were converted into accepting its system of medical treatment, others found it too difficult to do so. The Mission report of 1904 describes how, while these caste prejudices were slowly wearing away they had not been completely done away with.

> Prejudice is giving way to confidence, which is evidenced by the increasing number of female patients, accouchements, and especially the many house-visits, which amounted to 219, besides 181 made by the Hospital Assistants. This is the most important and interesting part of the work, and Dr. Zerweck has the impression that in families, where he has been a frequent visitor, the sick are more rationally treated, and even higher caste Hindus have the courage to follow his advice, without regard to caste prejudices, though he very often experiences the opposite. For instance, a young Brahmin woman came to the Hospital with inflammation of the hip-joint; she was bandaged and very soon felt relief. But the next day her father came and demanded the removal of the bandages, as his daughter refused to eat, unless according to the usual Brahmin custom she could bathe before and after meals. All persuasion and reasoning was in vain. The whole company disappeared during the night, taking the bandage with them. (RGEM 1904, p. 78)

14.6 Conclusion

The medical mission of the Basel Mission through appropriating pain into its evangelical enterprise gave rise to a new range of knowledges, practices, understandings, and cures of pain. Through their knowledge and treatment of pain, the missionaries were able to convert at least some of the heathens into new practices of bodily being. But for the missionaries, the Christian subjectivity of the newly converted native Christian was never completely free of the remnants of heathenism. For the indigenous converts their adopted faith involved a difficult disciplining. It also opened up for them enabling possibilities of bodily being which radically transformed their lives and in turn the world in which they lived. For both, pain became an important site for re-contouring the possibilities of corporeal being and re-imagining its significance.

References

Arnold, D. (2000). *The new Cambridge history of India: Science, technology and medicine in colonial India*. Cambridge: Cambridge University Press.

Asad, T. (1993). *Genealogies of religion: Discipline and reasons of power in Christianity and Islam*. London: Johns Hopkins University Press.

Foucault, M. (1995). *Discipline and punish: The birth of the prison*. (A. Sheridan. Trans.). New York: Vintage Books.

Foucault, M. (1994). *The birth of the Clinic: An archeology of medical perception*. (A.M. S. Smith, Trans.). New York: Vintage Books.

Morris, D. B. (1993). *The culture of pain*. Berkley, CA: University of California Press.

Panikkar, K. N. (2007). *Colonialism, culture and resistance*. New Delhi: Oxford University Press.

RGEM. (1841–1913). *The reports of the German evangelical mission*. Cited in text as RGEM. Mangalore, India: Basel Mission Press.

Sill, U. (2010). *Encounters in quest of Christian womanhood: The Basel mission in pre- and early colonial Ghana*. Leiden: Brill.

Index

© Springer India 2016
S.K. George and P.G. Jung (eds.), *Cultural Ontology of the Self in Pain*, DOI 10.1007/978-81-322-2601-7